Antimicrobial Alternatives Against Resilient Oral Biofilms

Antimicrobial Alternatives Against Resilient Oral Biofilms

Insights from In Vitro, Ex Vivo, and Clinical Studies

Aida Meto

MDPI

Basel • Beijing • Wuhan • Barcelona • Belgrade • Novi Sad • Cluj • Manchester

Author
Aida Meto
Department of Dentistry
Faculty of Dental Sciences
Aldent University
Tirana, Albania

Clinical Microbiology, Department of Surgery,
Medicine, Dentistry and Morphological
Sciences with Interest in Transplant, Oncology
and Regenerative Medicine
University of Modena and Reggio Emilia
Modena, Italy

Editorial Office
MDPI AG
Grosspeteranlage 5
4052 Basel, Switzerland

For citation purposes, cite as indicated below:

Lastname, A.A.; Lastname, B.B.; Lastname, C.C. *Book Title*. Series Title (optional). Year, Page Range.

ISBN 978-3-7258-2196-9 (Hbk)
ISBN 978-3-7258-2195-2 (PDF)
https://doi.org/10.3390/books978-3-7258-2195-2

Funding information: This monograph was generously supported by Humanchemie GmbH, Alfeld, Germany, and the Albanian Dental Association, Tirana, Albania.

Dedication

To my parents, Agron and Liza, and my son, Odin!

Content

Abbreviations

EPS	extracellular polymeric substances
S. mutans	*Streptococcus mutans*
P. gingivalis	*Porphyromonas gingivalis*
CLSM	confocal laser scanning microscopy
SEM	scanning electron microscopy
NGS	next-generation sequencing
S. sanguinis	*Streptococcus sanguinis*
S. gordonii	*Streptococcus gordonii*
F. nucleatum	*Fusobacterium nucleatum*
A. naeslundii	*Actinomyces naeslundii*
C. albicans	*Candida albicans*
HSV	Herpes Simplex Virus
HPV	Human Papillomavirus
M. oralis	*Methanobrevibacter oralis*
VSCs	volatile sulfur compounds
C. glabrata	*Candida glabrata*
C. tropicalis	*Candida tropicalis*
M. mazei	*Methanosarcina mazei*
P. intermedia	*Prevotella intermedia*
ANUG	acute necrotizing ulcerative gingivitis
CPC	cetylpyridinium chloride
IgA	immunoglobulin A
T. forsythia	*Tannerella forsythia*
S. salivarius	*Streptococcus salivarius*
S. pyogenes	*Streptococcus pyogenes*
T. denticola	*Treponema denticola*
BLIS	bacteriocin-kike inhibitory substance
NulOs	nonulosonic acids
FGFs	Fibroblast Growth Factors
BMPs	Bone Morphogenetic Proteins
QLF	Quantitative Light-Induced Fluorescence
OCT	Optical Coherence Tomography
CPP-ACP	Casein Phosphopeptide-Amorphous Calcium Phosphate
Bis-GMA	bisphenol-A glycidyl methacrylate
UDMA	urethane dimethacrylate
AGEs	advanced glycation end products
CBCT	cone-beam computed tomography
NSAIDs	Non-Steroidal Anti-Inflammatory Drugs
GERD	Gastroesophageal Reflux Disease
OLP	Oral Lichen Planus
GBR	Guided Bone Regeneration
IL-6	interleukin-6
TNF-α	tumor necrosis factor-alpha
CRP	C-reactive protein
ACPAs	anti-citrullinated protein antibodies
LPS	lipopolysaccharides
CVD	cardiovascular disease

LDL	low-density lipoproteins
COPD	chronic obstructive pulmonary disease
ICUs	intensive care units
RA	rheumatoid arthritis
PAD	peptidylarginine deiminase
AD	Alzheimer's disease
PD	Parkinson's disease
PDL	periodontal ligament
PDT	photodynamic therapy
E. faecalis	*Enterococcus faecalis*
ELISA	enzyme-linked immunosorbent assay
PCR	Polymerase Chain Reaction
MALDI-TOF MS	Matrix-Assisted Laser Desorption Ionization Time-of-Flight mass spectrometry
FISH	Fluorescence In Situ Hybridization
CLSM	confocal laser scanning microscopy
3D	three-dimensional
NaOCl	sodium hypochlorite
EDTA	Chelating Agents—Ethylenediaminetetraacetic Acid
CHX	chlorhexidine
MINST	minimally invasive non-surgical periodontal therapy
GTR	Guided Tissue Regeneration
RCT	root canal therapy
MTA	Mineral Trioxide Aggregate
CAPE	caffeic acid phenethyl ester
P. aeruginosa	*Pseudomonas aeruginosa*
S. aureus	*Staphylococcus aureus*
Cupral	copper–calcium hydroxide
Cu	copper
$Ca(OH)_2$	calcium hydroxide

About the Author

Dr. Aida Meto is a well-known dental specialist with a rich educational background and extensive experience in the field. She earned her dental degree from the Italian Catholic University "Our Lady of Good Counsel" in Tirana, Albania. Dr. Meto also holds a Master's degree in Orthodontics from the University of L'Aquila, Italy, and another in Endodontics from the University of Alma Mater Studiorum Bologna, Italy. Her specialization in Orthodontics was completed at Aldent University in Tirana, Albania.

Her academic journey led to a Ph.D. in Clinical and Experimental Medicine from the University of Modena and Reggio Emilia, Modena, Italy.

Dr. Meto has made substantial contributions to dental research, publishing numerous articles in high-impact journals. She serves as an editor and guest editor for several international journals and has reviewed more than 250 scientific articles. As of August 2025, Dr. Meto is the Editor-in-Chief of the Journal of Oral and Dental Approaches (JODA), published by ICCK (Spokane, United States). Her research achievements have been recognized with several awards, including first prize at the 18th Congress by the Balkan Association of Dentists (2013), at Harvard University—USA (2015), "Best Article of the Issue" award from the EC Dental Science Journal (2017), and the "Best Poster" award at the 28th National Congress of the Italian Dental School in Milan, Italy (2021).

Dr. Meto is the Senior Lecturer for Conservative Dentistry at the Aldent University, Tirana, Albania, and an Adjunct Lecturer in Clinical Microbiology at the University of Modena and Reggio Emilia, Modena, Italy.

In 2022, she joined the Department of Dental Research Cell at Dr. D.Y. Patil Dental College and Hospital in Pune, India, demonstrating her commitment to advancing global dental education and research.

In March 2025, she obtained the National Scientific Qualification (ASN) for the title of "Professore di II Fascia" in Italy.

Preface

The persistent challenge of managing resilient oral biofilms in dental and periodontal care has motivated the development of this book. Despite significant advancements in dental hygiene and treatment methodologies, oral biofilms remain a major obstacle to achieving optimal oral health. These complex microbial communities are not only responsible for common dental issues like caries and periodontal disease but also contribute to systemic health complications if left unchecked.

This book provides a comprehensive exploration of the pathogenic role of microorganisms in oral biofilms, with a particular focus on their resistance mechanisms and the limitations of current treatment options. By exploring the complexities of biofilm formation, its persistence, and the factors contributing to treatment failure, this work aims to deepen the understanding of biofilm ecology and its implications for disease progression. The inclusion of extensive references adds depth and reliability, offering readers a well-rounded perspective on the topic.

Combining insights from in vitro, ex vivo, and clinical studies, this book intends to integrate research findings with clinical practice. It provides valuable tools and knowledge for clinicians and researchers to enhance oral health outcomes. By going beyond conventional techniques, this book hopes to encourage new advances in antimicrobial solutions for oral biofilms that are difficult to eradicate.

Aida Meto
Author

Acknowledgments

First and foremost, I want to thank God for providing me with the strength, patience, and inspiration to bring this book to completion. My deepest thanks go to my parents, whose unwavering support and encouragement have been the foundation of all my achievements, and to my son, Odin, whose presence in my life has been a source of immense motivation and joy.

I extend my sincere appreciation to Prof. Elisabetta Blasi from UniMore, Italy. Her invaluable guidance and insightful advice significantly enriched this work, particularly from a microbiological perspective.

I am also immensely grateful to my student and future colleague, Nensi Kallfani, from the University of Aldent, Albania. Her creativity and dedication in producing the vibrant illustrations featured in this book have truly brought the content to life.

A special thanks to Ms. Sarah Hubert, Ms. Jelena Milojevic and Ms. Bojana Nadaždin for their support throughout the completion of this book.

I want to express my sincere gratitude to Mrs. Ursel Knappwost and Dr. Constanze Knappwost-Gieseke of HUMANCHEMIE GmbH (Alfeld, Germany) for their unwavering support and for giving me this invaluable opportunity.

I am also deeply grateful to the Albanian Dental Association, Tirana, for their invaluable assistance and sponsorship, which played an important role in the realization of this book.

1. Microbial Complex Ecosystems Influencing Oral Health: Oral Biofilms

1.1. Introduction

> *"One of Mother Nature's most surprising wonders exists right inside our mouths, oral biofilms. These complex microbial communities highlight the incredible adaptability and intelligence of microscopic life, reflecting the beauty and ingenuity of nature's design."*

Oral biofilms are organized in microbial communities that adhere to various surfaces in the mouth, including both biotic surfaces (teeth, gums, and the tongue), as well as abiotic surfaces (dental implants, orthodontic appliances, and prosthetic devices).

These communities are primarily composed of bacteria, fungi, viruses, and archaea, all embedded in a self-produced matrix called extracellular polymeric substance (EPS). The EPS provides both structural support and protection from damage, helping the biofilm attach to surfaces, retain nutrients, and resist antimicrobial agents and immune responses. Biofilm formation begins when free-floating microbes attach to a surface, followed by the accumulation of additional species and the secretion of EPS. Through mechanisms of communication, microbes within the biofilm coordinate activities such as growth, nutrient sharing, and defense. This organized structure helps the biofilm survive environmental challenges and persist over time.

Maintaining microbial balance in the oral cavity is vital for both oral and overall health. In a healthy state, biofilms contribute to oral homeostasis by supporting a stable and diverse microbial community. However, this balance can be disrupted by factors such as poor oral hygiene, an imbalanced diet, and changes in the host's immune response. Such disruptions can cause microbial dysbiosis, where harmful species compete with beneficial ones, increasing the risk of oral diseases like dental caries, periodontitis, and other oral infections that also affect systemic health.

Studying oral biofilms is important for understanding oral health and how microbial communities function throughout the body. Biofilms represent a common form of microbial life, found not only in the mouth but also in the gut, lungs, and other body systems, as well as in the environment. Over time, the focus in microbiology has evolved from studying single pathogens to examining complex microbial communities. This evolution has been supported by advances in microscopy, genetic sequencing, and analytical software, which allow scientists to study the detailed structure and function of biofilms and their impact on both health and disease.

This chapter offers an overview of oral biofilms, focusing on their role in health and disease. It explores how biofilms are formed, their microbial landscape, and the interactions that shape their behavior in the mouth.

1.2. Historical Perspective on Oral Biofilm Research

1.2.1. Early Discoveries and Theories

The exploration of oral biofilms has a rich history, dating back to the 17th century. An early contribution to this field came from the work of Antonie van Leeuwenhoek, often referred to as the father of microbiology. In the 1670s, using a simple, handmade microscope, Leeuwenhoek became the first person to observe and document microorganisms in dental plaque. He described these tiny life forms, which he called *"animalcules,"* following an analysis of samples taken from his own teeth. Leeuwenhoek's observations were revolutionary for the time, representing the first recorded identification of microorganisms in dental plaque [1].

In the 18th and 19th centuries, microbiology evolved from simple observation to identifying microbes linked to disease. The germ theory of disease, advanced by Louis Pasteur and Robert Koch in the mid-19th century, represented a significant moment in oral microbiology. It established that specific microorganisms cause specific illnesses, driving research into oral infections. This contributed to major advancements in the field, connecting certain bacteria to particular diseases and laying the foundation for the "*specific plaque hypothesis*" [2].

The specific plaque hypothesis, introduced in the early 20th century, proposed that certain bacteria, like *S. mutans* in dental caries and *P. gingivalis* in periodontitis, were the primary etiological agents responsible for these diseases. This view shaped dental research and practice, enabling precise antimicrobial treatments, developing preventive measures, such as the use of fluoride to inhibit the growth of cariogenic bacteria, and the promotion of good oral hygiene practices to reduce the accumulation of dental plaque [3].

Further research showed that dental plaque is not a homogeneous mass of bacteria but a complex, structured community of diverse microorganisms living in close association. This developed the "*nonspecific plaque hypothesis*", which proposed that the total amount of plaque, rather than specific pathogens, was the main factor of oral disease [4].

1.2.2. The Evolution of Biofilms and Their Role in Oral Disease

For most of the 20th century, bacteria were studied mainly as isolated cells grown in laboratory cultures, typically grown in liquid media under well-mixed conditions, leading to the formation of planktonic cells that were easily studied and manipulated. This view began to change in the late 1970s with the work of J. William Costerton, who introduced the concept of biofilms, organized microbial communities attached to surfaces and surrounded by a protective matrix. He and his colleagues showed that in natural environments, including the human body, bacteria typically live in these structured communities rather than as free-floating cells [5]. This discovery reshaped microbiology, revealing that bacteria in biofilms behave very differently from those in isolation. The evolved model influenced a new understanding that biofilms are the dominant form of bacterial life in both natural and clinical environments [5–7].

Within biofilms, bacteria communicate through quorum sensing, regulate gene expression collectively, and share nutrients and defense strategies [7,8]. The EPS matrix not only helps biofilms adhere to surfaces but also protects bacteria from antibiotics and immune attacks [8]. This explains why oral infections within biofilms are harder to treat and often become chronic [9]. Also, this explains better that diseases like dental caries and periodontitis are not caused by individual pathogens alone, but by imbalances within the entire microbial community [10]. Factors like poor oral hygiene, high sugar intake, and inflammation can disrupt this balance, allowing harmful bacteria to thrive and damage oral tissues [10].

1.2.3. Progress in Oral Microbiology

Technological progress has been important to the growth of biofilm research. In the 1990s, imaging tools like confocal laser scanning microscopy (CLSM) and scanning electron microscopy (SEM) enabled researchers to visualize biofilms in three dimensions for the first time. These imaging techniques offered new insights into the structure of biofilms, showing that they are highly organized communities with distinct layers where different microbes proliferate. This spatial organization is essential for functions like nutrient flow, waste removal, and protection against external threats [11,12].

Molecular biology techniques, especially 16S rRNA sequencing, have transformed the study of oral microbiology. Unlike traditional culture methods, which detected only a fraction of oral bacteria, 16S rRNA sequencing enabled the precise identification of a much broader range of microbial species. The findings showed that the oral microbiome is much more diverse than once thought, with hundreds of species living in balance. Rather than focusing on specific bacteria, the research emphasized that maintaining overall microbial harmony is key to oral health [13,14].

The 21st century marked a major advancement in oral microbiology with the introduction of metagenomic techniques, which allowed researchers to analyze the complete genetic material of microbial communities without the need for culturing. Metagenomics offered a deeper understanding of the functional capabilities of oral biofilms, uncovering the gene networks and metabolic mechanisms involved in their formation, maintenance, and pathogenic potential. This overall approach enabled the development of targeted therapies, including probiotics to support beneficial bacteria and antimicrobials that disrupt specific biofilm processes [15,16].

Complementing metagenomics, next-generation sequencing (NGS) technologies enabled high-performance sequencing of entire microbial communities. NGS demonstrated the extensive diversity of the oral microbiome, including previously undetected species, and provided new insights into how these microbes interact. Importantly, it also allowed researchers to compare microbial profiles in health and disease, monitoring alterations in composition and function linked to oral conditions [17].

These events show how research has progressed from simple observations to advanced studies that have shaped modern dentistry (Table 1). From Leeuwenhoek's early observations to the use of modern genetic tools, our understanding of the oral microbiome's complexity has greatly evolved.

Table 1. Significant milestones in oral biofilm research.

Years	Milestones/Events	Main Contributor(s)	Significance/Impact
1670s	Discovery of dental plaque microorganisms	Antonie van Leeuwenhoek	First observation of microorganisms in dental plaque, determining the basis of microbiology [1].
1850s	Germ theory of disease	Louis Pasteur, Robert Koch	Established the microbial cause of diseases, guiding the identification of specific oral pathogens [2].
1940s	Development of the specific plaque hypothesis	Various researchers	Identified key pathogens responsible for dental caries and periodontal disease, contributing to early therapeutic models [3,4].
1978	Biofilm concept development	J. William Costerton	Introduced the modern biofilm concept, emphasizing the structured nature of bacterial communities and their resistance to treatment [5].
1990s	Advances in imaging and molecular techniques	Various researchers	Enabled three-dimensional visualization of biofilms and detailed study of their spatial organization and microbial diversity [6,7,10,12].
2000s	Application of 16S rRNA sequencing in oral microbiology	Paster et al.	Revolutionized identification of microbial species in the oral cavity, demonstrating the rich complexity of the oral microbiome community [13,14].
2010s	Metagenomic analysis of oral microbiomes	Human Microbiome Project, National Research Council (US)	Provided knowledge about the genetic and functional potential of oral biofilms, resulting in novel therapeutic approaches [15,16].
2020s	Development of next-generation biofilm models and multi-omics integration	Rumbaugh & Whiteley; Cleaver & Garnett	Advanced clinical biofilm modeling and integrated microbiome analysis for improved translational applications [9,12,17].

Source: Table by author.

1.3. *Oral Biofilm Formation*

Biofilm development is a highly dynamic process influenced by a combination of microbial, environmental, and host-related factors. While the composition of oral biofilms depends on the types of microbial species present, it is also strongly shaped by mechanical forces, salivary chemistry, host immune responses, and the specific site within the oral cavity where the biofilm forms [10,18,19]. Among these factors, fluid dynamics play a particularly important role. Variations in fluid shear stress, such as those caused by salivary flow or chewing, can directly influence bacterial gene expression, thereby modifying behaviors like surface adhesion, EPS matrix production, and microbial competitiveness. For instance, *Streptococcus gordonii* has been shown to alter its transcriptional profile in response to changes in flow conditions, adjusting its biofilm-building capacity and ability to compete with other oral microbes [20].

Saliva plays a more active and regulatory role in biofilm development than previously recognized. Beyond its well-known functions in cleansing the oral cavity and buffering acids, saliva directly affects which bacterial species thrive, how they interact, and how the biofilm architecture evolves. Research by Choi et al. (2024) demonstrated that saliva significantly alters the growth patterns and competitive dynamics of oral streptococci, thereby influencing which strains become dominant in mature biofilms [21]. These interactions are essential, as the microbial composition of the biofilm directly impacts oral health.

When the natural microbial balance is disturbed, due to factors such as poor oral hygiene, high sugar intake, or chronic inflammation, opportunistic pathogens like *Streptococcus mutans* can proliferate. This shift often leads to the progression of dental caries and periodontal disease. For example, studies have shown that caries-active children tend to have reduced levels of beneficial bacteria such as *Rothia* and *Actinomyces*, and an overrepresentation of acidogenic and acid-tolerant species, including *S. mutans*, which contribute to enamel demineralization and lesion formation [22].

Central to the stability and resilience of these microbial communities is the EPS matrix. Much more than a simple barrier, the EPS serves as an organized scaffold that directs nutrient distribution, binds to antimicrobial compounds, and facilitates intercellular communication via quorum sensing. This coordinated communication allows bacteria within the biofilm to adapt collectively, regulate gene expression, and respond with effective resistance. These properties make biofilms notoriously resistant to both antimicrobial treatments and immune system attacks, presenting ongoing challenges for clinical management [23].

1.3.1. Stages of Oral Biofilm Formation

Oral biofilm formation is a highly coordinated, multi-stage process that begins with the attachment of pioneer microbial species and progresses toward the development of a mature, multi-species community (Figure 1). Each stage, from initial colonization to structural maturation, helps form a biofilm that is both stable and resistant to environmental challenges like antibiotics and the immune system.

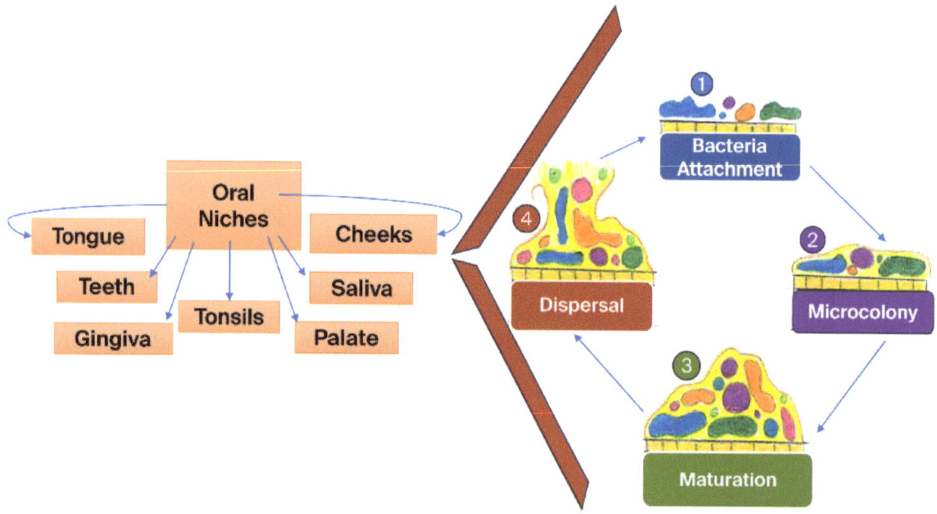

Figure 1. The biofilm life cycle in oral niches. This diagram illustrates the stages of the biofilm life cycle within various oral niches. (1) The biofilm life cycle begins with the initial attachment of microbial cells to surfaces within the oral cavity, such as the tongue, teeth, and gums. (2) This is followed by irreversible attachment and microcolony formation, namely, the cells firmly adhere, begin to produce EPS, and start to proliferate. (3) The biofilm then enters the maturation phase, during which the biofilm structure develops, expands, and allows the embedding of other microbial cells so that it acquires a complex, multispecies character. (4) Finally, in the dispersion stage, cells are released from the biofilm to spread towards other sites, including new surfaces, with the formation of new biofilms in the oral environment and elsewhere (oral niches). Credit: © Nensi Kallfani, used with permission.

Pellicle formation: The formation of oral biofilms begins rapidly after tooth cleaning with the development of the acquired pellicle, a thin, protein-rich film that coats the tooth surface within minutes. Although it measures only 0.1 to 1.0 μm in thickness (0.0001 to 0.001 mm), it plays an essential role in oral health and biofilm development. It acts as a substrate for initial bacterial adhesion, allowing pioneer species to attach to the tooth surface and initiate biofilm formation. The pellicle is a complex structure composed of glycoproteins, phosphoproteins, lipids, and enzymes, each contributing to its function. Glycoproteins bind to hydroxyapatite in enamel, providing anchor points for microbial colonization. Phosphoproteins, such as statherin and proline-rich proteins, help maintain enamel integrity by binding calcium ions, thereby preventing demineralization and promoting remineralization. Lipids reinforce the pellicle's structure, forming a hydrophobic barrier that shields the tooth surface from acids and environmental stressors. Embedded enzymes further modulate biochemical interactions, affecting how bacteria adhere and contributing to the biofilm's stability and composition. These enzymes can modify both the pellicle and the attached microbes, shaping the development and stability of the biofilm over time. Together, these molecular components form a dynamic and protective interface between the tooth and the oral environment, facilitating early bacterial colonization and influencing the long-term structure, function, and pathogenic potential of the biofilm [24,25].

Initial Bacterial adhesion: Following pellicle formation, pioneer bacterial species, particularly from the *Streptococcus* genus, initiate the first phase of biofilm development by adhering to the pellicle-coated tooth surface. This initial adhesion is mediated by a combination of nonspecific physical forces, such as van der Waals interactions and electrostatic attraction, alongside specific biochemical interactions. Central to this process are bacterial adhesins, surface proteins that recognize and bind to complementary receptors within the molecular structure of the pellicle. These interactions secure a stable attachment, forming the essential foundation for further colonization. Notably, species such as *Streptococcus sanguinis* and *Streptococcus gordonii* are among the key early colonizers. These organisms do more than simply adhere; they play active roles in structuring the early biofilm community. Through co-aggregation with other bacterial species and the production of extracellular substances, they help form the initial matrix that supports microbial stability. These early microbes help attract and support other, often more specialized, bacteria. Their actions are key in turning a simple biofilm into a more complex one, affecting how strong it becomes and whether it supports health or leads to disease, depending on the balance of microbes that follow [26].

Irreversible attachment and co-aggregation: As oral biofilms transition from early colonization to a mature, multi-species community, two key processes, irreversible attachment and co-aggregation, play essential roles in stabilizing the structure and supporting microbial diversity. Irreversible attachment represents an important transition from the initial, transitional adhesion phase. During this stage, bacteria form strong, permanent bonds with the acquired pellicle or with other microbial cells. These attachments are often mediated by high-affinity adhesins and surface proteins that reinforce the connection to the surface, anchoring the bacteria in place. This strong attachment is essential for biofilm stability and resistance to removal, making the microbial community more persistent and less susceptible to mechanical or chemical disruption. Following this, co-aggregation becomes an important mechanism for building a more complex and integrated biofilm community. Co-aggregation refers to species-specific interactions between different bacterial cells, allowing them to adhere to each other in a highly organized manner. This process facilitates the recruitment of secondary colonizers, which cannot directly attach to the pellicle but bind to already attached pioneer species. A key player in this stage is *Fusobacterium nucleatum*, a bacterium known for its role as a bridging organism. *F. nucleatum* can interact with both early and late colonizers, effectively connecting different microbial groups within the biofilm. Its unique ability to co-aggregate with a wide range of bacteria significantly enhances the structural complexity, microbial diversity, and stability of the biofilm. Together, irreversible attachment and co-aggregation lay the groundwork for a stable, mature biofilm capable of adapting to the constantly changing conditions in the oral environment [27,28].

Maturation and microbial succession: As biofilms continue to develop, they undergo significant changes in both microbial composition and structural organization. This process of maturation is driven by microbial succession, where early colonizers create favorable conditions for more diverse and specialized species to establish themselves in the community. One of the defining features of this stage is the increased production of EPS, a sticky, gel-like material secreted by bacteria that plays a central role in biofilm architecture and function. The EPS matrix acts as a biological "glue", binding cells together and anchoring the biofilm firmly to surfaces such as teeth, gums, and other oral tissues. It provides the structural scaffold necessary to support the biofilm's integrity, while also forming a protective barrier against external threats like antimicrobial agents, changes in pH or temperature, and the host's immune system. Beyond its defensive role, the matrix retains nutrients and forms microchannels that allow for the movement of water, waste, and signaling molecules, ensuring that the microbial community remains well-nourished, organized, and responsive to its environment. A critical element of biofilm coordination is quorum sensing, a form of microbial communication. Through this process, bacteria release and detect chemical signals that indicate population density. Once a certain threshold is reached, the community synchronizes its behavior, enhancing EPS production, increasing stress resistance, and sometimes initiating the release of virulence factors. This coordinated activity allows the biofilm to function not as isolated individual cells, but as a cooperative, resilient microbial community that can adapt to environmental pressures and persist within the host. During the maturation phase of biofilm development, the microbial composition undergoes a special change. Initial colonizers, such as *Streptococcus* species, establish the foundation of the biofilm and modify the local environment, paving the way for secondary colonizers like *Veillonella* and *Prevotella* species. These later arrivals play a crucial role in enhancing the diversity, stability, and functional complexity of the biofilm.

Veillonella species, for example, are known for metabolizing lactic acid produced by early *Streptococcus* species. This activity helps regulate pH levels within the biofilm, reducing local acidity and creating more favorable conditions for a broader range of microbes. *Prevotella* species contribute to the structural integrity and adaptability of the biofilm by breaking down complex carbohydrates and producing additional EPS. These actions not only reinforce the biofilm matrix but also support its long-term resilience. This process of microbial succession is essential for the development of a robust and balanced biofilm ecosystem, one that can adapt to environmental changes, resist external threats, and maintain functional cooperation among diverse microbial species within the oral cavity [29,30].

Biofilm dispersal: The final stage of biofilm development, known as biofilm dispersal, is a critical phase in the biofilm life cycle during which bacterial cells are released from the mature biofilm into the surrounding environment. This process enables bacteria to colonize new surfaces, expand their ecological niche, and initiate the formation of new biofilms. It does not just happen passively: dispersal is an active, highly regulated process driven by both internal genetic programs and external environmental signals. One of the main mechanisms of dispersal involves the enzymatic breakdown of the EPS matrix, which normally holds the biofilm together. Enzymes such as polysaccharide lyases and proteases degrade structural components of the EPS, weakening the matrix, and allowing individual cells or cell clusters to detach. In addition to biochemical triggers, physical forces, such as fluid shear, mechanical agitation, or temperature changes, can also disrupt the biofilm structure and promote cell release. Dispersal may also be triggered by nutrient limitations within the biofilm. When resources become limited, bacteria initiate a starvation response, activating genes that promote detachment and migration to more favorable environments. Another central mechanism is quorum sensing, a density-dependent signaling system that allows bacteria to coordinate gene expression related to dispersal. By synchronizing this process, the community ensures that dispersal occurs efficiently and at an optimal time [31]. The ability of biofilm-associated bacteria to disperse is a key contributor to their persistence and virulence. Dispersed cells can invade new tissues, evade immune defenses, and resist antimicrobial therapies, making infections harder to treat. This is especially relevant in chronic and recurrent infections, where dispersed cells reattach to surfaces and form new biofilms, undermining even aggressive treatment efforts and contributing to long-term disease progression [32].

Table 2 offers a detailed summary of the essential components, stages, and mechanisms involved in oral biofilm development, from initial formation to maturation and eventual dispersal. It outlines the role of the acquired pellicle as the foundational substrate for bacterial adhesion, followed by irreversible attachment and microbial co-aggregation, which establish the structural base of the biofilm. The table also describes key phases of biofilm maturation, including EPS production and microbial succession, as well as the mechanisms of dispersal that allow bacteria to colonize new sites. Each phase is paired with relevant microbial species and their specific contributions to biofilm dynamics.

Table 2. Components, processes, stages, and mechanisms in oral biofilm dynamics.

Stages	Description	Key Elements/ Processes	Examples Main Microbial Players/ Components
Acquired Pellicle Components	Substances involved in the initial formation of the biofilm on tooth surfaces [24,25].	- Salivary Glycoproteins - Phosphoproteins - Lipids - Enzymes	- Facilitate bacterial adhesion - Regulate mineralization - Provide structural stability - Modulate biochemical interactions
Irreversible Attachment & Co-Aggregation	Processes that solidify bacterial adhesion and establish inter-bacterial connections within the biofilm [26–28].	- Irreversible Attachment - Co-Aggregation	- *Streptococcus mutans* - *Actinomyces naeslundii* - *Fusobacterium nucleatum* - *Prevotella* spp.
Biofilm Maturation Stages	Phases of biofilm development characterized by increasing complexity and microbial diversity [29–31].	- Early Maturation - Late Maturation	- *Streptococcus mutans* - *Actinomyces naeslundii* - *Veillonella* spp. - *Prevotella* spp.
Biofilm Dispersal Mechanisms	Strategies by which biofilms disperse, allowing microorganisms to spread to new environments [32].	- Enzymatic Matrix Degradation - Physical Forces - Nutrient Limitation - Quorum Sensing	- *Pseudomonas aeruginosa* - *Streptococcus mutans*

Source: Table by author.

1.3.2. EPS Matrix and Biofilm Stability

More than structural support, the EPS matrix plays a central role in biofilm survival, antimicrobial resistance, and pathogenic potential. It provides both structural integrity and functional coordination within the biofilm, enabling microbial communities to persist in the dynamic and often hostile oral environment.

(A) Key Functions of the EPS Matrix in Biofilm Stability

1. Physical barrier: The EPS matrix forms a dense protective matrix that significantly restricts the penetration of antimicrobial agents. Antibiotics, antiseptics, and even immune cells like neutrophils and macrophages are often unable to reach bacteria embedded deep within the matrix. This physical separation contributes to the persistence of pathogens despite treatment.
2. Chemical defense: EPS components, such as charged polysaccharides, can bind and neutralize antimicrobial compounds. For instance, positively charged antibiotics may be sequestered by the negatively charged EPS, preventing them from reaching their bacterial targets and reducing their therapeutic effectiveness.
3. Nutrient retention and waste removal: The matrix contains fluid-filled channels that facilitate the distribution of nutrients and the removal of metabolic waste. This internal circulation supports metabolic cooperation among microbial species, enabling the biofilm to maintain vitality and self-sufficiency over time.
4. Immune evasion: The EPS helps the biofilm evade host immune defenses. It blocks immune cells from physically accessing bacteria and can cover antigenic structures, making it harder for the immune system to recognize and respond to pathogens. This evasion reduces immune-triggered tissue damage and supports long-term colonization.
5. Stress response: Within the protected microenvironment of the EPS, some bacterial cells enter a dormant or slow-growing state, becoming "persisted" cells. These cells are highly tolerant to antibiotics, primarily targeting actively dividing bacteria. Once treatment ends, persisting cells can reactivate, contributing to infection recurrence.

(B) Clinical Implications and Challenges

Due to the protective functions of the EPS matrix, biofilm-associated oral diseases, such as dental caries, chronic periodontitis, and peri-implantitis, are notoriously resistant to conventional treatments. Mechanical removal and repeated antibiotic therapy often fail to fully eliminate the biofilm, leading to chronic infection, inflammation, and frequent relapse.

Contemporary strategies for managing oral biofilms are evolving beyond the use of broad-spectrum antimicrobials in favor of more targeted and selective approaches. Rather than indifferently eliminating both harmful and beneficial microbes, modern therapies aim to precisely target pathogenic species, disrupt the structural integrity of the EPS matrix, and support the growth of beneficial, health-associated bacteria. This precision-based approach helps maintain the natural balance of the oral microbiome, reducing the risk of dysbiosis and promoting long-term oral health stability. Recent research emphasizes the value of integrating biocompatible materials with targeted drug delivery systems and host-modulating therapies to achieve more effective and sustainable biofilm control. These combined strategies enhance antimicrobial efficacy while simultaneously preserving soft tissue integrity and supporting immune function. This represents a significant shift toward site-specific, minimally disruptive interventions that align with the broader goals of precision medicine in oral healthcare [33,34].

These new methods try to solve the problems with regular treatments by targeting harmful bacteria more accurately, breaking down the biofilm structure, improving medicines' reach to the right place, and reducing damage to healthy tissue. Nanomaterials, thanks to their tiny size, large surface area, and ability to get through protective layers, offer great potential for removing biofilms in the mouth. To address these challenges, researchers are exploring novel therapeutic approaches, especially in nanotechnology, such as the following:

- Chitosan/nisin Z nanoparticles are biodegradable and biocompatible carriers that combine chitosan, a natural polysaccharide, with nisin Z, an antimicrobial peptide. This combination creates an efficient delivery system capable of penetrating deep into the EPS matrix of oral biofilms, reaching bacteria that are otherwise shielded from external agents. Chitosan enhances the nanoparticle's ability to adhere to negatively charged surfaces, such as biofilm components and oral tissues, which improves local retention. Meanwhile, nisin Z works by disrupting bacterial cell membranes, forming pores that cause the leakage of cellular contents and ultimately lead to bacterial death. The precision of this system allows it to effectively target pathogenic bacteria while minimizing harm to surrounding healthy tissues and beneficial microbes, making it a promising alternative to conventional broad-spectrum antimicrobials [35].
- Carboxymethyl chitosan-lysozyme nanogels are an advanced therapeutic system that combines carboxymethyl chitosan, which binds effectively to tooth surfaces and biofilms, with lysozyme, an enzyme capable of degrading bacterial cell walls. This formulation is particularly effective against *S. mutans*, the main bacteria involved in dental caries. Beyond its antibacterial action, the nanogel also promotes the remineralization of early enamel lesions, aiding in the reversal of initial tooth decay. Its dual function, eliminating harmful bacteria while supporting tissue repair, makes it especially well-suited for preventive care and the early management of carious lesions [36].
- Cargoless nanoparticles, unlike traditional drug-loaded systems, provide therapeutic benefits by interacting directly with host cells and modulating immune responses. In experimental models of periodontitis and peri-implantitis, these nanoparticles were shown to prevent bone loss by reducing inflammation and altering the host's response to biofilm-associated pathogens. Rather than killing bacteria directly, their effect lies in disrupting the harmful host–pathogen interactions and calming the inflammatory pathways triggered by biofilms. This approach highlights the promise of immune-targeted therapies that preserve the natural microbiome while still addressing the damaging effects of chronic infection [37].
- Sulforaphane is a natural compound found in cruciferous vegetables such as broccoli and kale. It has demonstrated notable antimicrobial activity, particularly against *S. mutans*, by interfering with bacterial metabolism and inhibiting biofilm formation. In addition to its antibacterial effects, sulforaphane possesses strong anti-inflammatory and antioxidant properties, which help reduce tissue damage linked to dental caries. Animal studies have shown that sulforaphane can significantly lower caries severity, highlighting its potential as a plant-based,

non-synthetic treatment option, especially appealing for individuals seeking natural alternatives to conventional therapies [38].

- Photosensitizing nanoliposomes loaded with Toluidine Blue O (TBO) represent an innovative photodynamic therapy (PDT) approach for managing oral biofilms. These nanoliposomes deliver an enhanced form of light-sensitive dye directly to the biofilm. Upon light activation, TBO produces reactive oxygen species (ROS) that effectively kill bacteria within the biofilm structure. This method is non-invasive and highly targeted, minimizing the risk of side effects often associated with systemic antibiotic use. It has shown particular effectiveness against cariogenic bacteria such as *Streptococcus mutans* and holds strong potential for minimally invasive, chairside applications in dental care [39].
- Next-generation imaging technologies, such as confocal laser scanning microscopy (CLSM) and scanning/transmission electron microscopy (SEM/TEM), have greatly enhanced our ability to visualize biofilms in high resolution and three dimensions. CLSM allows researchers to obtain real-time, layer-by-layer images of biofilm architecture using fluorescent dyes, making it possible to assess the spatial distribution of microbes and the structure of the EPS matrix. Electron microscopy, on the other hand, provides ultrastructural detail at the nanoscale, revealing fine surface and internal features of microbial cells and their surrounding matrix. These tools are essential not only for studying how biofilms form, grow, and mature, but also for evaluating their structural changes in response to antimicrobial treatments. By enabling the precise analysis of biofilm dynamics, these imaging methods have improved both diagnostic accuracy and research capabilities in oral microbiology [40].

Recent studies have confirmed that biofilm composition and behavior vary significantly depending on their location within the oral cavity. Different surfaces, such as supragingival (above the gumline), subgingival (below the gumline), and mucosal tissues like the tongue and cheeks, each provide unique environmental conditions that shape the microbial communities they host. For example, supragingival biofilms are typically exposed to oxygen and mechanical forces from chewing and brushing, favoring aerobic and facultative bacteria, while subgingival biofilms, protected within periodontal pockets, tend to harbor anaerobic and more pathogenic species associated with periodontitis. In contrast, mucosal surfaces support more dynamic and transient microbial populations due to epithelial cells and salivary flow. These site-specific differences influence not only the microbial diversity and ecology but also the host's immune response, the susceptibility to disease, and the efficacy of treatment strategies [41,42].

1.3.3. Microbial Composition and Health Implications

Having explored the formation of the oral biofilm, the next step is to explore the specific microorganisms that play important roles as the principal actors within these complex microbial communities. These microorganisms, each with unique characteristics and functions, are not merely passive inhabitants but active participants that drive the biofilm's formation, maturation, and pathogenic potential. Uncovering the roles of key microbial species, such as bacteria that initiate colonization, fungi that enhance biofilm stability, and viruses and archaea that influence biofilm dynamics, shows their combined impact on maintaining oral health and advancing oral diseases (Figure 2). This deeper understanding of the 'protagonists' of the biofilm will illuminate the intricate interactions that define the biofilm's behavior and impact, ultimately guiding more effective strategies for managing biofilm-related oral conditions.

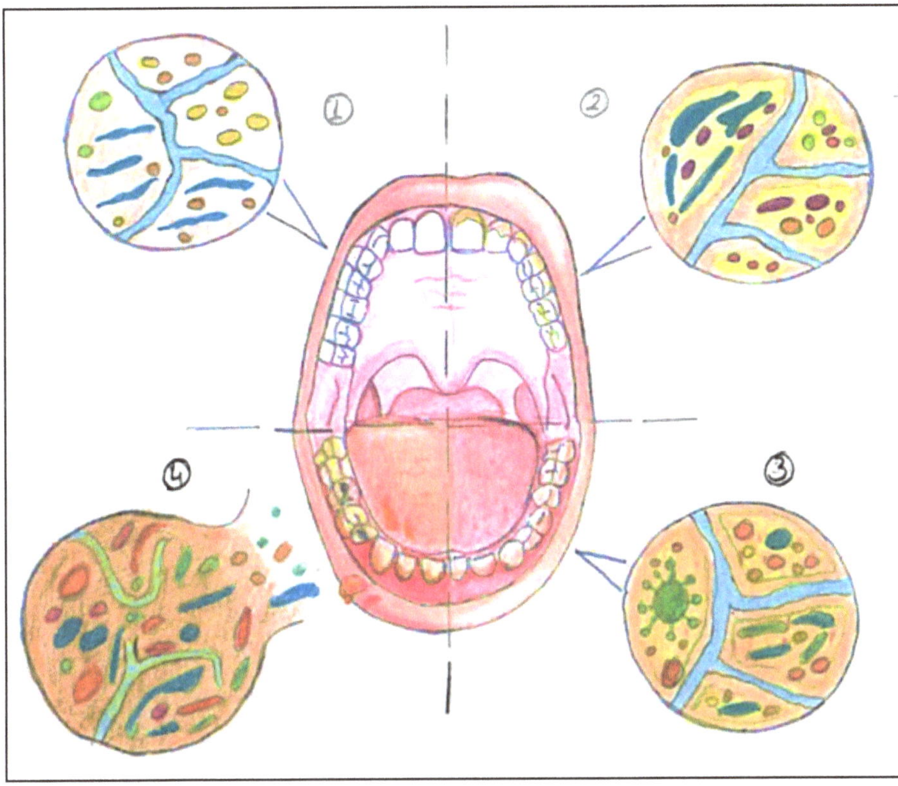

Figure 2. Microbial composition of oral biofilms, illustrating the interactions between bacteria, fungi, viruses, and archaea within an oral biofilm. The figure depicts how these interactions contribute to biofilm structure, stability, and the transition from health (1 & 2) to disease (3 & 4). Credit: © Nensi Kallfani, used with permission.

Bacteria: Single-celled microorganisms classified under the domain bacteria represent one of the three fundamental domains of life, alongside Archaea and Eukarya. These microorganisms are among the oldest and most diverse life forms on Earth, thriving in a vast array of environments, from soil, water, and air to the bodies of plants, animals, and humans. Within the oral cavity, bacteria are the most diverse and abundant constituents of biofilms, where they play crucial roles in maintaining oral health as well as in the development of diseases. Among these, *Streptococcus* species are particularly significant early colonizers that initiate the biofilm formation process. *S. mutans*, a primary species associated with dental caries, is highly acidogenic and aciduric, meaning it not only produces acid as a metabolic byproduct but also thrives in low-pH environments created by this acid production. This capability allows *S. mutans* to dominate in acidic conditions, leading to the demineralization of tooth enamel and the development of caries. The virulence of *S. mutans* is further enhanced by its ability to produce extracellular polysaccharides, which contribute to the biofilm's structural integrity and resistance to environmental stresses [43].

In contrast, other *Streptococcus* species, such as *S. sanguinis* and *S. gordonii*, play protective roles in maintaining oral health. These species are also early colonizers but are considered beneficial due to their ability to compete with pathogenic bacteria for adhesion sites and nutrients. *S. sanguinis* and *S. gordonii* contribute to a balanced microbial community by producing hydrogen peroxide and other antimicrobial substances that inhibit the growth of cariogenic bacteria like *S. mutans*. This competitive inhibition is a crucial factor in preventing the overgrowth of pathogenic species and maintaining oral microbial homeostasis [43].

Actinomyces species, particularly *A. naeslundii*, are also integral to the early stages of biofilm formation. These bacteria adhere strongly to the tooth surface and play a key role in the initial colonization process. *A. naeslundii* is known for its ability to form complex biofilm structures through co-aggregation with other microbial species. This structural complexity is critical for the stability of the biofilm and its resistance to physical and chemical disruption. Moreover, *A. naeslundii* is associated with the development of root caries, particularly in the presence of gingival recession, where the root surface is exposed. This bacterium is also implicated in periodontal disease, especially when the biofilm environment moves toward a pathogenic state dominated by anaerobic bacteria [44].

F. nucleatum is a key player in the maturation of the biofilm and the process of co-aggregation, which is the specific inter-bacterial interactions that link early colonizers with later-arriving species. It serves as a central bridge within the biofilm, facilitating the integration of various bacterial species into a cohesive community. *F. nucleatum* is particularly associated with periodontal disease progression due to its ability to induce inflammation and contribute to tissue destruction. It interacts with both pathogenic and commensal bacteria, promoting complex biofilm structures that are characteristic of advanced periodontal disease. The presence of *F. nucleatum* is often considered a marker of periodontal disease severity, as it is involved in the exacerbation of inflammatory responses and the degradation of periodontal tissues [45].

These bacterial species, with their distinct roles in biofilm formation, maturation, and pathogenicity, illustrate the complexity of microbial interactions within oral biofilms. Their activities not only influence the structural and functional integrity of the biofilm but also determine the balance between health and disease in the oral cavity.

Fungi: The diverse kingdom of fungi includes eukaryotic organisms such as yeasts, molds, and mushrooms. Unlike plants, fungi do not engage in photosynthesis; instead, they obtain nutrients by absorbing organic matter, often through the decomposition of dead organisms or parasitic relationships. Fungi are vital components of ecosystems, serving as decomposers, symbionts, and pathogens. Their roles are crucial in nutrient cycling, plant health, and the balance of natural environments. Additionally, fungi have significant implications for human health, agriculture, and industry due to their diverse functions and interactions. In the context of oral biofilms, fungi, particularly *Candida* species, are key players in biofilm composition and pathogenicity. *C. albicans*, the most prevalent fungal species in the oral cavity, is well known for its ability to form robust biofilms on various surfaces, including mucosal tissues and dental appliances, contributing to persistent infections and complications. These biofilms are characterized by a high degree of resistance to antifungal treatments, making infections caused by *C. albicans* particularly challenging to treat. This resistance is largely due to the biofilm's extracellular matrix, which acts as a protective barrier, shielding the fungal cells from antifungal agents and the host's immune defenses [45].

The biofilm-forming capability of *C. albicans* is a critical factor in the development of oral candidiasis, a condition that is especially prevalent among immunocompromised individuals. In such patients, the immune system's reduced capacity to control microbial growth allows *C. albicans* to proliferate and dominate the oral microbiome, leading to the establishment of persistent biofilms. These biofilms can cause significant discomfort and are often associated with complications such as mucosal inflammation and secondary bacterial infections.

Moreover, the presence of *C. albicans* within oral biofilms has broader implications for the microbial community as a whole. Fungal cells within the biofilm can interact with bacterial species, influencing the overall composition and behavior of the biofilm. For instance, *C. albicans* can engage in synergistic relationships with certain bacteria, such as *S. mutans*, enhancing the biofilm's pathogenic potential. These interactions can lead to more complex biofilm structures that are more resilient and difficult to eradicate, thereby contributing to the persistence of oral infections and the progression of disease [46].

Viruses: Microscopic infectious agents, viruses, occupy a unique position at the interface between living and non-living systems. Significantly smaller than bacteria, they consist of genetic material, either DNA or RNA, encased in a protein shell known as a capsid. Some viruses also possess an outer lipid envelope derived from the host cell membrane. Unlike living organisms, viruses lack the cellular machinery required for metabolism, energy production, and independent reproduction, making them entirely dependent on a host cell for replication.

These enigmatic entities challenge our conventional understanding of life, serving as pivotal agents in both health and disease, and influencing a wide range of biological processes across all domains of life. In the context of oral biofilms, viruses play an essential role in shaping microbial communities. Bacteriophages, which are viruses that specifically target bacteria, act as key regulators of bacterial populations within biofilms, maintaining balance and diversity. Meanwhile, human viruses like HSV and HPV also contribute to the dynamics of oral biofilms, impacting both the structure and pathogenicity of these complex microbial ecosystems. By lysing bacterial cells, bacteriophages control the abundance and diversity of bacterial species, thereby shaping the overall composition of the biofilm. This lytic activity not only helps maintain microbial balance but also influences the evolutionary pressures within the biofilm, potentially driving the selection of more resilient bacterial strains. Additionally, bacteriophages can facilitate horizontal gene transfer among bacteria, contributing to the spread of antibiotic resistance and virulence factors, which can enhance the pathogenic potential of the biofilm [47].

Human viruses such as HSV-1 are significant in terms of their direct impact on the host and their indirect influence on the microbial communities within oral biofilms. HSV-1 is known for causing mucosal infections, including herpes labialis (cold sores) and herpetic gingivostomatitis. These infections can disrupt the integrity of oral tissues and alter the local immune response, creating an environment that may favor the colonization and persistence of pathogenic microbes. HSV-1 can modulate the host's immune system, potentially weakening the body's defenses and allowing for more aggressive bacterial and fungal growth within the biofilm. This modulation can lead to changes in the microbial composition, further complicating the clinical management of oral diseases [48].

HPV, particularly high-risk types like HPV-16 and HPV-18, is strongly associated with the development of oropharyngeal cancers. These viruses can integrate into the host's genome and induce oncogenic transformations in epithelial cells, leading to malignancies. Beyond its role in cancer development, HPV also alters the local immune environment, which can affect the composition and virulence of oral biofilms. The presence of HPV in the oral cavity may disrupt the natural balance of microbial communities, promoting the overgrowth of certain pathogenic species and contributing to a more virulent biofilm state. This interaction between HPV and the oral microbiome underscores the complex interplay between viral infections and microbial dynamics in the development of oral diseases [47,48].

Archaea: A distinct domain of single-celled microorganisms, Archaea, like bacteria, lack a nucleus and other membrane-bound organelles, classifying them as prokaryotes. However, they differ significantly from bacteria in their genetic, biochemical, and structural attributes, making them a unique group within the microbial world. Initially discovered in extreme environments such as hot springs and salt lakes, archaea are now known to inhabit a broad range of ecosystems, including soils, oceans, and various parts of the human body, particularly the gut and oral cavity. This connects the microbial worlds of bacteria and eukaryotes, highlighting unique adaptations that are important for the environment and human health.

In the oral cavity, archaea, especially methanogens, play a particular role within the biofilm ecosystem. *M. oralis*, the most frequently identified archaeal species in this environment, is noted for its methanogenic activity, a process that involves the production of methane through the reduction in carbon dioxide using hydrogen as the electron donor. This activity not only contributes to the metabolic dynamics of oral biofilms but also highlights the specialized functions that archaea perform in various ecosystems. The methanogenic activity of *M. oralis* is crucial for maintaining the redox balance within the oral biofilm, which in turn supports the overall metabolic efficiency of the microbial community. By consuming hydrogen, methanogens prevent the accumulation of this gas, which could otherwise inhibit the metabolic processes of other microbes within the biofilm. This interspecies interaction highlights the cooperative nature of microbial communities in the oral cavity, where the byproducts of one species serve as substrates for others, enhancing the stability and functionality of the biofilm [49].

The presence of *M. oralis* has been increasingly associated with periodontal disease, where their interactions with other microorganisms contribute to disease progression. In particular, methanogens collaborate with sulfate-reducing bacteria within the biofilm to produce VSCs, such as hydrogen sulfide and methyl mercaptan. These compounds are not only responsible for the characteristic malodor of halitosis but also contribute to the destruction of periodontal tissues. The production of VSCs exacerbates inflammation and tissue damage, which are hallmarks of periodontal disease. The ability of methanogens to influence both the chemical environment of the biofilm and the host's response underscores their role in the pathogenesis of oral diseases [49].

The involvement of archaea, particularly methanogens, in oral health and disease is a growing area of research that highlights the complexity of the oral microbiome. Their unique metabolic capabilities, interactions with other microbes, and contribution to conditions like halitosis and periodontal disease suggest that archaea are not just passive inhabitants but active participants in the dynamics of oral biofilms.

Table 3 summarizes the main microbial groups, bacteria, fungi, viruses, and archaea, involved in oral biofilm development.

Table 3. Microbial species in oral biofilms, roles, and health implications.

Microbial Groups	Key Species	Role in Biofilm	Health Implications
Bacteria	*S. mutans*	Acid production, biofilm formation [43].	Dental caries
	S. sanguinis	Initial colonization, pathogen competition [43].	Oral health maintenance
	A. naeslundii	Early colonization, structural integrity [44].	Root caries, periodontal disease
	F. nucleatum	Biofilm maturation, co-aggregation [45].	Periodontal disease
Fungi	*C. albicans*	Biofilm formation, interaction with bacteria [46].	Oral candidiasis, increased biofilm resistance.
	C. glabrata	Biofilm formation, antifungal resistance [46].	Oral candidiasis in immunocompromised patients.
	C. tropicalis	Biofilm formation, invasive infections [46].	Higher risk of systemic infections.
Viruses	Bacteriophages	Regulation of bacterial populations, gene transfer [47].	Modulation of biofilm composition, antibiotic resistance.
	HSV-1	Infection of epithelial cells, immune modulation [48].	Herpes labialis, gingivostomatitis.
	HPV	Oncogenic transformation, immune modulation [48].	Oropharyngeal cancers, benign oral lesions.
Archaea	*M. oralis*	Methanogenesis, interaction with bacteria [49].	Periodontal disease, contribution to halitosis.
	M. mazei	Broad substrate utilization for methanogenesis [49].	Modulation of microbial ecology in biofilms.

Source: Table by author.

1.4. *Factors Influencing Microbial Composition of Oral Biofilms*

Many things affect the types of microbes in our mouths, like diet, brushing habits, saliva, genetics, and the mouth's environment. These factors help decide whether microbes support health or cause disease. Knowing how they work can help us prevent dental problems and support general well-being.

1.4.1. Diet: Carbohydrate Intake and Fermentable Substrates

The impact of diet on the microbial composition of oral biofilms is profound, with fermentable carbohydrates such as sugars and starches being key drivers of this influence [50]. For example, foods and beverages high in sucrose, glucose, fructose, and other fermentable sugars, such as candies, sugary drinks, pastries, and bread, provide ample substrates for acidogenic bacteria like *S. mutans* and *Lactobacillus* species.

When these bacteria metabolize these sugars, they produce lactic acid, which significantly lowers the pH in the oral environment. A sustained acidic environment (pH below 5.5) promotes the demineralization of tooth enamel, which can lead to dental caries. For instance, frequent consumption of sugary snacks or drinks throughout the day can result in prolonged periods of low pH in the mouth, giving cariogenic bacteria an advantage over other, non-cariogenic species. To illustrate, *S. mutans* is particularly efficient at converting sucrose into lactic acid and also uses sucrose to produce extracellular polysaccharides, which enhances its ability to adhere to the tooth surface and form biofilms. This dual function of sucrose in both acid production and biofilm stability underscores why high-sugar diets are so detrimental to dental health.

Additionally, other fermentable carbohydrates like starches found in refined foods such as white bread, crackers, and chips can also contribute to acid production. Although starches are less readily fermentable than simple sugars, they can still be broken down by amylase, an enzyme in saliva, into simpler sugars that can then be fermented by bacteria.

In contrast, diets that are lower in fermentable carbohydrates and higher in fibrous foods like vegetables and whole grains can help maintain a more neutral pH in the oral cavity. Fibrous foods stimulate saliva production, which acts as a natural buffer, neutralizing acids and washing away food particles and bacteria, thereby reducing the risk of caries. Moreover, certain foods, such as cheese and other dairy products, contain calcium and phosphate, which can help remineralize enamel and counteract the effects of acidic conditions, further emphasizing the role of diet in oral health [50].

Protein and fat intake: While sugars and starches are primary contributors to dental caries, diets rich in protein and fat influence the oral environment in a different way, supporting the growth of bacteria associated with periodontal disease. These nutrients do not fuel acid-producing bacteria that cause cavities; instead, they promote the proliferation of proteolytic and lipolytic microorganisms, such as *Porphyromonas gingivalis* and *Prevotella intermedia*, which thrive on proteins and fats.

Protein-rich foods, such as red meat, poultry, fish, eggs, and dairy products, provide a continuous source of amino acids and peptides. These are utilized by proteolytic bacteria as energy sources. *P. gingivalis*, a well-recognized keystone pathogen in periodontitis, is particularly adept at degrading host proteins. During this process, it produces harmful metabolic byproducts, including volatile sulfur compounds (VSCs) such as hydrogen sulfide and methyl mercaptan. These compounds are not only responsible for halitosis (bad breath) but also contribute to tissue irritation and inflammation in the periodontal environment.

Additionally, *P. gingivalis* secretes potent proteolytic enzymes, most notably gingipains, which degrade structural proteins like collagen, undermining the integrity of the periodontal tissues. This enzymatic destruction weakens the gums and periodontal ligaments, and supports alveolar bone, ultimately contributing to the development and progression of periodontal disease.

Fat-rich foods, such as those high in saturated fats, oils, butter, and processed snacks, also influence the oral microbiota. Lipolytic bacteria metabolize fats into fatty acids and glycerol, altering the local environment. An accumulation of fatty acids can lower oxygen availability, fostering anaerobic conditions that favor the growth of pathogenic bacteria commonly found in periodontal pockets.

This dietary pattern, high in proteins and fats, encourages microbial communities adapted to deep, low-oxygen environments rich in host-derived nutrients. Over time, such conditions can disrupt oral microbial balance (dysbiosis) and elevate the risk of chronic periodontitis. *P. intermedia* is another proteolytic bacterium implicated in periodontal conditions, including acute necrotizing ulcerative gingivitis (ANUG). Like *P. gingivalis*, it thrives on protein-rich substrates and contributes to soft tissue destruction and inflammatory responses.

Although proteins and fats do not directly contribute to tooth decay, they play a significant role in shaping the subgingival microbiome. By supporting the growth of proteolytic and anaerobic pathogens, these nutrients increase the risk of periodontal tissue breakdown and gum disease [51].

Vitamins and micronutrients: The microbial composition of oral biofilms and overall oral health are significantly influenced by the roles of vitamins and micronutrients. This can be demonstrated as follows:

- Vitamin C (ascorbic acid) is not only crucial for the synthesis of collagen and the maintenance of healthy gingival tissues but also possesses antimicrobial properties that can influence the balance of microbial communities within the oral cavity. Adequate intake of vitamin C helps fortify the connective tissues of the gums, making them more resistant to infection and inflammation. Conversely, a deficiency in vitamin C can lead to gingival inflammation, bleeding, and a weakened periodontal structure, creating an environment conducive to the proliferation of pathogenic bacteria. This deficiency can exacerbate conditions such as gingivitis and periodontitis, where the inflammatory response further disrupts the microbial balance, favoring the overgrowth of harmful species.
- Similarly, Vitamin D is critical for calcium homeostasis and bone health, playing an indirect essential role in supporting the structural integrity of the periodontium, which includes the gums, periodontal ligament, and alveolar bone. Adequate levels of Vitamin D are necessary for the proper mineralization of bone, which helps maintain the strength and density of the jawbone that supports teeth. In addition, Vitamin D has been shown to possess anti-inflammatory and antimicrobial properties, potentially inhibiting the growth of periodontopathogens. A deficiency in Vitamin D can lead to decreased bone density and a compromised periodontal structure, increasing the susceptibility to periodontal diseases as the supporting tissues around the teeth become more vulnerable to bacterial invasion.

- Vitamin A also plays a crucial role in maintaining the health of mucosal barriers within the oral cavity. This vitamin is essential for the differentiation and maintenance of epithelial tissues, which form the first line of defense against microbial invasion. A deficiency in Vitamin A can impair the immune response, weakening the mucosal barriers and allowing for increased colonization by pathogenic species. This can lead to a higher incidence of oral infections and an imbalance in the microbial community that favors disease progression.
- In addition to these key vitamins, other micronutrients such as zinc and iron are also vital for oral health. Zinc, for example, is known for its role in immune function and wound healing and has been shown to have direct antimicrobial effects on oral pathogens. Iron, while essential for various bodily functions, must be carefully regulated, as both deficiency and excess can influence the composition of the oral microbiome, potentially fostering environments that support pathogenic bacteria.

Overall, the adequate intake of these vitamins and micronutrients is essential, not only for general health but also for maintaining a balanced oral microbiome (Figure 3). Their roles in immune function, tissue integrity, and microbial modulation highlight the intricate connections between nutrition and oral health [52].

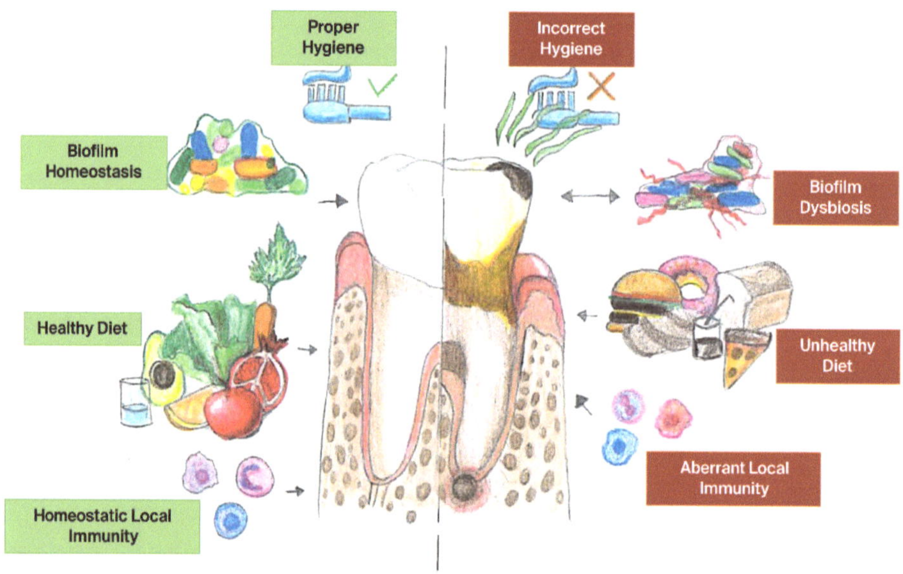

Figure 3. Impact of diet on oral biofilm composition illustrates how various dietary components (carbohydrates, proteins, fats, and vitamins) influence the composition and health outcomes of oral biofilms. The figure demonstrates pathways from nutrient intake to changes in microbial communities and subsequent health implications, such as caries and periodontal disease. Credit: © Nensi Kallfani, used with permission.

1.4.2. Oral Hygiene Practices

The regular mechanical disruption of oral biofilms through brushing and flossing is crucial for maintaining oral health. These practices effectively remove dental plaque, a bacterial biofilm that begins forming on teeth shortly after cleaning, and help reduce the overall microbial load in the mouth. If not adequately removed, plaque can mature into more complex and pathogenic biofilms, increasing the risk of dental caries and periodontal disease. Brushing and flossing physically disrupt these biofilms, preventing their progression into harmful states. Proper brushing technique, as detailed in Table 4, plays a crucial role in managing plaque and supporting long-term oral health.

Table 4. Main oral hygiene practices and recommendations for effective plaque control.

Practice	Recommendations	Details
Brushing Frequency	Brush at least twice a day [52,53].	Morning and night brushing are critical to remove accumulated plaque.
Brushing Duration	Brush for a minimum of two minutes [52].	Ensures thorough cleaning of all tooth surfaces.
Toothbrush Type	Use a soft-bristled toothbrush [52].	Prevents gum irritation and enamel wear.
Toothpaste	Use fluoride toothpaste (1000–1500 ppm fluoride) [52].	Strengthens enamel and prevents demineralization.
Brushing Technique	Use small circular motions or hold the toothbrush at a 45° angle to the gumline [53].	Effective for cleaning and avoiding gum damage.
Additional Oral Hygiene	Include flossing and mouthwash [53].	Flossing removes plaque between teeth; antimicrobial mouthwash helps reduce bacterial load.
Tongue Cleaning	Brush or scrape the tongue daily [52,53].	Reduces bacterial presence and improves breath.
Timing After Meals	Wait 30 min to brush after consuming acidic foods [52].	Prevents enamel erosion by allowing saliva to neutralize pH before brushing.
Toothbrush Replacement	Replace toothbrush every 3–4 months [52,53].	Worn bristles lose efficacy in disrupting biofilm and can harbor microorganisms.
Professional Cleanings	Visit a dental professional every 6 months (or as recommended) [53].	Conducting scaling procedures and evaluating oral health indicators.

Source: Table by author.

Brushing not only effectively clears dental plaque from the tooth surfaces and gum line but also prevents the development of an anaerobic environment that favors the growth of pathogenic bacteria, such as *Fusobacterium* and *Prevotella*, commonly associated with periodontitis. These bacteria thrive in low-oxygen conditions and contribute to the inflammatory processes that damage the gums and supporting structures of the teeth. Inadequate oral hygiene practices allow plaque to accumulate, creating an environment favorable to these harmful bacteria. Incorporating additional oral hygiene measures, such as the use of antimicrobial mouthwash and brushing the tongue, can further enhance the effectiveness of routine brushing and flossing. Together, these practices are fundamental to maintaining optimal oral hygiene, reducing the risk of oral diseases, and promoting overall oral health [53]. The use of antimicrobial mouthwashes and toothpaste plays a significant role in shaping the microbial composition of oral biofilms. These products typically contain active ingredients designed to eliminate or inhibit bacteria, thereby reducing overall bacterial counts and helping to prevent oral diseases such as gingivitis and periodontitis.

Mouthwashes, in particular, are commonly used as an adjunct to mechanical cleaning methods like brushing and flossing. Recognizing the differences between various types of mouthwashes enables individuals to make informed, personalized choices that best support their oral health. Each type of mouthwash offers distinct benefits and limitations, and selecting the most appropriate one depends on specific oral health goals and conditions. Chlorhexidine-based mouthwashes are highly effective in controlling gingival inflammation and are often used in the short-term management of gingivitis. However, they are not recommended for prolonged use. Long-term or excessive use can lead to tooth and tongue staining, taste alterations, and the disruption of the oral microbiome, potentially increasing the risk of microbial imbalance and other side effects. In comparison, essential oil-based mouthwashes, formulated with active ingredients such as eucalyptol, thymol, and menthol, are generally milder and less disruptive to the oral microbial community. While they minimize the potential for bacterial resistance and are well-tolerated for daily use, they may be less potent than chlorhexidine in managing active periodontal disease. Fluoride mouthwashes are primarily used to strengthen enamel and prevent dental caries, making them an ideal daily option for individuals at risk of tooth decay. These rinses typically exert minimal influence on the oral microbiome, allowing for routine use without disturbing microbial balance. Incorporating the appropriate mouthwash into a comprehensive oral hygiene routine, which includes brushing, flossing, and regular dental visits, can help control dental plaque (biofilm), support gum and tooth health, and minimize potential side effects or microbiome disruption [54,55]. Table 5, below, summarizes the common types of mouthwashes and their respective impacts.

Table 5. Types of mouthwashes and their impact on oral biofilms.

Types of Mouthwash	Active Ingredients	Primary Effects	Potential Side Effects
Chlorhexidine	Chlorhexidine gluconate	Exhibits strong and broad-spectrum antimicrobial action against Gram-positive and Gram-negative bacteria; considered the gold standard for short-term plaque control [54,55].	Overuse may lead to microbial resistance, altered oral microbiota (dysbiosis), tooth staining, and taste disturbance [54,55].
Essential Oils	Thymol, eucalyptol, menthol, methyl salicylate	Demonstrates antiplaque and antigingivitis effects through disruption of bacterial cell walls; less potent than chlorhexidine but suitable for long-term use [54].	Possible mucosal irritation or allergic reactions in sensitive individuals [54,55].
Fluoride	Sodium fluoride, stannous fluoride	Strengthens enamel, reduces caries risk [54,55].	Typically well-tolerated, minimal microbial disruption [54,55].
Cetylpyridinium chloride (CPC)-based	Cetylpyridinium chloride	Antimicrobial action, reduces plaque and gingivitis [54,55].	Potential staining of teeth, altered taste [54,55].
Hydrogen Peroxide	Hydrogen peroxide	Antiseptic and mild whitening effects by releasing reactive oxygen species that disrupt biofilm structure [54].	Overuse can irritate oral tissues, disrupt beneficial bacteria [54].
Herbal Mouthwashes	Aloe vera, tea tree oil, green tea extract	Antimicrobial properties, generally milder than chemical counterparts [54,55].	Limited clinical evidence; efficacy may vary between formulations [54,55].

Source: Table by author.

1.4.3. Saliva and Biofilm Pathogenicity

Saliva serves as one of the body's most effective natural defenses against harmful microbes in the oral cavity. Beyond its role in lubrication and digestion, saliva contains a diverse array of antimicrobial molecules that collectively regulate the microbial population, helping to maintain a stable, health-supporting oral biofilm. These components act synergistically, meaning their combined effects are more powerful than individual actions, forming a comprehensive line of defense against bacterial, fungal, and viral colonization.

Among the most crucial antimicrobial agents in saliva are as follows:

- Lysozyme, an enzyme that breaks down the peptidoglycan layer of bacterial cell walls, especially in Gram-positive bacteria, compromises their integrity and enhances their susceptibility to other immune defenses.
- Lactoferrin is a multifunctional protein that sequesters iron, an essential nutrient for bacterial growth. By limiting iron availability, lactoferrin slows microbial proliferation and also exhibits direct antimicrobial and antifungal effects, including activity against *Candida albicans*.

- Secretory immunoglobulin A (sIgA), an antibody that binds to microbial surfaces, blocking pathogens from adhering to teeth and mucosal surfaces. sIgA also facilitates the clearance of microbes through swallowing, reducing their ability to colonize and form biofilms.
- Histatins are a family of antimicrobial peptides particularly effective against fungal pathogens like *Candida* species. They also promote wound healing and maintain mucosal health.
- Peroxidases (such as salivary peroxidase and myeloperoxidase) catalyze the formation of reactive oxygen species (ROS). These compounds inhibit microbial metabolism and can damage bacterial membranes, contributing to pathogen elimination.
- Bicarbonate and phosphate ions buffer acids produced by bacterial metabolism, helping to maintain a neutral pH that inhibits acidogenic and aciduric bacteria such as *S. mutans* and *Lactobacillus* spp.
- Calcium and phosphate ions support remineralization of enamel, counteracting the effects of dietary and microbial acids.

Together, these agents form a multilayered, adaptive antimicrobial system. Rather than indiscriminately eliminating all microbes, saliva's components selectively suppress pathogenic organisms while supporting the growth of beneficial, commensal bacteria. When saliva is rich in antimicrobial proteins (like lysozyme, lactoferrin, and secretory IgA), buffers (like bicarbonate), and minerals (like calcium and phosphate), it helps maintain a stable environment.

The Role of Saliva in Oral Biofilm Regulation and Xerostomia-Associated Imbalances

The effectiveness of saliva in maintaining a healthy oral environment is largely determined by its composition, flow rate, and buffering capacity. These factors directly influence the formation, composition, and pathogenicity of oral biofilms, which are complex communities of microorganisms that adhere to the teeth and other oral surfaces [56].

Research has shown that when people suffer from xerostomia, or dry mouth, these protective functions of saliva are weakened. This condition can be caused by diseases like Sjögren's syndrome, medications, aging, or radiation therapy. In such cases, there is less saliva, and its quality also changes, which allows harmful bacteria to thrive and disrupt the natural balance of the mouth's microbial ecosystem [57,58].

Several clinical studies highlight that changes in saliva affect not only how biofilms form but also how aggressive they become. For example, Babanouri et al. (2025) demonstrated that using xylitol and fluoride varnishes in orthodontic patients helped reduce biofilm buildup and improve saliva quality [59]. Similarly, Souza et al. (2024) showed that artificial saliva products can protect tooth roots from demineralization when natural saliva is lacking [60].

Older adults and denture wearers are particularly affected by xerostomia. Mhatre et al. (2024) and Müller et al. (2023) report that dry mouth in these groups leads to more frequent dental problems, changes in diet, and a drop in quality of life [61, 62]. Managing xerostomia, therefore, is not only about comfort; it is crucial for preventing disease.

In addition, researchers are exploring both traditional and innovative treatments to manage dry mouth and restore oral balance. These include non-drug approaches like topical gels, sprays, and acupuncture, and even advanced lubricants that mimic saliva's natural flow and feel [63,64].

Saliva's Role in Oral Biofilm Management

Saliva plays a central role in regulating the behavior and pathogenic potential of oral biofilms through several interconnected mechanisms. One important function is the modulation of microbial metabolism. Salivary mucins, particularly MUC5B, have been shown to influence glucose metabolism in early biofilm communities, helping maintain microbial balance and reducing the risk of cariogenic activity [65]. Beyond metabolic regulation, saliva also impacts the structural architecture of biofilms. Studies demonstrate that human saliva alters the growth patterns and spatial organization of oral streptococci, affecting their stability and competitive behaviors, factors critical to biofilm maturation and virulence [21]. In addition to shaping biofilm composition and structure, saliva provides innate antimicrobial protection. It contains a range of bioactive molecules, including enzymes, peptides, and antibodies, that inhibit the adhesion and growth of pathogens. Notably, its antifungal properties help control *Candida* species, thereby preventing fungal overgrowth and contributing to the overall stability of the oral microbiome [66]. These combined effects underscore saliva's essential role as both a physical medium and a biochemical regulator in oral biofilm management.

Saliva-Based Diagnostics: Emerging Applications

Recent advances in salivary diagnostics are revolutionizing disease detection by offering a non-invasive, accessible, and cost-effective alternative to traditional testing methods. Saliva is an attractive diagnostic fluid due to its ease of collection and its complex composition, which includes proteins, enzymes, nucleic acids, hormones, and microbial metabolites. These characteristics make it a valuable medium for identifying biomarkers associated with both oral and systemic conditions. For example, salivary analysis is being explored for the early detection of oral cancers, metabolic disorders, and even neurodegenerative diseases, expanding the potential of personalized medicine [67].

Innovative technologies are driving the development of novel diagnostic tools that utilize saliva in real time. One such advancement includes saliva-sensing dental floss, which integrates molecularly imprinted polymers with microfluidic threads to detect salivary cortisol. This device enables on-demand monitoring of stress levels, reflecting broader health states without the need for invasive procedures or laboratory infrastructure [68].

Despite the growing interest and technological progress, regulatory barriers remain. Currently, no saliva-based diagnostic tests have received FDA approval specifically for assessing risks of periodontal disease, dental caries, or head and neck cancers. This regulatory gap highlights the need for continued validation, the standardization of collection protocols, and large-scale clinical trials to confirm diagnostic accuracy and reproducibility [69].

Additional studies continue to enrich the understanding of salivary diagnostics. For instance, shifts in the salivary microbiome following dental scaling in children [70] and the use of salivary biomarkers to monitor biofilm composition and dietary influences [71] demonstrate the diverse applications of saliva-based tools. Furthermore, research into compounds like usnic acid has shown promise in controlling polymicrobial biofilms in artificial saliva environments, adding antimicrobial relevance to diagnostic contexts [72].

As outlined by Constantin et al. (2025) and Javaid et al. (2016), the field continues to progress with both standard and emerging technologies, ranging from lateral flow immunoassays and biosensors to next-generation sequencing platforms [73,74]. These developments underscore the evolving role of saliva not only as a diagnostic fluid but also as a window into the oral and systemic health of the individual.

1.4.4. Host Genetics

Genetic variation also affects salivary composition, including levels of antimicrobial peptides, enzymes, and immunoglobulins. Differences in the genetic regulation of these components can lead to reduced salivary flow, weakened antimicrobial activity, or lower buffering capacity, all of which promote conditions favorable to cariogenic and periodontopathogenic species. This is particularly relevant in the development of caries and periodontal diseases [75].

Additionally, host genetics can influence the expression of glycoproteins and receptors on oral epithelial cells, which serve as adhesion sites for bacteria. Variations in these receptors can change bacterial binding efficiency, thereby shaping early biofilm formation and microbial community structure. For instance, enhanced binding of *P. gingivalis* in genetically predisposed individuals increases their risk of periodontal disease.

Local Environment and Oral Cavity Niches

The structure and behavior of the oral microbiome are profoundly shaped by the diverse microenvironments within the oral cavity. Factors such as pH, oxygen levels, temperature, and moisture create distinct ecological niches, each favoring the colonization of specific microbial communities based on their environmental tolerances and metabolic needs.

For example, supragingival tooth surfaces frequently experience pH fluctuations due to the consumption of fermentable carbohydrates. These dietary sugars are metabolized by acidogenic bacteria like *Streptococcus mutans* and *Lactobacillus* spp., leading to acid production and localized enamel demineralization. In contrast, the dorsum of the tongue presents a low-oxygen, moist environment ideal for anaerobic species such as *Fusobacterium* and *Porphyromonas*, organisms commonly associated with halitosis and periodontal disease [76].

1.5. Conclusions

Oral biofilms represent complex, highly structured microbial ecosystems composed of bacteria, fungi, viruses, and archaea. When in balance, these communities play a protective role by supporting enamel remineralization and modulating immune defenses. However, the disruption of this equilibrium, known as dysbiosis, can drive the onset of oral diseases such as dental caries, gingivitis, and periodontitis.

The formation of biofilms follows a stepwise process, beginning with microbial adhesion to oral surfaces, progressing to community maturation within a self-produced extracellular polymeric substance (EPS) matrix. This matrix not only stabilizes the biofilm but also enhances microbial survival by conferring resistance to antimicrobial treatments and host immune responses.

Multiple factors shape the composition and pathogenic potential of biofilms, including diet, saliva flow, oral hygiene practices, genetic predispositions, and the surrounding microenvironment. Conditions such as frequent sugar consumption, reduced salivary secretion, or impaired immunity can tip the balance toward pathogenic states, whereas beneficial microbial species help maintain oral homeostasis.

Because mature biofilms are inherently resistant to conventional therapies, research is shifting toward innovative approaches that target biofilm structure and restore ecological balance. Promising strategies include enzymatic agents that degrade the EPS matrix, nanotechnology-based drug delivery, photodynamic therapy, and the use of probiotics. At the same time, advances in genomic and proteomic technologies are paving the way for personalized treatments tailored to an individual's unique microbial profile.

Looking ahead, oral healthcare must evolve from eradication-based strategies to the precision modulation of biofilms. By focusing on restoring microbial harmony rather than indiscriminate elimination, clinicians may achieve more effective, sustainable, and patient-specific outcomes. As innovations in DNA sequencing and personalized medicine continue to advance, the prospect of individualized, biofilm-centered therapies holds the potential to transform not only oral health management but also reduce the broader systemic consequences linked to oral dysbiosis.

References

1. van Leewenhoeck, A. Observations, communicated to the publisher by Mr. Antony van Leewenhoeck, in a Dutch letter of the 9th of Octob. 1676. Here English'd: Concerning little animals by him observed in rain-well-sea. And snow water; as also in water wherein pepper had lain infused. *Philos Trans.* **1677**, *12*, 821–831. [CrossRef]
2. Smith, K.A. Louis Pasteur, the father of immunology? *Front. Immunol.* **2012**, *3*, 68. [CrossRef]
3. Rosier, B.T.; De Jager, M.; Zaura, E.; Krom, B.P. Historical and contemporary hypotheses on the development of oral diseases: Are we there yet? *Front. Cell. Infect. Microbiol.* **2014**, *4*, 92. [CrossRef]
4. Loesche, W.J. Chemotherapy of dental plaque infections. *Oral. Sci. Rev.* **1976**, *9*, 65–107. [PubMed]
5. Costerton, J.W.; Geesey, G.G.; Cheng, K.J. How bacteria stick. *Sci. Am.* **1978**, *238*, 86–95. [CrossRef] [PubMed]
6. Costerton, J.W.; Lewandowski, Z.; Caldwell, D.E.; Korber, D.R.; Lappin-Scott, H.M. Microbial biofilms. *Annu. Rev. Microbiol.* **1995**, *49*, 711–745. [CrossRef]
7. Stoodley, P.; Sauer, K.; Davies, D.G.; Costerton, J.W. Biofilms as complex differentiated communities. *Annu. Rev. Microbiol.* **2002**, *56*, 187–209. [CrossRef] [PubMed]

8. Flemming, H.C.; Wingender, J.; Szewzyk, U.; Steinberg, P.; Rice, S.A.; Kjelleberg, S. Biofilms: An emergent form of bacterial life. *Nat. Rev. Microbiol.* **2016**, *14*, 563–575. [CrossRef]
9. Rumbaugh, K.P.; Whiteley, M. Towards improved biofilm models. *Nat. Rev. Microbiol.* **2024**, *23*, 57–66. [CrossRef]
10. Marsh, P.D. Dental plaque as a biofilm and a microbial community—Implications for health and disease. *BMC Oral Health* **2006**, *6*, S14. [CrossRef]
11. Berger, D.; Rakhamimova, A.; Pollack, A.; Loewy, Z. Oral Biofilms: Development, Control, and Analysis. *High-Throughput* **2018**, *7*, 24. [CrossRef]
12. Cleaver, L.; Garnett, J.A. How to study biofilms: Technological advancements in clinical biofilm research. *Front. Cell. Infect. Microbiol.* **2023**, *13*, 1335389. [CrossRef]
13. Ames, N.J.; Ranucci, A.; Moriyama, B.; Wallen, G.R. The Human Microbiome and Understanding the 16S rRNA Gene in Translational Nursing Science. *Nurs. Res.* **2017**, *66*, 184–197. [CrossRef]
14. Benn, A.; Heng, N.; Broadbent, J.M.; Thomson, W.M. Studying the human oral microbiome: Challenges and the evolution of solutions. *Aust. Dent. J.* **2018**, *63*, 14–24. [CrossRef]
15. National Research Council (US) Committee on Metagenomics: Challenges and Functional Applications. *The New Science of Metagenomics: Revealing the Secrets of Our Microbial Planet*; National Academies Press (US): Washington, DC, USA, 2007; Bookshelf ID: NBK54006. [CrossRef] [PubMed]
16. Human Microbiome Project Consortium. A framework for human microbiome research. *Nature* **2012**, *486*, 215–221. [CrossRef]
17. Wensel, C.R.; Pluznick, J.L.; Salzberg, S.L.; Sears, C.L. Next-generation sequencing: Insights to advance clinical investigations of the microbiome. *J. Clin. Investig.* **2022**, *132*, e154944. [CrossRef] [PubMed]
18. Kolenbrander, P.E.; Palmer, R.J., Jr.; Rickard, A.H.; Jakubovics, N.S.; Chalmers, N.I.; Diaz, P.I. Bacterial interactions and successions during plaque development. *Periodontol 2000* **2006**, *42*, 47–79. [CrossRef]
19. Darveau, R.P.; Curtis, M.A. Oral biofilms revisited: A novel host tissue of bacteriological origin. *Periodontol 2000* **2021**, *86*, 8–13. [CrossRef] [PubMed]
20. Nairn, B.L.; Lima, B.P.; Chen, R.; Yang, J.Q.; Wei, G.; Chumber, A.K.; Herzberg, M.C. Effects of fluid shear stress on oral biofilm formation and composition and the transcriptional response of Streptococcus gordonii. *Mol. Oral. Microbiol.* **2024**, *39*, 477–490. [CrossRef]
21. Choi, A.; Dong, K.; Williams, E.; Pia, L.; Batagower, J.; Bending, P.; Shin, I.; Peters, D.I.; Kaspar, J.R. Human saliva modifies growth, biofilm architecture, and competitive behaviors of oral streptococci. *mSphere* **2024**, *9*, e0077123. [CrossRef] [PubMed]
22. Boisen, G.; Brogårdh-Roth, S.; Neilands, J.; Mira, A.; Carda-Diéguez, M.; Davies, J.R. Oral biofilm composition and phenotype in caries-active and caries-free children. *Front. Oral Health* **2024**, *5*, 1475361. [CrossRef]
23. Almatroudi, A. Biofilm Resilience: Molecular Mechanisms Driving Antibiotic Resistance in Clinical Contexts. *Biology* **2025**, *14*, 165. [CrossRef]

24. Hannig, M.; Joiner, A. The structure, function and properties of the acquired pellicle. *Monogr. Oral Sci.* **2006**, *19*, 29–64. [CrossRef]
25. Enax, J.; Ganss, B.; Amaechi, B.T.; Schulze Zur Wiesche, E.; Meyer, F. The composition of the dental pellicle: An updated literature review. *Front. Oral Health* **2023**, *4*, 1260442. [CrossRef] [PubMed]
26. Berne, C.; Ellison, C.K.; Ducret, A.; Brun, Y.V. Bacterial adhesion at the single-cell level. *Nat. Rev. Microbiol.* **2018**, *16*, 616–627. [CrossRef] [PubMed]
27. Brennan, C.A.; Garrett, W.S. Fusobacterium nucleatum—Symbiont, opportunist and oncobacterium. *Nat. Rev. Microbiol.* **2019**, *17*, 156–166. [CrossRef] [PubMed]
28. Katharios-Lanwermeyer, S.; Xi, C.; Jakubovics, N.S.; Rickard, A.H. Mini-review: Microbial coaggregation: Ubiquity and implications for biofilm development. *Biofouling.* **2014**, *30*, 1235–1251. [CrossRef]
29. Boisen, G.; Davies, J.R.; Neilands, J. Acid tolerance in early colonizers of oral biofilms. *BMC Microbiol.* **2021**, *21*, 45. [CrossRef]
30. Samaranayake, L.; Matsubara, V.H. Normal Oral Flora and the Oral Ecosystem. *Dent. Clin. N. Am.* **2017**, *61*, 199–215. [CrossRef]
31. Verma, D.; Garg, P.K.; Dubey, A.K. Insights into the human oral microbiome. *Arch. Microbiol.* **2018**, *200*, 525–540. [CrossRef] [PubMed]
32. Sauer, K.; Stoodley, P.; Goeres, D.M.; Hall-Stoodley, L.; Burmølle, M.; Stewart, P.S.; Bjarnsholt, T. The biofilm life cycle: Expanding the conceptual model of biofilm formation. *Nat. Rev. Microbiol.* **2022**, *20*, 608–620. [CrossRef]
33. Yin, I.X.; Udduttulla, A.; Xu, V.W.; Chen, K.J.; Zhang, M.Y.; Chu, C.H. Use of Antimicrobial Nanoparticles for the Management of Dental Diseases. *Nanomaterials* **2025**, *15*, 209. [CrossRef] [PubMed]
34. Xu, K.; Huang, R.; Li, X.; Jin, L.; Ko, C.N.; Li, M.; Wong, H.M.; Leung, K.C. Nanomaterial-based synergistic strategies for combating dental caries: Progress and perspectives. *Nanoscale* **2025**, *17*, 1874–1888. [CrossRef] [PubMed]
35. Rajan, B.; Abdelmoneim, D.; Salem, A.S.; Belibasakis, G.N.; Phemister, R.; Chen, C.; Coates, D. Nanoencapsulation, biocompatibility and antibiofilm properties of chitosan/nisin Z spheres. *Arch. Oral. Biol.* **2025**, *173*, 106193. [CrossRef]
36. Zhou, J.; Zhou, L.; Chen, Z.Y.; Sun, J.; Guo, X.W.; Wang, H.R.; Zhang, X.Y.; Liu, Z.R.; Liu, J.; Zhang, K.; et al. Remineralization and bacterial inhibition of early enamel caries surfaces by carboxymethyl chitosan lysozyme nanogels loaded with antibacterial drugs. *J. Dent.* **2025**, *152*, 105489. [CrossRef]
37. Saleh, M.H.A.; Roh, A.; Martin, K.; Mianecki, M.; Tariq Sheikh, A.; Singh, P.; Akorede, K.; Saunders, M.N.; Shea, L.D.; Decker, A.; et al. Cargo-less Nanoparticles Prevent Bone Loss in Periodontitis and Peri-implantitis. *J. Dent. Res.* **2025**. [CrossRef]
38. Yu, M.; Chen, Y.; Dong, S.; Chen, Z.; Jiang, X.; Wang, Y.; Zhang, L. Sulforaphane as a promising anti-caries agents: Inhibitory effects on Streptococcus mutans and caries control in a rat model. *Front. Microbiol.* **2025**, *15*, 1427803. [CrossRef] [PubMed]
39. Panda, S.; Rout, L.; Mohanty, N.; Satpathy, A.; Sankar Satapathy, B.; Rath, S.; Gopinath, D. Exploring the photosensitizing potential of Nanoliposome Loaded Improved Toluidine Blue O (NLITBO) Against Streptococcus mutans: An in-vitro feasibility study. *PLoS ONE* **2024**, *19*, e0312521. [CrossRef]

40. Gerardi, D.; Bernardi, S.; Bruni, A.; Falisi, G.; Botticelli, G. Characterization and morphological methods for oral biofilm visualization: Where are we nowadays? *AIMS Microbiol.* **2024**, *10*, 391–414. [CrossRef]
41. Yang, Z.; Khan, S.A.; Walsh, L.J.; Ziora, Z.M.; Seneviratne, C.J. Classical and Modern Models for Biofilm Studies: A Comprehensive Review. *Antibiotics* **2024**, *13*, 1228. [CrossRef]
42. Ray, R.R. Biofilm architecture and dynamics of the oral ecosystem. *BioTechnologia* **2024**, *105*, 395–402. [CrossRef]
43. Abranches, J.; Zeng, L.; Kajfasz, J.K.; Palmer, S.R.; Chakraborty, B.; Wen, Z.T.; Richards, V.P.; Brady, L.J.; Lemos, J.A. Biology of Oral Streptococci. *Microbiol. Spectr.* **2018**, *6*. [CrossRef]
44. Dige, I.; Raarup, M.K.; Nyengaard, J.R.; Kilian, M.; Nyvad, B. Actinomyces naeslundii in initial dental biofilm formation. *Microbiology* **2009**, *155*, 2116–2126. [CrossRef]
45. Krieger, M.; AbdelRahman, Y.M.; Choi, D.; Palmer, E.A.; Yoo, A.; McGuire, S.; Kreth, J.; Merritt, J. Stratification of Fusobacterium nucleatum by local health status in the oral cavity defines its subspecies disease association. *Cell Host Microbe* **2024**, *32*, 479–488.e4. [CrossRef]
46. Hu, L.; He, C.; Zhao, C.; Chen, X.; Hua, H.; Yan, Z. Characterization of oral candidiasis and the Candida species profile in patients with oral mucosal diseases. *Microb. Pathog.* **2019**, *134*, 103575. [CrossRef]
47. Naureen, Z.; Dautaj, A.; Anpilogov, K.; Camilleri, G.; Dhuli, K.; Tanzi, B.; Maltese, P.E.; Cristofoli, F.; De Antoni, L.; Beccari, T.; et al. Bacteriophages presence in nature and their role in the natural selection of bacterial populations. *Acta Biomed.* **2020**, *91*, e2020024. [CrossRef]
48. Fatahzadeh, M.; Schwartz, R.A. Human herpes simplex virus infections: Epidemiology, pathogenesis, symptomatology, diagnosis, and management. *J. Am. Acad. Dermatol.* **2007**, *57*, 737–763. [CrossRef] [PubMed]
49. Mohammadzadeh, R.; Mahnert, A.; Duller, S.; Moissl-Eichinger, C. Archaeal key-residents within the human microbiome: Characteristics, interactions and involvement in health and disease. *Curr. Opin. Microbiol.* **2022**, *67*, 102146. [CrossRef] [PubMed]
50. Santonocito, S.; Giudice, A.; Polizzi, A.; Troiano, G.; Merlo, E.M.; Sclafani, R.; Grosso, G.; Isola, G. A Cross-Talk between Diet and the Oral Microbiome: Balance of Nutrition on Inflammation and Immune System's Response during Periodontitis. *Nutrients* **2022**, *14*, 2426. [CrossRef] [PubMed]
51. Gondivkar, S.M.; Gadbail, A.R.; Gondivkar, R.S.; Sarode, S.C.; Sarode, G.S.; Patil, S.; Awan, K.H. Nutrition and oral health. *Dis. Mon.* **2019**, *65*, 147–154. [CrossRef]
52. Rowińska, I.; Szyperska-Ślaska, A.; Zariczny, P.; Pasławski, R.; Kramkowski, K.; Kowalczyk, P. The Influence of Diet on Oxidative Stress and Inflammation Induced by Bacterial Biofilms in the Human Oral Cavity. *Materials* **2021**, *14*, 1444. [CrossRef] [PubMed]
53. Kurtzman, G.M.; Horowitz, R.A.; Johnson, R.; Prestiano, R.A.; Klein, B.I. The systemic oral health connection: Biofilms. *Medicine* **2022**, *101*, e30517. [CrossRef]

54. Takenaka, S.; Ohsumi, T.; Noiri, Y. Evidence-based strategy for dental biofilms: Current evidence of mouthwashes on dental biofilm and gingivitis. *Jpn. Dent. Sci. Rev.* **2019**, *55*, 33–40. [CrossRef]
55. Brookes, Z.; Teoh, L.; Cieplik, F.; Kumar, P. Mouthwash Effects on the Oral Microbiome: Are They Good, Bad, or Balanced? *Int. Dent. J.* **2023**, *73*, S74–S81. [CrossRef]
56. Uchida, H.; Ovitt, C.E. Novel impacts of saliva with regard to oral health. *J. Prosthet. Dent.* **2022**, *127*, 383–391. [CrossRef]
57. Muszyński, D.; Kucharski, R.; Marek-Trzonkowska, N.; Kalinowska, M.; Brzóska, A.; Bolcewicz, M.; Kalinowski, L.; Kaźmierczak-Siedlecka, K. Treatment of xerostomia in Sjögren's syndrome—What effect does it have on the oral microbiome? *Front. Cell. Infect. Microbiol.* **2025**, *15*, 1484951. [CrossRef]
58. Pei, X.M.; Zhou, L.X.; Tsang, M.W.; Tai, W.C.; Wong, S.C. The Oral Microbial Ecosystem in Age-Related Xerostomia: A Critical Review. *Int. J. Mol. Sci.* **2024**, *25*, 12815. [CrossRef]
59. Babanouri, N.; Sahmeddini, S.; Khadang, S.; Bazargani, A. Effect of Xylitol and Fluoride Varnish on Biofilm and Saliva in Orthodontic Patients: A Triple-Blind Randomized Clinical Trial. *Clin. Exp. Dent. Res.* **2025**, *11*, e70062. [CrossRef]
60. de Souza, B.M.; Braga, A.S.; Vertuan, M.; Sassaki, S.; Araújo, T.T.; Santos, P.S.D.S.; Buzalaf, M.A.R.; Magalhães, A.C. Influence of irradiated dentin, biofilm and different artificial saliva formulations on root dentin demineralization. *Heliyon* **2024**, *10*, e36334. [CrossRef] [PubMed]
61. Mhatre, S.; Srichand, R.; Sethumadhavan, J.; Mishra, P.B.; Patil, S.D.; Chavan, R.S.; Joshi, M.; Shetty, U. Dry Mouth Dilemma: A Comprehensive Review of Xerostomia in Complete Denture Wearers. *Cureus* **2024**, *16*, e58564. [CrossRef] [PubMed]
62. Müller, F.; Chebib, N.; Maniewicz, S.; Genton, L. The Impact of Xerostomia on Food Choices-A Review with Clinical Recommendations. *J. Clin. Med.* **2023**, *12*, 4592. [CrossRef]
63. Sardellitti, L.; Filigheddu, E.; Serralutzu, F.; Bortone, A.; Bandiera, E.; Milia, E. Nonpharmacological Interventions in the Management of Xerostomia: A Review on Topical Treatments, Alternative Medicine, and Innovative Therapies. *Oral* **2024**, *4*, 616–638. [CrossRef]
64. Austin, W.; Hdeib, M.; Fraser, P.; Goldchtaub, M.; Shams, E.; Han, T.; Michaud, P.-L.; Adibnia, V. Oral Lubrication, Xerostomia, and Advanced Macromolecular Lubricants for Treatment of Dry Mouth. *Lubricants* **2024**, *12*, 126. [CrossRef]
65. Robertsson, C.; Davies, J.; Svensäter, G.; Nord, A.B.; Norrström, N.; Wickström, C. MUC5B modulation of early oral biofilm glucose metabolism. *Front. Oral Health* **2025**, *6*, 1516025. [CrossRef]
66. Tamai, R.; Kiyoura, Y. *Candida* Infections: The Role of Saliva in Oral Health—A Narrative Review. *Microorganisms* **2025**, *13*, 717. [CrossRef]
67. Cosaert, M.; Hold, N.; Kifle, F.; Mar, J.; Powell, S.; Oyoyo, U.; Kwon, S.R. Awareness and Perception of Salivary Diagnostics of Dental Students and Faculty: A Pilot Study. *J. Calif. Dent. Assoc.* **2024**, *52*, 2438955. [CrossRef]

68. Sharma, A.; Hossain, N.I.; Thomas, A.; Sonkusale, S. Saliva-Sensing Dental Floss: An Innovative Tool for Assessing Stress via On-Demand Salivary Cortisol Measurement with Molecularly Imprinted Polymer and Thread Microfluidics Integration. *ACS Appl. Mater. Interfaces* **2025**, *17*, 25083–25096. [CrossRef] [PubMed]
69. Adami, G.R.; Li, W.; Green, S.J.; Kim, E.M.; Wu, C.D. Ex vivo oral biofilm model for rapid screening of antimicrobial agents including natural cranberry polyphenols. *Sci. Rep.* **2025**, *15*, 6130. [CrossRef]
70. Octaricha, T.; Ilmiawati, C.; Kasuma, N. Salivary microbiome profile shifts after scaling in stunted children. *BMC Res. Notes* **2025**, *18*, 69. [CrossRef] [PubMed]
71. Superdock, D.K.; Johnson, L.M.; Ren, J.; Khan, A.; Eno, M.; Man, S.; Poole, A.C. The Impact of Human Salivary Amylase Gene Copy Number and Starch on Oral Biofilms. *Microorganisms* **2025**, *13*, 461. [CrossRef] [PubMed]
72. Tabassum, N.; Khan, F.; Jeong, G.J.; Oh, D.K.; Kim, Y.M. Controlling Oral Polymicrobial Biofilm Using Usnic Acid on the Surface of Titanium in the Artificial Saliva Media. *Antibiotics* **2025**, *14*, 115. [CrossRef]
73. Constantin, V.; Luchian, I.; Goriuc, A.; Budala, D.G.; Bida, F.C.; Cojocaru, C.; Butnaru, O.-M.; Virvescu, D.I. Salivary Biomarkers Identification: Advances in Standard and Emerging Technologies. *Oral* **2025**, *5*, 26. [CrossRef]
74. Javaid, M.A.; Ahmed, A.S.; Durand, R.; Tran, S.D. Saliva as a diagnostic tool for oral and systemic diseases. *J. Oral. Biol. Craniofacial Res.* **2016**, *6*, 66–75. [CrossRef] [PubMed]
75. Li, P.; Zhang, Y.; Chen, D.; Lin, H. Investigation of a novel biofilm model close to the original oral microbiome. *Appl. Microbiol. Biotechnol.* **2024**, *108*, 330. [CrossRef] [PubMed]
76. Radaic, A.; Kapila, Y.L. The oralome and its dysbiosis: New insights into oral microbiome-host interactions. *Comput. Struct. Biotechnol. J.* **2021**, *19*, 1335–1360. [CrossRef]

2. Significant Impact of Oral Biofilms on Systemic Health

2.1. Introduction

To fully appreciate the impact of oral biofilms on systemic health, it is essential to first understand the intricate processes of tooth formation, homeostasis, and repair, as these foundational elements are crucial in maintaining oral health and preventing disease. Tooth development, known as odontogenesis, is a highly regulated and complex process that begins early in embryogenesis and continues postnatally (Figure 4a).

The initiation of tooth development involves the interaction between epithelial and mesenchymal cells, leading to the formation of the dental lamina, a critical epithelial structure from which tooth buds arise. This early stage is driven by various signaling pathways, including Wingless/Integrated signaling pathway (Wnt), Fibroblast Growth Factors (FGFs), and Bone Morphogenetic Proteins (BMPs), which coordinate cell proliferation and differentiation, setting the stage for the intricate architecture of the tooth [1–3].

As development progresses, the tooth bud evolves into the cap and bell stages, where the enamel organ, dental papilla, and dental follicle differentiate. The enamel organ, which consists of the inner and outer enamel epithelium, stellate reticulum, and stratum intermedium, plays a key role in the formation of enamel, the highly mineralized outer layer of the tooth. Simultaneously, the dental papilla, composed of ectomesenchymal cells, differentiates into odontoblasts, which are responsible for dentin formation. The dental follicle surrounds these structures and will later give rise to the supporting tissues of the tooth, including the periodontal ligament, cementum, and alveolar bone. The intricate interplay of these tissues ensures that the tooth forms correctly, with each layer contributing to the overall function and longevity of the tooth [2].

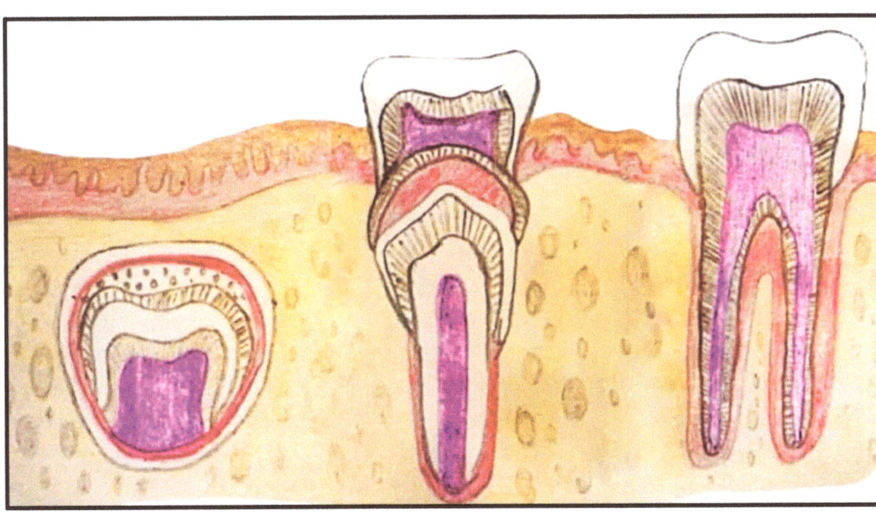

(a)

Figure 4. *Cont.*

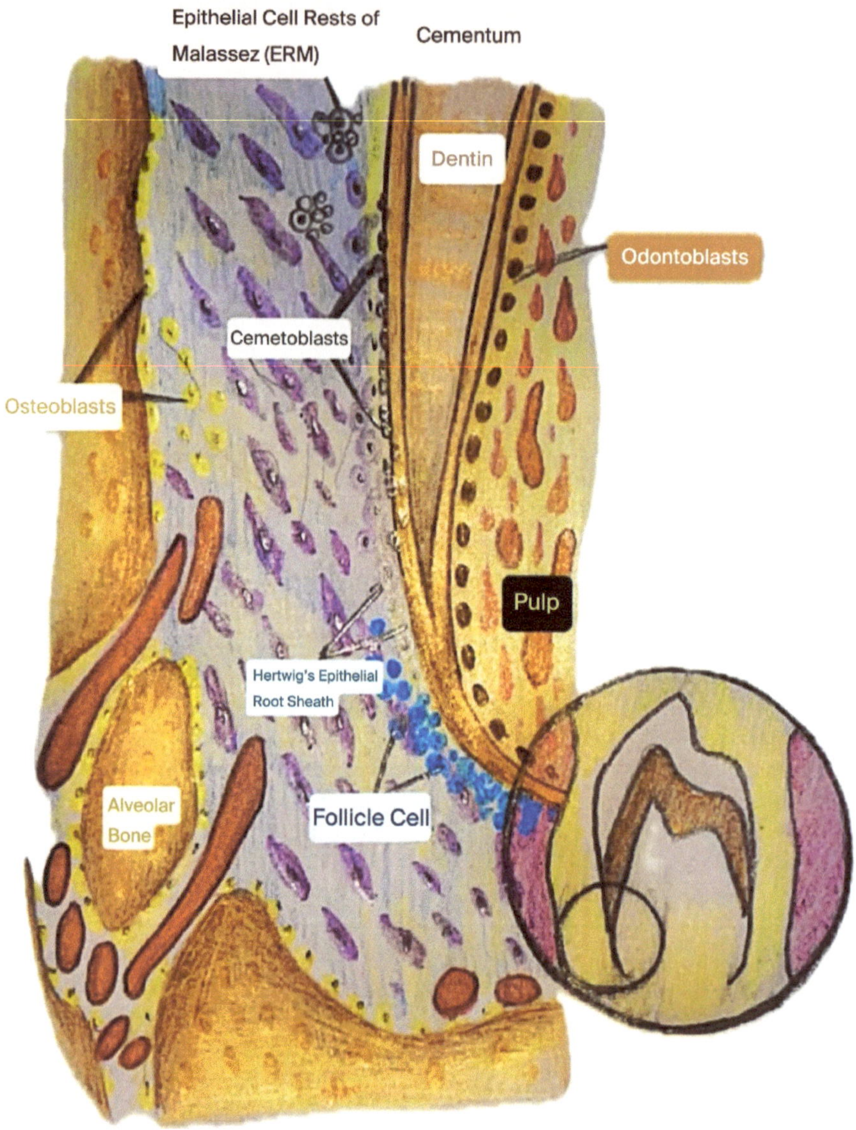

(**b**)

Figure 4. (**a**) Illustration of human tooth development showing a cross-sectional view of teeth at different stages of eruption through the gingiva and underlying alveolar bone. (**b**) Histologic illustration of root development showing the interaction of Hertwig's epithelial root sheath with dental papilla and follicle cells, highlighting the formation of dentin, cementum, and alveolar bone along with associated cells such as odontoblasts, cementoblasts, osteoblasts, and epithelial cell rests of Malassez. Credit: © Nensi Kallfani, used with permission.

The bell stage marks the final stage of crown development, where the cells of the inner enamel epithelium differentiate into ameloblasts, the cells that secrete enamel matrix proteins, which later mineralize to form the hard enamel (Figure 4b).

This stage is characterized by reciprocal signaling between ameloblasts and odontoblasts, ensuring the synchronized formation of the enamel and dentin layers. Disruptions in these signaling processes can lead to developmental defects, such as enamel hypoplasia or dentin dysplasia, underscoring the importance of these pathways in tooth morphogenesis [4].

Following crown formation, the development of the tooth root begins, involving the formation of Hertwig's epithelial root sheath, which guides root elongation and the differentiation of cementoblasts. Cementoblasts deposit cementum, a mineralized tissue that covers the tooth root and anchors the periodontal ligament fibers. The periodontal ligament itself is a dynamic structure that not only connects the tooth to the alveolar bone but also plays a crucial role in tooth homeostasis and repair by providing nutrients and sensory feedback. The maintenance of these supporting structures is vital for the overall health of the tooth, as they enable the tooth to resist the mechanical forces of mastication [1].

Tooth homeostasis, the maintenance of tooth structure and function throughout life, relies on the continued activity of various cell populations, particularly those in the dental pulp. The dental pulp, housed within the pulp chamber, contains stem cells that can differentiate into odontoblast-like cells, contributing to the production of reparative dentin in response to injury or disease. This process is critical for the tooth's defense against caries and other forms of damage, though it is limited in scope compared to the regenerative capacities of other tissues. The balance between tissue homeostasis and repair is finely regulated by molecular signaling pathways, including those involved in inflammation and cellular stress responses, which can influence the longevity of dental tissues [2,3].

The ability to harness stem cells for tooth regeneration is an area of significant research interest, offering the potential to restore lost or damaged dental tissues biologically rather than through synthetic materials. Stem cell-based therapies aim to regenerate enamel, dentin, and even entire teeth by leveraging the inherent regenerative properties of dental stem cells. This approach holds promise for addressing the limitations of traditional dental restorations, which often lack the durability and functionality of natural teeth. The use of stem cells for tooth regeneration is still in the experimental stages but represents a promising future direction in dental medicine. Ongoing research, particularly into the Wnt signaling pathway, is crucial for advancing these regenerative strategies, as it plays a key role in stem cell activation and tissue repair [1,3].

Table 6 highlights the different structures of the tooth, their composition, and their specific roles in maintaining tooth integrity and function.

Table 6. Composition and function of tooth structures.

Tooth Structures	Compositions	Functions
Enamel	96% hydroxyapatite (crystalline calcium phosphate), 4% water and organic material [1,2].	Protects the tooth from mechanical forces, chemical erosion, and temperature changes [1,2].
Dentin	70% hydroxyapatite, 20% organic material (primarily collagen), 10% water [1,2].	Forms the bulk of the tooth; transmits sensory stimuli and supports the enamel [1,2].
Cementum	45–50% hydroxyapatite, 50–55% organic material and water [1,2].	Anchors the periodontal ligament to the tooth, covering the root and providing support [1,2].
Pulp	Connective tissue, blood vessels, nerves, and stem cells [1,2].	Provides nutrients, sensory feedback, and plays a role in tooth repair through the production of dentin [1,2].
Periodontal Ligament	Dense connective tissue composed of collagen fibers, cells, and extracellular matrix [1,2].	Connects the tooth to the alveolar bone, absorbs shock, and supports tooth mobility [1,2].

Source: Table by author.

Each layer contributes to the overall health and resilience of the tooth, making it capable of resisting the various challenges it faces throughout life. Understanding these components is crucial for seeing how disruptions, such as those caused by oral biofilms, can lead to oral diseases and affect overall health. These biofilms, which form on the surfaces of teeth, are not only a key factor in the development of oral diseases like dental caries and periodontitis but also have broader implications for systemic health. Oral biofilms, composed of complex microbial communities, facilitate the accumulation of pathogenic bacteria that produce acids and toxins, eroding enamel, penetrating dentin, and triggering inflammation in surrounding tissues. As discussed in Chapter 1, these microbial communities play a significant role in the onset and progression of oral diseases. However, their impact extends beyond the oral cavity, as recent research underscores their potential influence on systemic health. Pathogens within these biofilms can enter the bloodstream, leading to systemic inflammation that is closely associated with the development of various chronic conditions, including cardiovascular diseases, diabetes, and respiratory infections. This connection highlights the critical link between oral health and overall bodily health, emphasizing the importance of managing oral biofilms to prevent broader systemic repercussions.

Immune Resistance by Oral Biofilms

A critical aspect of the persistence and pathogenicity of oral biofilms lies in their ability to evade host immune responses. This immune evasion is a major reason why biofilm-associated oral infections, such as periodontitis and peri-implantitis, often become chronic and resistant to conventional treatments.

Oral biofilms develop structured microbial communities encased in an EPS matrix. This matrix acts as a physical barrier, shielding the resident bacteria from both innate and adaptive immune mechanisms. For instance, neutrophils, the first line of defense, are often rendered ineffective against mature biofilms. Studies show that biofilm EPS can impede neutrophil chemotaxis and phagocytosis, while also suppressing the release of antimicrobial peptides and reactive oxygen species (ROS) [5].

Furthermore, periodontal pathogens such as *P. gingivalis* have evolved sophisticated strategies to manipulate the host immune system. *P. gingivalis* can subvert Toll-like receptor (TLR) signaling, skewing the immune response from a protective to a permissive one, promoting microbial persistence and tissue destruction [6,7]. This manipulation leads to a state of "para-inflammation", where low-grade, non-resolving inflammation promotes disease progression without effectively clearing the infection.

Biofilms can also interfere with adaptive immunity. The antigenic variation in constituent microbes, combined with suppression of dendritic cell activation, compromises the development of effective T- and B-cell responses. Chronic exposure to microbial antigens in the context of immune dysregulation can also lead to immune tolerance or exhaustion, contributing to the recalcitrant nature of these infections [8].

These immune resistance mechanisms help explain why standard treatments, including mechanical debridement and antimicrobials, often fail to fully eradicate biofilms or prevent recurrence [9,10].

2.2. Impact of Oral Biofilms on Oral Health

This section will explain the role that biofilms play in the development and progression of various oral health conditions. It will provide an in-depth analysis of the pathogenesis of major diseases such as dental caries, gingivitis, and periodontitis, all of which are closely linked to the presence and activity of oral biofilms. The intricate interactions within these microbial communities contribute to tissue damage, inflammation, and the disruption of normal oral homeostasis. Additionally, the clinical implications of biofilm-related diseases will be discussed, highlighting the challenges they pose for treatment, as well as the importance of early intervention and prevention strategies.

2.2.1. Dental Caries

Let us begin with dental caries, commonly known as tooth decay or cavities, which is a multifactorial and progressive disease characterized by the destruction of the tooth's hard tissues, enamel, dentin, and cementum. This destruction is the result of a complex interplay between cariogenic bacteria within the oral biofilm (dental plaque), fermentable dietary sugars, and the host's dental tissues [11]. The caries process begins when these bacteria metabolize fermentable carbohydrates, particularly sugars from the diet, producing organic acids such as lactic acid. These acids lower the pH within the biofilm, creating an acidic environment that leads to the demineralization of enamel and dentin [12].

In the past decade, dental caries has expanded to emphasize its nature as a dynamic and chronic condition. It is now recognized not just as the presence of cavities but as a continuous process that can range from early, reversible stages of enamel demineralization to severe, irreversible damage if left untreated. This broader definition highlights the disease's dependency on a balance between demineralization and remineralization processes, influenced by biological, behavioral, and environmental factors, including the composition of the oral microbiome, dietary habits, saliva flow, fluoride exposure, and socio-economic factors. If dental caries is not addressed, it can progress deeper into the tooth structure, reaching the dentin and potentially the pulp, leading to pain, infection, and, in severe cases, tooth loss. The modern approach to managing dental caries focuses on early detection, risk assessment, and individualized preventive strategies aimed at maintaining this balance and preventing the progression of the disease.

Etiology and Pathogenesis

The development and progression of dental caries are influenced by a complex interplay of factors, including the oral microbiome, dietary habits, and host-specific conditions. Traditionally, *S. mutans* has been considered the primary bacterial cause in caries development. However, recent research expands this paradigm, emphasizing the role of a diverse microbiome in caries etiology [13]. Beyond *S. mutans*, other bacterial species, including *Streptococcus sobrinus* and various *Lactobacilli*, contribute to the cariogenic process. These bacteria, thriving in the acidic environment of biofilms, work synergistically to enhance the production of acids that demineralize tooth enamel. Chen et al. (2020) further explored the microbial etiology of dental caries, pointing out that cariogenic bacteria produce extracellular polysaccharides that not only help in adhering to the tooth surface but also in creating a protective matrix around the biofilm [14]. This matrix shields the bacteria from external threats, including antimicrobial agents and mechanical removal, making biofilms resilient and challenging to eradicate. The pathogenic potential of these biofilms is heightened by their ability to maintain a low-pH environment, which is conducive to enamel demineralization.

Dietary sugars, particularly sucrose, are central to the pathogenic process of dental caries, as highlighted by van Loveren (2019) and Lagerweij and van Loveren (2020) [15,16]. The amount and frequency of sugar intake are critical factors in caries development. Sucrose is fermented by cariogenic bacteria, producing organic acids that lower the pH in the oral cavity. When sugar consumption exceeds 10% of total daily caloric intake, the risk of caries significantly increases. Frequent sugar intake prevents the pH from returning to neutral, prolonging the acidic environment that promotes enamel demineralization. This sustained acid attack is the primary mechanism through which dietary sugars contribute to caries formation.

Host-related factors also significantly influence susceptibility to dental caries [17]. These factors include the composition and flow rate of saliva, which are essential in neutralizing acids and providing the minerals necessary for enamel remineralization. Variations in enamel composition, influenced by genetic and environmental factors, also play a role in an individual's vulnerability to caries. Additionally, behavioral factors such as oral hygiene practices and fluoride exposure are critical in modulating the risk of caries.

Clinical Manifestations

The clinical manifestations of dental caries represent a spectrum of changes in tooth structure, beginning with the earliest sign of demineralization and potentially progressing to more severe stages of decay. One of the initial clinical signs of caries is the formation of white spot lesions on the enamel surface. These lesions, as detailed by Lopes et al. (2024), are indicative of subsurface demineralization, where the enamel loses its translucency and appears chalky or opaque [18]. White spot lesions are reversible with appropriate treatment, such as fluoride application, which can promote remineralization and restore the enamel's integrity. However, these lesions also serve as a critical warning sign, signaling the need for immediate intervention to prevent further progression.

As demineralization continues unchecked, these white spots can evolve into cavitated lesions (Figure 5a). Roberts et al. (2022) describe how the acidic environment maintained by cariogenic bacteria leads to the breakdown of enamel and subsequent cavitation [19]. The cavity formation process begins when the demineralized enamel surface collapses under mechanical stress, creating a visible hole or pit. At this stage, the carious process becomes irreversible without restorative intervention. The decay progresses into the underlying dentin, which, in turn, is less mineralized and more organic, more susceptible to rapid destruction.

If the caries process is not arrested, it can further progress into the pulp of the tooth, causing significant pain and potentially leading to pulpitis, a painful inflammation of the tooth's nerve tissue. The infection can spread beyond the tooth, leading to abscess formation and even involvement of the surrounding bone [19].

Diagnosis and Assessment

The detection, diagnosis, and monitoring of dental caries are critical aspects of modern dental care, with an increasing focus on individualized approaches to patient management. Recent advancements in diagnostic technologies have significantly enhanced the ability to identify carious lesions at their earliest stages, thereby improving the potential for preventive and minimally invasive interventions.

Denis et al. (2013) highlighted the critical role of differential diagnosis in accurately identifying and managing white enamel lesions, given the varied etiologies and distinct characteristics of these defects [20]. White lesions can generally be categorized into two primary types: hypomineralization and hypoplasia. Hypomineralization is defined as enamel with normal thickness but decreased mineral content, resulting in opaque, chalky, and often poorly defined white spots. These lesions are usually due to systemic conditions during enamel formation, such as excessive fluoride exposure (fluorosis) or childhood illnesses. On the other hand, hypoplasia refers to areas where enamel is reduced in quantity, leading to thinner or pitted surfaces that can appear as white, yellow, or brown. Hypoplastic defects are often well-defined and localized, typically resulting from trauma or localized infection during tooth development. The differential diagnosis of these lesions is important because the treatment approach varies depending on the underlying cause and type of defect.

Hypomineralized lesions may require remineralization strategies or restorative interventions, while hypoplastic defects might need more extensive restorative work or even prosthetic solutions. Denis et al. underline the necessity of combining clinical examination with a thorough understanding of the lesion's optical properties, patient history, and possible etiological factors to accurately diagnose and effectively treat these white enamel lesions [20]. This careful diagnostic process helps clinicians navigate the "optical maze" of these defects and ensures that the chosen treatment aligns with the specific type and severity of the lesion. Also, the authors delve into the concept of the "optical maze" associated with white enamel lesions, a term they use to describe the complex and often misleading visual characteristics of these defects. This complexity arises because the visual presentation of white enamel lesions can vary widely depending on several factors, such as the depth of the defect, the degree of mineralization, and the structural integrity of the enamel. The optical properties of enamel are primarily influenced by the way light interacts with the tooth's surface and subsurface layers. In healthy enamel, light passes through and reflects uniformly due to the high degree of mineralization and the regular arrangement of enamel crystals. However, in the case of white lesions, this optical clarity is disrupted. Hypomineralization, for instance, results in areas of enamel where the mineral content is reduced, causing these areas to scatter light rather than allowing it to penetrate. This scattering effect creates the characteristic opaque, chalky white appearance of hypomineralized lesions. These lesions are typically less reflective and appear dull compared to the surrounding healthy enamel, making them visually distinct but sometimes difficult to accurately assess in terms of depth and severity without additional diagnostic tools.

Conversely, hypoplasia presents a different optical challenge. Since hypoplasia involves a reduction in enamel thickness, the affected areas might allow light to pass through, leading to a translucent or even brownish appearance, depending on the severity and the extent of the defect. The thinner enamel in these regions can create a contrast with the adjacent healthier enamel, but this contrast might not always be apparent, especially under different lighting conditions or when viewed from various angles. This variability adds to the complexity of the "optical maze", as what might seem like a minor surface defect could be a significant structural issue requiring a more in-depth examination.

Moreover, the authors highlight that the visual diagnosis of white lesions can be further complicated by the presence of multiple types of defects on the same tooth or within the same oral environment. For instance, a tooth might exhibit both hypomineralized and hypoplastic lesions, each contributing differently to the overall appearance [20]. This overlapping of optical properties can mislead even experienced clinicians, leading to potential misdiagnosis or inappropriate treatment planning. They suggest the use of complementary diagnostic tools such as radiographs, which can help assess the depth of enamel defects, or fluorescence-based techniques, which can provide additional insights into the mineral content of the enamel. By integrating these tools with a detailed clinical examination and patient history, clinicians can more accurately identify the type and extent of white enamel lesions, thus avoiding the pitfalls of the "optical maze" and ensuring more effective treatment outcomes.

According to Abdelaziz (2023), the future of dental care lies in the early detection and personalized monitoring of caries, which allows for tailored treatment strategies that can halt or even reverse the progression of early lesions [21]. This individualized approach is supported by advanced diagnostic tools, such as

Quantitative Light-Induced Fluorescence (QLF), Optical Coherence Tomography (OCT), and digital radiography, which provide detailed insights into the extent and activity of carious lesions. These technologies not only detect demineralization before it becomes clinically visible but also monitor changes over time, offering a more dynamic understanding of the disease process.

Ghodasra and Brizuela (2023) emphasize the importance of combining traditional diagnostic methods with these newer technologies to achieve a comprehensive assessment of caries [22]. Standard clinical examination techniques, such as visual inspection and tactile exploration with dental instruments, remain foundational for caries diagnosis. However, their accuracy is significantly enhanced when complemented by radiographic imaging, which is particularly useful for detecting interproximal and subsurface lesions that are not visible to the naked eye. Bitewing radiographs, for instance, are the gold standard for identifying caries between teeth, while periapical radiographs provide detailed images of the tooth structure and surrounding bone, aiding in the detection of deeper carious lesions.

Prevention and Management

The landscape of dental caries prevention and management is rooted in both biological and behavioral strategies aimed at reducing the incidence and progression of this common oral disease. Fluoride remains a cornerstone of caries prevention, extensively supported by evidence for its efficacy in enhancing enamel remineralization and inhibiting demineralization. Fluoride works by promoting the formation of fluorapatite, a mineral more resistant to acid attacks than hydroxyapatite, thus strengthening the tooth structure against cariogenic bacteria [23]. The use of fluoride is personalized according to age and individual caries risk.

In pediatric populations, the European Academy of Paediatric Dentistry provides clear guidelines for fluoride use, emphasizing that it should be tailored to the child's risk level. For instance, children at higher risk of caries may require more frequent fluoride applications, such as biannual fluoride varnish treatments and the use of fluoride supplements in non-fluoridated areas. These guidelines are critical in ensuring that children receive appropriate levels of fluoride for effective caries prevention while minimizing the risk of dental fluorosis [24].

The effective management of caries also involves advances in oral care products, particularly kinds of toothpaste. Modern formulations now include high-concentration fluoride for individuals at high risk, along with additional technologies such as calcium phosphate complexes and biomimetic materials like hydroxyapatite, which provide enhanced protection and remineralization benefits. The use of these advanced formulations, alongside consistent oral hygiene practices and dietary management, plays a crucial role in reducing caries incidence and maintaining overall oral health. The following table summarizes the recommended guidelines for the use of fluoride and various toothpaste formulations based on different age groups and specific dental needs (Table 7).

Table 7. Fluoride and toothpaste guidelines by age and dental needs.

Age Groups	Fluoride Application	Recommended Toothpastes	Key Considerations
Infants (0–2 years)	Fluoridated water; fluoride varnish every 6 months for high-risk [23,24].	Fluoridated toothpaste (smear size) [23,24].	Supervise brushing to prevent swallowing; start brushing when the first teeth appear [23,24].
Children (3–6 years)	Fluoride varnishes every 6 months; fluoride supplements in non-fluoridated areas [23,24].	Fluoridated toothpaste (pea size) [23,24].	Supervise brushing; consider supplements if in a non-fluoridated area and at high risk for caries [23,24].
Children (7–18 years)	Biannual professional fluoride treatments for high-risk [23,24].	Regular fluoridated toothpaste [23,24].	Add fluoride mouth rinses for those with high caries risk (e.g., braces, frequent cavities) [23,24].
Adults	Periodic professional fluoride treatments if at high risk [23,24].	Fluoridated toothpaste; fluoride mouth rinse [23,24].	Incorporate fluoride mouth rinses, especially for those with reduced salivary flow or high caries risk [23,24].
Elderly	High-concentration fluoride gels/varnishes for increased caries risk [23,24].	Fluoridated toothpaste [23,24].	Focus on fluoride to prevent root caries and manage dry mouth (xerostomia) [23,24].
High-Risk Individuals	Use high-fluoride products (~5000 ppm fluoride) [23,24].	High-fluoride toothpaste [23,24].	Recommended for those with frequent cavities, orthodontic treatment, or xerostomia; use under dental supervision [23,24].
Sensitive Teeth/ Fluoride-Free	Not typically needed [23,24].	Hydroxyapatite toothpaste [23,24].	Ideal for those seeking fluoride-free options; helps with sensitivity and enamel remineralization [23,24].
Probiotic Users	Not typically needed [23,24].	Probiotic toothpaste [23,24].	Supports oral microbiome balance; can be used alongside regular fluoride toothpaste [23,24].

Table 7. *Cont.*

Age Groups	Fluoride Application	Recommended Toothpastes	Key Considerations
Plaque Control	Not typically needed [23,24].	Enzyme-based toothpaste [23,24].	Breaks down biofilm for easier plaque removal; useful for individuals with difficulty maintaining oral hygiene [23,24].
Whitening with Protection	Not typically needed [23,24].	Whitening toothpaste with fluoride/calcium phosphates [23,24].	Combines esthetic benefits with protection; suitable for regular use in non-sensitive teeth [23,24].
Antibacterial Needs	Not typically needed [23,24].	Antibacterial toothpaste [23,24].	Contains agents like triclosan or natural antimicrobials; suitable for those at high risk for periodontal disease [23,24].

Source: Table by author.

The pathogenesis of dental calculus and developing strategies to prevent its formation were critical in maintaining oral health and preventing caries. Recent research has shed light on the complex mechanisms underlying dental calculus formation and highlighted innovative approaches to prevent this common oral health issue [25]. Dental calculus, which forms when dental plaque becomes mineralized, is a significant contributor to periodontal disease and caries. The study emphasized the importance of targeting the early stages of plaque formation to prevent calculus buildup, suggesting that novel preventive strategies could play a crucial role in improving oral health outcomes. Wei et al. (2024) discussed various advanced prevention strategies, including the use of biofilm-disrupting agents and novel pharmaceutical approaches that target the calcification process [25]. These strategies aimed to inhibit the initial formation of plaque, thereby reducing the likelihood of it becoming calcified into dental calculus. The research also explored the potential of using probiotics and other biological agents to maintain a balanced oral microbiome, which can naturally resist the formation of pathogenic biofilms that lead to calculus and caries.

Complementing this, the review by Kalesinskas et al. (2014) provided a comprehensive overview of current methods for reducing dental plaque formation and caries development, with an emphasis on the role of pharmaceuticals in oral care [26]. The review highlighted traditional mechanical methods of plaque removal, such as toothbrushing and flossing, but also points to the limitations of these methods in preventing the formation of biofilms that contribute to plaque and calculus. Also, they emphasized the potential of novel pharmaceuticals, including antimicrobial agents and inhibitors of plaque biofilm formation, as promising tools for reducing the risk of caries and periodontal disease. The integration of these pharmaceutical approaches with conventional oral hygiene practices could significantly enhance the prevention of plaque formation and the subsequent development of calculus.

Moreover, these strategies are especially important for individuals who are at higher risk of caries due to factors such as poor oral hygiene, genetic predisposition, or other health conditions that affect saliva production and oral microbiome balance.

However, recent developments have expanded the role of toothpaste beyond just fluoride delivery. Modern formulations now incorporate a variety of active ingredients tailored to address specific dental needs, offering a more targeted and effective approach to oral care. For instance, high-fluoride toothpastes, with fluoride concentrations significantly higher than standard formulations, are designed for individuals at higher risk of caries, such as those with frequent cavities or orthodontic appliances. These formulations provide enhanced protection by promoting more robust enamel remineralization [27].

A study by Walsh et al. (2019) offered an in-depth analysis of how different fluoride concentrations in toothpaste influence the effectiveness of caries prevention [28]. The review highlighted those toothpastes with higher fluoride concentrations, particularly those exceeding the standard 1000–1500 ppm (parts per million), provide significantly greater protection against dental caries. Specifically, concentrations of 2800 ppm or 5000 ppm are particularly advantageous for high-risk groups, including children and adults with a history of frequent cavities, orthodontic patients, and individuals with xerostomia. These elevated fluoride levels enhance the remineralization process and promote the formation of fluorapatite, a more acid-resistant mineral, thereby offering superior defense against acid attacks from cariogenic bacteria. For populations at low to moderate caries risk, standard fluoride concentrations (1000–1500 ppm) generally suffice for effective caries prevention. However, in individuals with heightened risk, the use of higher fluoride concentrations is strongly recommended to achieve optimal prevention outcomes. The review underscored the importance of tailoring fluoride use to individual risk profiles, enabling dental professionals to provide more personalized and effective care. Moreover, the study highlighted the crucial role of fluoride concentration in toothpaste in caries prevention, advocating for the use of higher concentrations in those at greater risk.

Nanotechnology has revolutionized the formulation of toothpaste, offering significant advancements in the prevention and management of dental caries. Nanoparticles, due to their extremely small size, possess unique properties that allow them to interact with tooth enamel at the molecular level, thereby improving the efficacy of active ingredients. One of the key benefits of incorporating nanotechnology into toothpaste is the enhanced bioavailability and stability of remineralizing agents, such as calcium phosphate. These nanoparticles can penetrate deeper into the enamel, promoting more effective remineralization and repair of early carious lesions. Additionally, nanoparticles help in forming a stronger and more durable protective layer on the tooth surface, which is more resistant to acid attacks from cariogenic bacteria. The trends in nanotechnology indicate the increasing use of materials like nano-hydroxyapatite, silver nanoparticles, and zinc oxide nanoparticles in toothpaste formulations. Nano-hydroxyapatite, for instance, is a biomimetic material that mimics the natural composition of tooth enamel, making it particularly effective in repairing microscopic defects and reducing tooth sensitivity. Silver nanoparticles, known for their antimicrobial properties, help in controlling the bacterial load in the oral cavity, thus preventing plaque formation and reducing the risk of periodontal disease [29]. Regulatory bodies are increasingly focusing on ensuring that these products are safe for daily use, with studies indicating that, when used within recommended guidelines, nanotechnology-based toothpastes are both effective and safe.

Furthermore, fluoride-free calcium-phosphate-based biomimetic toothpastes have emerged as a promising alternative in the field of oral care, particularly for individuals looking for fluoride-free options. The study by Limeback et al. (2023) provided an updated review of the clinical evidence supporting the effectiveness of these toothpastes in preventing dental caries and promoting overall oral health [30]. These biomimetic toothpastes utilize calcium and phosphate compounds, which are naturally occurring minerals in tooth enamel, to enhance the remineralization and repair of the enamel surface. One of the primary advantages of calcium-phosphate-based toothpastes is their ability to mimic the natural processes of enamel formation and repair. By delivering bioavailable calcium and phosphate ions directly to the tooth surface, these toothpastes facilitate the deposition of hydroxyapatite, the mineral that forms the bulk of tooth enamel. This process not only repairs early carious lesions but also strengthens the enamel, making it more resistant to acid attacks from cariogenic bacteria. The review underlined the use of specific calcium-phosphate technologies, such as CPP-ACP and nano-hydroxyapatite. CPP-ACP, for instance, stabilizes calcium and phosphate ions in a form that is readily available to the teeth, thereby enhancing remineralization. Nano-hydroxyapatite, a biomimetic material that closely resembles the natural mineral content of enamel, is particularly effective in filling microscopic defects in the enamel and reducing tooth sensitivity. The study also emphasizes that these fluoride-free formulations are well-suited for individuals who are either sensitive to fluoride, concerned about fluoride exposure, or simply prefer fluoride-free products. The safety profile of these biomimetic toothpastes is another significant advantage, as they pose no risk of fluorosis, a condition caused by excessive fluoride intake, particularly in children.

Another study by O'Hagan-Wong et al. (2022) provided a detailed examination of the efficacy of hydroxyapatite, a biomimetic material that closely resembles the natural mineral composition of tooth enamel [31]. The primary advantage of hydroxyapatite is its ability to bind to the enamel surface, filling in microscopic defects and creating a protective layer that is resistant to acid attacks from cariogenic bacteria. This action not only prevents demineralization but also promotes the remineralization of early carious lesions. Unlike fluoride, which strengthens teeth primarily by forming a more acid-resistant mineral layer (fluorapatite), hydroxyapatite directly contributes to the restoration of the enamel's original mineral structure, making it particularly beneficial for individuals with sensitivity to fluoride or those seeking fluoride-free oral care options. The authors highlighted the growing body of evidence supporting the effectiveness of hydroxyapatite toothpaste in both caries prevention and the reduction in tooth sensitivity. The study notes that hydroxyapatite is especially useful for patients who experience sensitivity due to enamel erosion or for those with existing carious lesions, as the material's reparative properties help to rebuild the enamel and relieve discomfort. Moreover, the safety profile of hydroxyapatite toothpaste is excellent, with no known adverse effects associated with its use. This makes it a suitable option for a wide range of individuals, including children, pregnant women, and others who may be concerned about fluoride exposure.

The increasing interest in natural and alternative ingredients for oral care has driven the development of innovative toothpastes incorporating probiotics, neem, and advanced biomimetic technologies. These formulations are gaining attention for their potent antimicrobial properties, particularly in targeting harmful oral bacteria such as *S. mutans*.

A study by Selvaraj et al. (2020) provided in vivo evidence of the antimicrobial efficacy of toothpastes containing probiotics and neem as primary ingredients, focusing on a population in Melmaruvathur [32]. The study demonstrated that both probiotic and neem-based toothpastes significantly reduced levels of *S. mutans* in saliva, underscoring their potential as effective alternatives to traditional fluoride toothpastes [32]. Neem, a natural antibacterial agent, has been recognized in traditional medicine for its ability to combat oral pathogens and improve overall oral health. Furthermore, newer formulations also incorporate other plant-based antimicrobial compounds, such as tea tree oil, which is known for its broad-spectrum antimicrobial activity, helping to reduce plaque formation and prevent gum disease. These natural ingredients not only offer significant antibacterial properties but also provide a viable option for individuals seeking to avoid synthetic chemicals in their oral care routine while effectively maintaining dental hygiene. The promising results from studies like those by Selvaraj et al. (2020) and Abedi et al. (2024) suggest that these natural alternatives can play a vital role in oral health, offering consumers safe and effective ways to support oral hygiene and reduce the risk of dental diseases [29,32]. In a complementary study, Meto et al. (2020) explored the antibacterial effects of MicroRepair®BIOMA-based toothpaste and chewing gum on orthodontic elastics contaminated with saliva in an in vitro setting [33]. MicroRepair®BIOMA technology incorporates zinc-substituted hydroxyapatite particles, which not only aid in remineralization but also exhibit potent antibacterial properties. The study found that MicroRepair®BIOMA-based products were effective in reducing bacterial contamination on orthodontic elastics, suggesting that these formulations could play a crucial role in maintaining oral hygiene, particularly in orthodontic patients. The zinc-substituted hydroxyapatite particles help to restore the natural mineral balance of the teeth while simultaneously inhibiting the growth of bacteria, thus offering the dual action of remineralization and antimicrobial protection.

Whitening toothpastes are widely used for their ability to remove surface stains and enhance the esthetic appearance of teeth. However, their impact on the structural integrity of dentin and enamel has been the subject of ongoing research. The study by Dionysopoulos et al. (2023) provides valuable insights into how different active agents in whitening toothpastes affect the abrasive wear of dentin [34]. Using a tooth-brushing simulation, the study evaluated the degree of wear caused by various formulations, highlighting the potential risks associated with the long-term use of these products. They found that while whitening toothpastes are effective in reducing surface stains, they can also contribute to increased dentin wear, particularly when they contain high levels of abrasives or bleaching agents. The study emphasizes the importance of formulating whitening toothpastes that balance efficacy with safety, ensuring that they do not compromise the underlying dentin or lead to excessive abrasion over time. The findings suggest that consumers should be cautious in their selection of whitening toothpastes, especially those with sensitive teeth or pre-existing dental conditions. In a related investigation, Jamwal et al. (2022) conducted a systematic review and meta-analysis to assess the effects of whitening toothpastes on the surface roughness and microhardness of human teeth [35]. The review included multiple studies that measured changes in enamel and dentin properties following the use of whitening products. The analysis revealed that while whitening toothpastes are generally effective in improving tooth esthetics, they can also lead to an increase in surface roughness and a decrease in microhardness, particularly with prolonged use. Jamwal et al. (2022) highlight that the impact of whitening toothpastes on tooth structure is influenced by the type and concentration of active agents used, as well as the duration of use [35]. The review underscores the need for further research to develop whitening formulations that minimize potential adverse effects on enamel and dentin while maintaining their whitening efficacy. Moreover, the study suggests that dental professionals should guide patients in choosing whitening products that are both safe and effective, particularly for those with compromised enamel or dentin integrity.

Diet and nutrition play a pivotal role in the prevention of dental problems, including dental caries, periodontal disease, and enamel erosion. The consumption of a balanced diet rich in essential nutrients is crucial for maintaining oral health and preventing the onset of dental issues. The frequent consumption of fermentable carbohydrates, particularly sugars, is a primary driver of dental caries. These sugars are metabolized by oral bacteria to produce acids, which then demineralize tooth enamel, leading to cavities. To mitigate this risk, it is recommended to substitute fermentable sugars with non-cariogenic sweeteners such as xylitol, which not only reduces acid production by bacteria but also enhances saliva flow, thereby aiding in the natural remineralization of enamel. Additionally, a diet high in fiber, fruits, and vegetables is beneficial as these foods stimulate saliva production, which is a natural protective factor against tooth decay [36]. Also, the importance of adequate intake of calcium, phosphorus, and vitamin D, are essential for maintaining strong teeth and bones. These nutrients help in the remineralization process, fortifying the tooth structure and making it more resistant to acid attacks. Dairy products, leafy greens, nuts, and fish are excellent sources of these vital nutrients. The frequent consumption of acidic items such as citrus fruits, sodas, and certain sports drinks can lead to the gradual wear of enamel, making teeth more susceptible to decay and sensitivity. To prevent enamel erosion, it is advised to limit the intake of acidic foods and to rinse the mouth with water after consuming such items to neutralize the acids.

Maintaining excellent oral hygiene is essential for preventing common dental issues like cavities at any age (Figure 5a), gum disease, and bad breath. While traditional practices such as brushing twice daily and flossing are effective, they may not fully eliminate harmful bacteria, especially in hard-to-reach areas. Dental plaque, a sticky biofilm formed by bacteria and food particles, is the main cause of tooth decay and gum disease. When plaque is not removed promptly, it hardens into tartar, leading to further oral health complications (Figure 5b).

To address the limitations of traditional oral hygiene, Chhaliyil et al. (2020) introduced a novel oral cleaning methodology [37]. This novel approach emphasizes the importance of simplicity and frequency, focusing on the continuous removal of plaque and bacteria throughout the day before they can cause damage. The study revealed that adopting this frequent cleaning routine significantly reduces harmful bacteria, such as *S. mutans* and *P. gingivalis*, which are key contributors to dental caries and periodontal disease. By consistently lowering bacterial load and disrupting plaque formation, this method significantly enhances overall oral hygiene and provides a more effective means of preventing common dental problems. The key steps of this new methodology are outlined in the following table (Table 8), making it easy to implement and follow.

Table 8. Step-by-step guide for the simple and frequent oral cleaning method.

Steps	Description
1. Post-Meal Cleaning	Gently brush your teeth for 1–2 min with soft-bristled toothbrush or interdental brush, after every meal or snack, focusing on areas where food particles accumulate [37].
2. Interdental Cleaning	Use an interdental brush or floss to clean between teeth, removing debris from hard-to-reach areas [37].
3. Rinse with Water	Rinse your mouth thoroughly with water to wash away dislodged food particles and bacteria [37].
4. Optional Antimicrobial Rinse	For those at higher risk, use an antimicrobial mouth rinse to further reduce bacterial load [37].
Frequency	Repeat this method after every meal or snack, ideally 3–5 times a day, depending on meal frequency [37].

Source: Table by author.

Dental sealants are a highly effective tool in the prevention and management of tooth decay, particularly in younger populations where the risk of cavities is highest [38]. These thin, protective coatings are applied to the chewing surfaces of the back teeth, specifically, the premolars and molars, which are most vulnerable to decay due to their deep grooves and crevices. Sealants work by creating a physical barrier that prevents food particles and bacteria from accumulating in these hard-to-clean areas, thereby reducing the likelihood of cavities. The application of dental sealants is a simple and non-invasive procedure that can significantly decrease the incidence of dental caries. This preventive measure is especially beneficial for children and adolescents, providing long-lasting protection during the years when they are most prone to developing cavities. In addition to preventing new cavities, sealants can also halt the progression of early signs of decay, helping to avoid more extensive dental treatments later on. Different types of sealants are available, including resin-based and glass ionomer sealants, each offering distinct benefits. Resin-based sealants are known for their strong adherence to tooth enamel, making them particularly effective in preventing decay. Glass ionomer sealants, on the other hand, release fluoride, which adds an extra layer of protection by strengthening the enamel and further reducing the risk of cavities. Incorporating dental sealants into routine dental care, especially for children and adolescents, is a highly recommended strategy for maintaining oral health and preventing tooth decay. Sealants offer a straightforward, cost-effective solution that can greatly reduce the prevalence of cavities, supporting long-term dental health [38].

Dental resin composites have become a cornerstone in restorative dentistry, offering versatile and effective solutions for repairing and restoring damaged teeth. These materials are widely used due to their ability to closely mimic the appearance and function of natural tooth structure, making them ideal for both esthetic and functional restorations. Over the years, significant advancements have been made in the development of dental resin composites, improving their performance, durability, and applicability in various dental procedures [39]. Modern dental resin composites are engineered to provide excellent mechanical properties, such as high strength and wear resistance, which are crucial for withstanding the forces of chewing and biting. These composites are composed of a polymer matrix, typically made of Bisphenol A-Glycidyl Methacrylate (Bis-GMA) or Urethane Dimethacrylate (UDMA), reinforced with fillers such as silica or zirconia. The inclusion of these fillers enhances the composite's physical properties, making it more resilient and durable over time. In addition to their mechanical benefits, dental resin composites offer superior esthetic qualities. They can be color-matched to the patient's natural teeth, providing a seamless and visually appealing restoration. This is particularly important in anterior restorations, where appearance is a key consideration (Figure 5c).

Furthermore, advancements in nanotechnology have led to the development of nanocomposites, which offer improved polish-ability and a more natural luster, further enhancing the esthetic outcomes. The versatility of dental resin composites extends to their application in various types of restorations, from small fillings to complex full-coverage restorations. They are also used in minimally invasive procedures, preserving more of the natural tooth structure compared to traditional amalgam fillings. Additionally, the ability to bond directly to the tooth structure enhances the retention and longevity of the restoration.

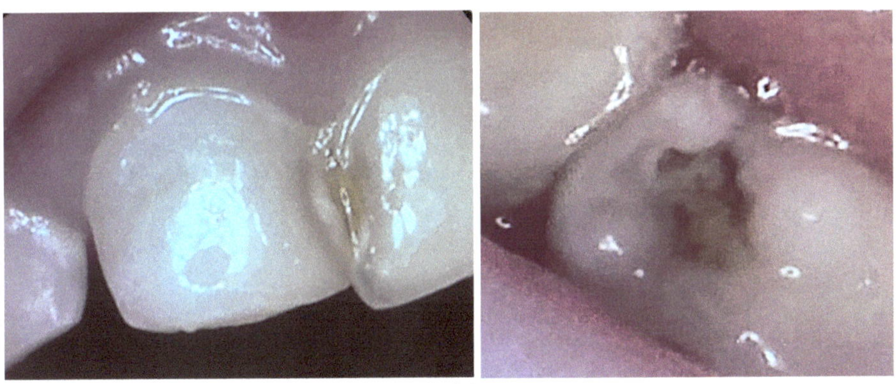

(**a**)

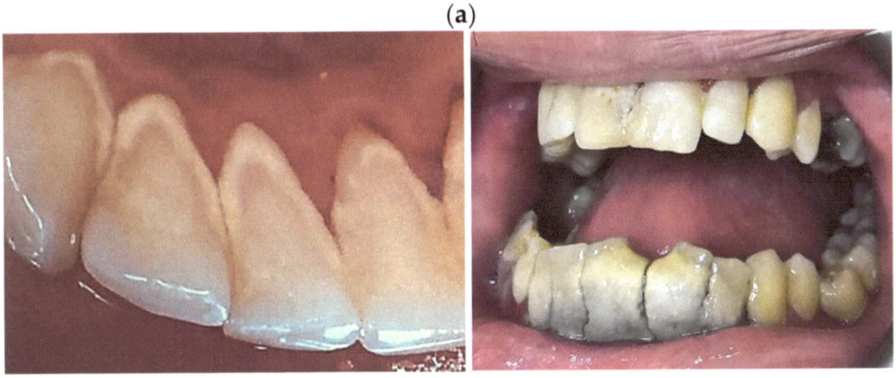

(**b**)

Figure 5. *Cont.*

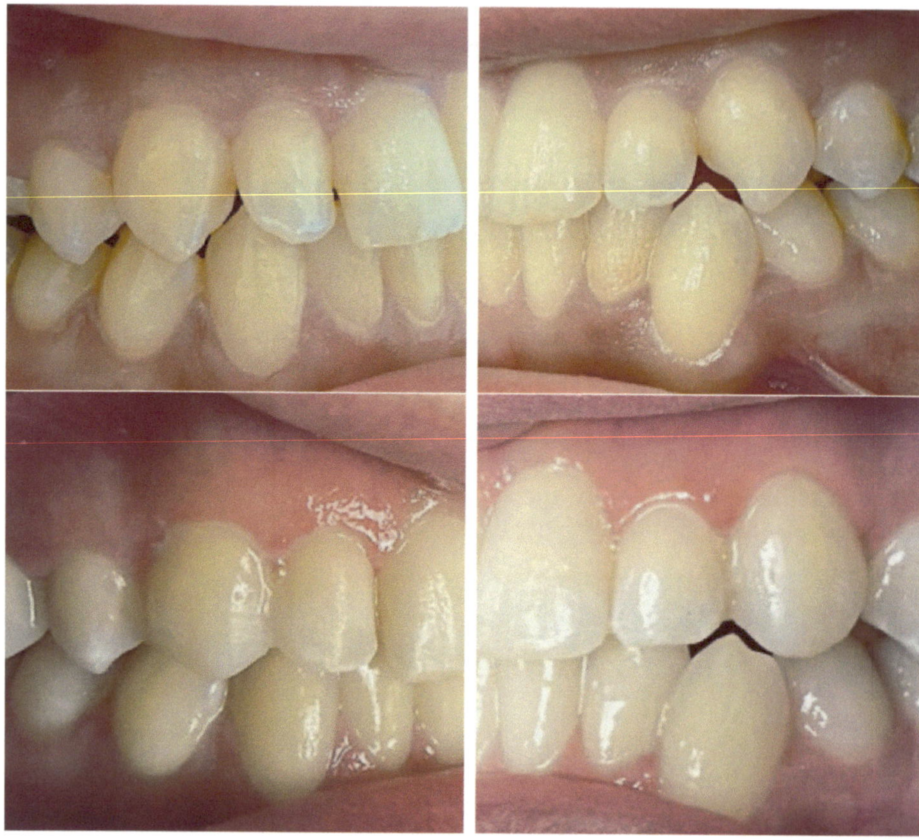

(c)

Figure 5. (**a**) Oral condition of a 34-month-old child displaying pronounced caries lesions in the deciduous teeth of both the upper teeth (#51 & #62) (left) and lower teeth (#74) (right). (**b**) Left: A 20-year-old male presents with dental plaque that has calcified on the lower front teeth. Right: A 35-year-old male showing advanced generalized dental disease characterized by heavy calculus and plaque accumulation, particularly on the mandibular teeth. The image demonstrates discolored crowns, caries, gingival inflammation, and severe oral neglect. (**c**) Esthetic restoration of the upper canines and lateral incisors (#1.3, #1.2, #2.3, #2.2) in a 25-year-old female patient following the completion of orthodontic treatment. The upper panel shows the teeth before restoration with dental resin composites, and the lower panel displays the esthetic outcome after the composite application. Source: Photos by author.

2.2.2. Periodontal Disease: Pathogenesis, Systemic Links, and Advances in Diagnosis and Treatment

Periodontal disease is a prevalent inflammatory condition of the oral cavity with significant local and systemic health implications. Periodontitis, the more severe form, involves the chronic inflammation of the supporting tooth structures, leading to progressive alveolar bone loss, increased tooth mobility, and eventual tooth loss if left untreated (Figure 6). Once considered a localized dental issue, it is now widely recognized as a complex immuno-inflammatory disease with systemic manifestations.

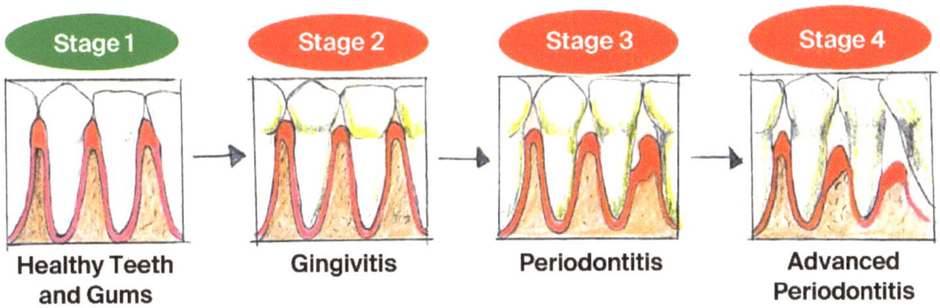

Figure 6. Stages of gingival inflammation, illustrating the progression from initial inflammation to advanced bone loss, increased tooth mobility, and eventual tooth loss if left untreated. Credit: © Nensi Kallfani, used with permission.

The disease typically begins with gingivitis, an inflammatory response to dental plaque biofilms. If untreated, gingivitis may progress to periodontitis, characterized by an aggressive immune response that damages the periodontal ligament and alveolar bone. This transition is largely driven by microbial dysbiosis, a shift from a symbiotic to a pathogenic oral microbiome. In health, commensal bacteria support tissue homeostasis and immune tolerance. However, in disease, pathogens such as *P. gingivalis*, *T. forsythia*, and *T. denticola* dominate, evading immune surveillance and actively subverting host defenses to promote chronic inflammation [40–42].

These pathogens manipulate host immune responses through virulence mechanisms that promote immune evasion, oxidative stress, and the sustained release of pro-inflammatory cytokines. As a result, the immune system's attempts to clear infection result in collateral damage to host tissues, contributing to the progressive destruction seen in periodontitis. Genetic predispositions also influence disease susceptibility; polymorphisms in cytokine-related genes, such as IL-1, TNF-α, and IL-6, can amplify host responses to microbial stimuli and accelerate tissue breakdown [42].

Periodontitis is now established as a chronic inflammatory condition with systemic effects. Ulcerated periodontal pockets provide a portal for pathogens and their components, such as lipopolysaccharides (LPS), to enter the bloodstream. Once disseminated, these microbial elements activate immune and endothelial cells via pattern recognition receptors, especially Toll-like receptors, resulting in elevated systemic inflammatory markers like C-reactive protein (CRP), IL-6, and TNF-α.

This low-grade systemic inflammation plays a contributory role in the pathogenesis of multiple chronic conditions. Numerous intrinsic and extrinsic factors influence disease susceptibility and progression. Smoking is among the most significant environmental risk factors; it alters the subgingival microbiome, suppresses immune function, and impairs healing. Other modifiable factors include stress and poor oral hygiene. Systemic diseases, especially diabetes, further increase risk by inducing a pro-inflammatory, hyperglycemic environment that favors tissue breakdown. Together, these variables shape individual disease trajectories and treatment responses [41–43].

Advances in diagnosis: Traditional periodontal diagnosis has relied on probing depth measurements, bleeding on probing, and radiographs [44]. While useful, these tools often detect disease at a relatively advanced stage. Recent innovations, particularly cone-beam computed tomography (CBCT) and digital radiography, are transforming diagnostic capabilities. CBCT offers high-resolution 3D imaging of alveolar bone, enabling clinicians to assess complex defects and anatomical structures with greater precision. Digital radiography enhances image quality, reduces radiation exposure, and supports longitudinal disease monitoring through image storage and manipulation [45].

These technologies allow earlier diagnosis, better risk assessment, and more targeted interventions, shifting periodontal care toward a more proactive and personalized model.

Host-modulation therapy aims to temper destructive immune responses using agents such as NSAIDs or cytokine inhibitors. These interventions can mitigate tissue damage while allowing natural healing processes to proceed [41].

Regenerative therapies, including the application of growth factors, stem cells, and biocompatible scaffolds, aim to restore lost periodontal structures. These biologically based strategies show promise in reversing damage and restoring function in patients with severe disease [46,47].

Importantly, these advances align with the broader movement toward personalized periodontal care. By considering each patient's unique genetic, microbial, and systemic profile, clinicians can tailor treatment strategies to improve outcomes and long-term oral–systemic health.

2.2.3. Halitosis: Etiology, Diagnosis, and Treatment Approaches

In Chapter 1, halitosis is discussed in the context of bacterial aspects; this section will explore the topic in greater depth. Halitosis affects a significant portion of the population and can have profound social and psychological implications. For many individuals, it leads to embarrassment, reduced self-esteem, and social anxiety, which can negatively impact their quality of life. The causes of halitosis can be categorized into intra-oral and extra-oral sources, with intra-oral causes being the most common. These include issues related to oral hygiene, dental health, and the microbiota of the mouth. Effectively diagnosing and managing halitosis requires a comprehensive understanding of its multifaceted nature [48,49].

The etiology of halitosis is complex and involves a variety of factors that contribute to the development of this condition. Intra-oral causes, which account for about 90% of halitosis cases, are primarily related to the metabolic activity of anaerobic bacteria in the mouth. These bacteria thrive in oxygen-deprived environments, such as periodontal pockets, the surface of the tongue, and areas with heavy plaque accumulation. They metabolize proteins from food particles, dead cells, and blood, producing VSCs like hydrogen sulfide, methyl mercaptan, and dimethyl sulfide. These VSCs are the primary contributors to the foul odor associated with halitosis. The surface of the tongue, particularly the dorsum, provides an ideal environment for these bacteria due to its rough texture and the presence of papillae, which trap debris and create a haven for bacterial growth. Periodontal disease, characterized by inflamed and receding gums, further exacerbates halitosis by creating deep pockets around teeth where bacteria can thrive and produce VSCs. Additionally, factors such as dry mouth (xerostomia) reduce the natural cleansing effect of saliva, allowing bacteria to multiply and contribute to bad breath. Extra-oral causes of halitosis, though less common, are equally important to consider. These can include systemic conditions such as gastrointestinal disorders, including GERD, respiratory tract infections, liver or kidney diseases, and metabolic disorders like diabetes, where the production of ketones can lead to a characteristic fruity odor [50].

Diagnosing halitosis involves a multifaceted approach, combining subjective and objective methods to accurately assess the presence and severity of bad breath. The subjective method primarily involves self-reporting by patients, who may notice the issue themselves or be informed by others. However, self-assessment can be unreliable due to the adaptation of olfactory receptors, leading to a diminished perception of one's own breath odor. Objective diagnostic methods include organoleptic assessments, where a clinician directly smells the patient's breath and rates the odor on a scale. While considered the gold standard for halitosis diagnosis, organoleptic assessment can be subjective and may vary between practitioners. To complement this, more precise tools such as halitometers are used to measure the concentration of VSCs in the breath. Halitometers provide a quantitative analysis of VSCs, offering a more objective and reproducible method of diagnosis. However, recent studies have shown that organoleptic and halitometric assessments do not always correlate well, particularly in cases of intra-oral halitosis. This discrepancy may arise because organoleptic assessments capture a broader range of odors, including non-VSC-related smells, whereas halitometers specifically measure VSCs. Therefore, a comprehensive diagnostic approach often involves using both methods in conjunction to ensure the accurate identification of the cause and extent of halitosis. Additionally, advanced diagnostic tools such as gas chromatography can identify and quantify specific compounds in the breath, providing detailed insights into the underlying causes of halitosis. Microbial analysis of plaque samples can also help identify the presence of odor-producing bacteria, guiding targeted treatment strategies. A thorough diagnostic process is essential for developing an effective treatment plan and addressing both intra-oral and extra-oral causes of halitosis [51,52].

The management of halitosis: For intra-oral halitosis, improving oral hygiene practices is fundamental. This includes brushing teeth at least twice a day with fluoride toothpaste, flossing to remove interdental plaque, and using tongue scrapers to reduce bacterial load on the tongue. Regular professional dental cleanings are crucial, especially for patients with periodontal disease, as they help remove plaque and tartar that contribute to the formation of VSCs. In addition to mechanical cleaning, antimicrobial mouthwashes can be effective in reducing the bacterial population in the mouth, particularly those responsible for VSC production. Mouthwashes containing chlorhexidine, cetylpyridinium chloride, or essential oils have been shown to significantly reduce halitosis. However, these should be used with caution, as overuse can lead to side effects such as staining of the teeth and disruption of the natural oral microbiome. When halitosis is linked to extra-oral causes, such as gastrointestinal disorders or respiratory infections, managing the underlying condition is essential. Collaboration with medical professionals is often necessary to address these systemic issues. For instance, treating GERD with appropriate medications or managing diabetes effectively can help reduce associated halitosis. Moreover, novel therapeutic approaches are emerging in the management of halitosis. Probiotics, which aim to alter the oral microbiome by promoting the growth of beneficial bacteria, have shown promise in reducing bad breath. These probiotics work by competing with odor-producing bacteria, thereby reducing the production of VSCs. Enzyme-based products that break down proteins before they can be metabolized by bacteria are also being explored as a way to prevent the formation of malodorous compounds. In some cases, psychological counseling may be necessary, particularly for patients who suffer from pseudohalitosis (perceived halitosis without objective evidence) or halitophobia (an irrational fear of having bad breath). Addressing the psychological aspects of halitosis is important for improving the overall quality of life for these individuals [53].

2.2.4. Oral Candidiasis: Etiology, Diagnosis, and Treatment Approaches

Oral candidiasis, commonly known as oral thrush, is a fungal infection in the mouth primarily caused by *Candida* species, with *C. albicans* being the most prevalent. This condition typically manifests as creamy white lesions on the tongue, inner cheeks, gums, tonsils, or the roof of the mouth. While *Candida* organisms are part of the normal oral flora, they can overgrow and lead to infection under certain conditions, particularly in individuals who are immunocompromised or have disrupted oral microflora. The overgrowth of *Candida* can lead to discomfort, pain, and in severe cases, difficulty in eating and swallowing, impacting the quality of life of those affected [54].

The etiology of oral candidiasis is multifactorial, with several predisposing factors contributing to the overgrowth of *Candida* species. These factors include immunosuppression (such as in HIV/AIDS or cancer therapy), the use of broad-spectrum antibiotics, diabetes mellitus, xerostomia (dry mouth), and the wearing of dentures. Each of these factors creates an environment in the oral cavity that favors the proliferation of *Candida*, disrupting the balance between the host immune defenses and the microbial flora. The pathogenesis of oral candidiasis involves the adherence of *Candida* to the epithelial cells of the oral mucosa, followed by the colonization and invasion of the tissues. *Candida* possesses several virulence factors, including the ability to form biofilms, produce hydrolytic enzymes, and switch between yeast and hyphal forms, which enhance its pathogenic potential. The formation of biofilms on mucosal surfaces and medical devices like dentures is particularly problematic, as biofilms protect *Candida* from antifungal agents and host immune responses, making infections more difficult to treat. The pathophysiological microenvironments within the oral cavity, such as pH alterations, oxygen levels, and nutrient availability, also play crucial roles in the development and persistence of oral candidiasis [55].

Several clinical forms can be observed, each defined by specific characteristics. The most common form is pseudomembranous candidiasis, characterized by white, curd-like plaques that can be wiped off to reveal an erythematous, often bleeding, mucosa underneath. Erythematous candidiasis presents as red, inflamed areas, typically on the palate or tongue, and is often associated with denture wearers. Hyperplastic candidiasis, or candidal leukoplakia, presents as persistent white plaques that cannot be wiped off and is more commonly seen in immunocompromised patients. Angular cheilitis, another form, manifests as inflammation and cracking at the corners of the mouth, often in conjunction with other forms of candidiasis [56,57].

The diagnosis of oral candidiasis is primarily clinical, based on the characteristic appearance of lesions in the oral cavity. These lesions are typically white and creamy, and can be scraped off to reveal an underlying red and sometimes bleeding mucosa. While clinical examination is often sufficient for diagnosis, confirmatory tests can be employed to ensure accuracy, especially in atypical cases. These tests include potassium hydroxide preparation, which involves scraping a lesion and examining it under a microscope to detect yeast cells. Culture tests can also be used to identify the specific *Candida* species involved, which can guide targeted therapy. In more complex cases, histopathological examination of biopsy samples may be required to differentiate oral candidiasis from other conditions that present similarly, such as oral leukoplakia or lichen planus. Additionally, molecular techniques, including PCR, can be used for species identification and to detect resistance markers, particularly in cases where there is suspicion of antifungal resistance [58].

The treatment of oral candidiasis involves both eliminating the fungal infection and addressing the underlying predisposing factors to prevent recurrence. The primary approach to treatment is the use of antifungal agents. Topical antifungals, such as nystatin and clotrimazole, are commonly used as first-line treatments, particularly in mild to moderate cases. These medications are available in various forms, including lozenges, mouthwashes, and creams, making them versatile in managing different presentations of the disease. For more severe cases or in patients with systemic involvement, systemic antifungal therapy with agents like fluconazole or itraconazole may be necessary. These drugs are effective in eradicating the infection but must be used cautiously due to potential side effects and drug interactions. In addition to pharmacological treatment, addressing underlying risk factors is crucial for the long-term management of oral candidiasis. This includes managing conditions like diabetes, improving oral hygiene, minimizing the use of broad-spectrum antibiotics, and ensuring proper denture care. Denture wearers, in particular, should be advised to remove their dentures at night, clean them thoroughly, and, if necessary, use antifungal treatments on the denture surfaces to reduce the risk of recurrence. Emerging therapeutic strategies are also being explored, including the use of probiotics to restore the balance of the oral microbiota, phytotherapy involving plant-derived antifungal compounds, and PDT, which uses light-activated compounds to kill *Candida* cells. These novel approaches offer promising alternatives or adjuncts to traditional antifungal therapy, especially in cases of recurrent or resistant infections [59,60].

2.2.5. Oral Lichen Planus: Etiology, Diagnosis, and Treatment Approaches

OLP is a chronic inflammatory condition that affects the mucous membranes inside the mouth, presenting as white, lacy patches; red, swollen tissues; or open sores. This condition is considered an autoimmune disorder, where the body's immune system mistakenly attacks the mucosal tissues, leading to inflammation and damage. Although OLP is not contagious, it can cause significant discomfort, pain, and potential complications if left untreated. Managing OLP requires a comprehensive understanding of its etiology, clinical manifestations, diagnostic criteria, and available treatment options to effectively alleviate symptoms and prevent further complications [61].

The etiology of OLP is complex and not entirely understood, but it is widely recognized as an autoimmune condition. In OLP, the immune system targets the keratinocytes in the oral mucosa, leading to a chronic inflammatory response. Several factors are believed to contribute to the development of OLP, including genetic predisposition, stress, systemic diseases (such as diabetes and hepatitis C), and exposure to certain medications or dental materials. These factors may trigger or exacerbate the immune response, leading to the characteristic lesions seen in OLP. The pathogenesis of OLP involves a T-cell-mediated immune response, where cytotoxic T cells (CD8+) attack the basal cells of the oral epithelium. This immune attack results in the apoptosis (cell death) of these basal cells, leading to the formation of the lesions characteristic of OLP. Additionally, the inflammatory process in OLP involves the release of various cytokines and chemokines, which further perpetuate the immune response and contribute to the chronic nature of the disease [62].

OLP can manifest in several clinical forms, each with distinct features. The most common form is the reticular type, which presents as white, lacy, web-like patterns on the buccal mucosa. These patterns, known as Wickham's striae, are often asymptomatic and may go unnoticed by the patient. However, OLP can also present in more symptomatic forms, such as the erosive type, where painful ulcers or erosions develop on the mucosal surfaces. This form is associated with significant discomfort, particularly during eating or speaking. Other forms of OLP include the atrophic type, characterized by erythematous (red) and inflamed areas, and the plaque type, which resembles leukoplakia with raised white patches that may be mistaken for other conditions. The bullous type is less common and involves the formation of fluid-filled vesicles that can rupture, leaving behind painful erosions. Recognizing these various clinical presentations is essential for the accurate diagnosis and appropriate management of the condition [63].

The diagnosis of OLP is primarily clinical, based on the characteristic appearance of the lesions. However, because OLP can resemble other oral conditions, a definitive diagnosis often requires histopathological examination of a biopsy sample. Histopathology typically reveals a band-like lymphocytic infiltrate in the subepithelial layer, the degeneration of the basal cell layer, and saw-tooth rete ridges, which are diagnostic features of OLP. Direct immunofluorescence may also be used to detect specific immunoreactants, such as fibrinogen, at the basement membrane zone, which can help differentiate OLP from other similar conditions like lupus erythematosus or chronic ulcerative stomatitis [64]. Given the chronic nature of OLP and its potential to transform into oral squamous cell carcinoma, regular monitoring and follow-up are crucial components of managing the disease. Patients diagnosed with OLP should be educated about the importance of maintaining regular dental visits to monitor for any changes in their condition.

The management of OLP focuses on relieving symptoms, controlling inflammation, and preventing complications, as there is currently no cure for the condition. The primary goal of treatment is to reduce pain and discomfort, particularly in symptomatic cases such as the erosive or atrophic forms of OLP. Topical corticosteroids are the mainstay of treatment and are effective in reducing inflammation and promoting healing of the lesions. In cases where topical treatment is insufficient, systemic corticosteroids may be prescribed. Other immunosuppressive agents, such as cyclosporine, tacrolimus, or azathioprine, can be used in patients who do not respond adequately to corticosteroids. These agents work by suppressing the immune response that drives the disease. However, their use must be carefully monitored due to potential side effects, including increased susceptibility to infections. In addition to pharmacological treatments, patients are advised to maintain good oral hygiene and avoid potential triggers that could exacerbate their condition, such as spicy foods, alcohol, and tobacco. Stress management techniques may also be beneficial, as stress is a known trigger for OLP flare-ups. Recently, there has been interest in exploring alternative therapies, such as low-level laser therapy and PDT, which show promise in reducing inflammation and promoting healing with fewer side effects compared to traditional treatments [65].

Although OLP is a benign condition, it carries a small but significant risk of malignant transformation into oral squamous cell carcinoma. This risk underscores the importance of regular monitoring and follow-up for patients with OLP, particularly those with erosive or atrophic forms, which are more prone to malignant transformation. Any persistent lesions or changes in the appearance of the lesions should be biopsied to rule out malignancy. In addition to the risk of malignancy, OLP can significantly impact a patient's quality of life due to chronic pain, discomfort, and difficulty in eating and speaking. Therefore, a multidisciplinary approach involving dental specialists, dermatologists, and, if necessary, oncologists, is often required to manage the condition effectively and to address any complications that arise [66].

2.2.6. Peri-Implantitis: Etiology, Diagnosis, and Treatment Approaches

Peri-implantitis is a pathological condition characterized by inflammation around dental implants, leading to the destruction of peri-implant tissues, including both soft tissue inflammation and the progressive loss of supporting bone around an osseointegrated implant. This condition shares similarities with periodontitis but specifically affects dental implants rather than natural teeth. The progressive nature of peri-implantitis can lead to significant complications, including implant failure if left untreated, making early diagnosis and effective management crucial for maintaining peri-implant health and the longevity of dental implants [67].

The etiology and pathogenesis of peri-implantitis are multifactorial, involving a complex interplay between microbial, host, and environmental factors. The primary initiating factor is the formation of a bacterial biofilm on the implant surface, similar to the biofilms that cause periodontitis around natural teeth. However, the response of peri-implant tissues to biofilm formation differs due to the absence of the periodontal ligament and the direct contact between the implant and bone, which makes peri-implant tissues more susceptible to rapid and severe destruction. The biofilm-mediated inflammation around the implant leads to an immune response that results in the release of pro-inflammatory cytokines and enzymes, which degrade the peri-implant bone. This process is compounded by factors such as poor oral hygiene, smoking, a history of periodontitis, and systemic conditions like diabetes, all of which can exacerbate the inflammatory response and accelerate bone loss. Additionally, mechanical factors such as implant overload due to occlusal forces, as well as the design and positioning of the implant, can contribute to the development and progression of peri-implantitis [68,69].

Peri-implantitis can present with a range of clinical signs and symptoms that may vary depending on the severity of the condition. Early signs include bleeding on probing and suppuration, which indicate soft tissue inflammation. As the disease progresses, more pronounced symptoms such as peri-implant pocket formation, swelling, redness, and pain may develop. Radiographic evidence of bone loss around the implant is a critical diagnostic criterion and typically indicates more advanced disease. Patients with peri-implantitis may also report discomfort, a sensation of mobility in the implant (in severe cases), and an unpleasant taste. The impact of these symptoms on the patient's quality of life can be significant, affecting their ability to chew, speak, and maintain oral hygiene effectively. Moreover, peri-implantitis can lead to esthetic concerns, particularly if the inflammation and bone loss are visible in the anterior regions of the mouth. Recognizing these clinical signs early is crucial for prompt intervention and the successful management of the disease [70].

The diagnosis of peri-implantitis involves a combination of clinical and radiographic assessments to evaluate the health of the peri-implant tissues and the extent of bone loss. Clinically, peri-implantitis is diagnosed by the presence of bleeding on probing, increased probing depths around the implant, and suppuration. These clinical signs are often accompanied by symptoms of inflammation, such as erythema and the swelling of the peri-implant mucosa. Radiographic assessment is essential for detecting bone loss, which is a hallmark of peri-implantitis. Periapical radiographs and, in more complex cases, CBCT is used to assess the amount and pattern of bone loss around the implant. CBCT offers a three-dimensional view, providing detailed information about the extent of bone destruction and the proximity of vital anatomical structures. Regular radiographic monitoring is recommended for the early detection of bone changes, allowing for timely intervention before significant damage occurs [71].

The treatment of peri-implantitis aims to control infection, halt the progression of bone loss, and restore peri-implant health. The therapeutic approach depends on the severity of the disease and may range from non-surgical interventions to more advanced surgical procedures. Non-surgical treatments typically include the mechanical debridement of the implant surface to remove biofilm and calculus, often combined with the use of antimicrobial agents such as chlorhexidine or systemic antibiotics to reduce bacterial load [72]. In cases where non-surgical methods are insufficient, surgical interventions may be necessary. These can include flap surgery to gain access to the affected area, the decontamination of the implant surface using laser therapy or chemical agents, and bone grafting procedures to regenerate lost bone. The use of GBR techniques, involving barrier membranes and bone substitutes, has shown promise in restoring peri-implant bone support. Additionally, implantoplasty, the process of smoothing the implant surface, may be employed to reduce plaque retention and improve long-term outcomes. Prevention plays a critical role in managing peri-implantitis, emphasizing the importance of maintaining excellent oral hygiene, regular dental check-ups, and professional cleaning. For patients at higher risk, such as those with a history of periodontitis or smokers, more frequent monitoring and preventive measures are recommended. Patient education on proper oral care techniques and the importance of avoiding risk factors is essential in preventing the onset and recurrence of peri-implantitis [73,74].

2.3. Mechanisms and Systemic Impact of Oral Biofilms

The pathogenic potential of oral biofilms lies in their capacity to harbor microorganisms that can penetrate the bloodstream and contribute to the initiation or progression of systemic diseases through multiple biological mechanisms. Understanding how these biofilms, particularly those dominated by periodontal pathogens, influence systemic health is essential for both prevention and treatment. The following section outlines the major systemic diseases associated with oral biofilms (Figure 7).

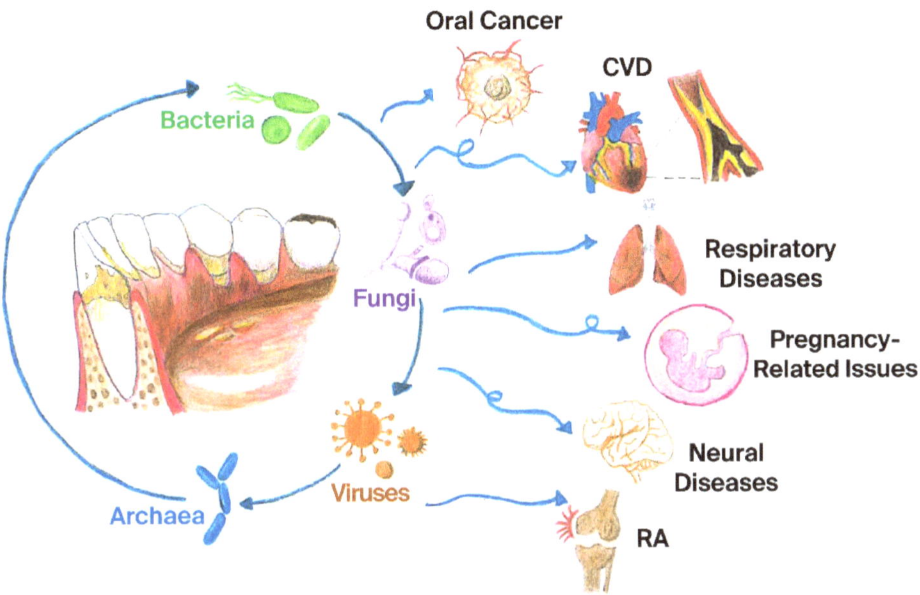

Figure 7. Oral biofilms are associated with oral diseases and significantly impact systemic health by contributing to the pathogenesis and progression of various systemic conditions. Credit: © Nensi Kallfani, used with permission.

Cardiovascular disease: Oral biofilms have emerged as significant contributors to cardiovascular disease (CVD), with periodontal pathogens influencing vascular health through systemic inflammation, immune dysregulation, and direct microbial interactions with endothelial tissues. During routine activities such as brushing, flossing, or dental procedures, bacteria from inflamed periodontal sites can enter the bloodstream, leading to bacteremia, a process facilitated by the compromised epithelial barriers present in periodontitis [75]. Once in circulation, pathogens such as *S. mutans* and *P. gingivalis* disseminate to distant organs, where they can colonize tissues and exacerbate systemic disease. A well-documented example is the role of *S. mutans* in infective endocarditis, where the bacterial colonization of damaged or prosthetic heart valves induces vegetation formation and severe cardiovascular complications [76]. Beyond direct colonization, periodontal pathogens release virulence factors, particularly lipopolysaccharides (LPS) from *P. gingivalis*, which are potent endotoxins capable of breaching epithelial barriers and entering systemic circulation [77]. Circulating LPS activates Toll-like receptors, especially TLR4, on endothelial and immune cells, triggering NF-κB signaling and the release of cytokines such as IL-6, TNF-α, and IL-1β, which drive systemic inflammation and insulin resistance, thereby linking periodontal infections not only to CVD but also to broader cardiometabolic disorders [77]. Once bacteria or their products reach the vasculature, they adhere to endothelial surfaces, causing localized inflammation, endothelial dysfunction, and the initiation of atherosclerotic plaque formation. The chronic low-grade inflammation sustained by these pathogens elevates systemic levels of C-reactive protein (CRP), a biomarker consistently associated with atherosclerosis and cardiovascular risk; CRP itself is not merely a marker but actively contributes to endothelial dysfunction and plaque progression [78]. Moreover, bacterial LPS and other virulence factors promote oxidative stress and the oxidation of low-density lipoproteins (LDL), accelerating lipid deposition within vessel walls and further fueling plaque growth. Critically, periodontal pathogens can destabilize pre-existing atherosclerotic plaques by enhancing local inflammation and matrix degradation, increasing the likelihood of plaque rupture, thrombus formation, and acute cardiovascular events such as myocardial infarction or stroke. In addition, alterations in lipid metabolism induced by chronic periodontal infection can increase circulating levels of atherogenic lipids, compounding cardiovascular risk. Large-scale epidemiological and meta-analytic studies confirm that individuals with periodontal disease have a significantly higher risk of developing CVD, and clinical evidence suggests that maintaining periodontal health may reduce systemic inflammation and mitigate cardiovascular burden [79]. These insights have led major organizations such as the American Heart Association to acknowledge the potential role of periodontal disease in cardiovascular risk, reinforcing the view that oral health must be considered a vital component of cardiovascular prevention and management strategies [80].

Diabetes mellitus: The relationship between periodontal disease and diabetes mellitus is bidirectional, with each condition worsening the other through tightly interconnected inflammatory and metabolic mechanisms. Periodontal infection initiates a chronic systemic inflammatory state, driven by oral biofilm pathogens such as *P. gingivalis* and *S. mutans*, which can enter the circulation and stimulate the release of cytokines, including interleukin-6 (IL-6) and tumor necrosis factor-alpha (TNF-α) [81]. These cytokines activate intracellular pathways such as NF-κB, leading to the increased expression of pro-inflammatory mediators that interfere with insulin receptor signaling by impairing the phosphorylation of insulin receptor substrates, thereby reducing glucose uptake by target cells and promoting insulin resistance [82]. Elevated systemic markers such as C-reactive protein (CRP), produced in the liver in response to cytokine stimulation, further reflect and reinforce this pro-inflammatory state, with high CRP levels strongly correlated with both poor glycemic control and the progression of vascular complications [83]. Persistent low-grade inflammation and oxidative stress also alter pancreatic β-cell function, reducing insulin secretion and further destabilizing glucose homeostasis. Conversely, diabetes mellitus exacerbates periodontal disease by creating a hyperglycemic environment that weakens innate immunity and promotes tissue destruction. Hyperglycemia impairs neutrophil chemotaxis and phagocytic capacity, compromising host defense against periodontal pathogens, while simultaneously enhancing the formation of advanced glycation end products (AGEs) that accumulate in periodontal tissues [82,84]. Engagement of AGEs with their receptors (RAGEs) on endothelial and immune cells stimulates the production of additional cytokines and reactive oxygen species, perpetuating a cycle of inflammation, collagen degradation, and alveolar bone loss that defines severe periodontitis. This reciprocal relationship explains why poorly controlled diabetes is associated with higher prevalence and severity of periodontal disease, while periodontal infection, in turn, aggravates glycemic dysregulation and accelerates systemic complications [82]. Importantly, clinical trials demonstrate that effective periodontal therapy, including scaling and root planing, reduces systemic inflammatory markers and improves insulin sensitivity, with HbA1c reductions of approximately 0.4%, an effect comparable to certain second-line antidiabetic medications [82,85].

Adverse pregnancy outcomes: Periodontal disease has been increasingly recognized as a significant risk factor for adverse pregnancy outcomes, including preterm birth, low birth weight, and preeclampsia, with mounting evidence suggesting that maternal oral health is closely linked to fetal well-being through systemic inflammatory and microbial pathways [86]. The pathophysiological connection begins with the ability of oral pathogens, particularly *P. gingivalis*, to enter the maternal circulation via inflamed periodontal tissues and translocate to the placenta, where they stimulate localized immune responses and inflammation [86]. This inflammatory cascade can disrupt the tightly regulated intrauterine environment necessary for sustaining pregnancy, leading to adverse consequences for both mother and child. One key mechanism involves the elevation of inflammatory mediators such as prostaglandins, interleukins, and tumor necrosis factor-alpha (TNF-α), which play central roles in the initiation of labor; when abnormally increased due to periodontal infection, these mediators can prematurely trigger uterine contractions and cervical ripening, resulting in preterm birth [86]. Preterm birth remains one of the leading causes of neonatal morbidity and mortality, and its association with periodontal infection highlights the systemic impact of maternal oral health on pregnancy outcomes. Beyond inducing preterm labor, maternal periodontal infection may also provoke placental inflammation and dysfunction, impairing nutrient and oxygen transfer to the fetus, thereby restricting fetal growth and contributing to low birth weight [87]. Low birth weight is not only linked to immediate developmental complications but is also associated with long-term risks, including cardiovascular disease, diabetes, and impaired cognitive development in later life, demonstrating how maternal periodontal disease can influence health trajectories across the lifespan [87]. Furthermore, systemic inflammation and bacterial dissemination associated with periodontal disease have been implicated in the development of preeclampsia, a severe pregnancy complication characterized by hypertension and multi-organ dysfunction, which further underscores the systemic burden imposed by maternal oral infections [87]. Importantly, clinical research has shown that treating periodontal disease during pregnancy can reduce systemic inflammatory markers and is associated with lower rates of preterm birth and improved neonatal birth weights, providing evidence for the direct benefit of periodontal therapy on maternal–fetal outcomes [88,89]. This underscores the necessity of integrating oral healthcare into standard prenatal protocols, where interventions such as scaling, root planing, and antimicrobial therapies can decrease oral bacterial load and mitigate systemic inflammation. In addition, emerging therapeutic strategies, including the use of dental stem cells, are being explored as innovative tools to enhance oral health and reduce pregnancy-related risks, offering novel avenues for maternal and fetal protection [89]. Collectively, these findings highlight the critical role of maternal oral health in pregnancy, emphasizing that effective prevention and management of periodontal disease may serve not only to safeguard oral health but also to reduce the burden of adverse pregnancy outcomes and improve both immediate and long-term health for mother and child.

Respiratory diseases: Respiratory diseases are increasingly recognized as being influenced by oral health, with oral biofilms playing a crucial role in the development and progression of conditions such as chronic obstructive pulmonary disease (COPD), pneumonia, and asthma, particularly among elderly individuals, immunocompromised patients, and those with pre-existing respiratory conditions [90]. Oral biofilms serve as reservoirs for pathogenic bacteria, including

Streptococcus pneumoniae, Haemophilus influenzae, and *P. gingivalis,* which can be aspirated into the lower respiratory tract during sleep, in individuals with swallowing difficulties, or in patients requiring mechanical ventilation, where they colonize the lungs and trigger infections [91]. Once established in the respiratory tract, these pathogens stimulate local immune responses, inducing the release of pro-inflammatory cytokines such as interleukin-6 (IL-6) and tumor necrosis factor-alpha (TNF-α), which amplify airway inflammation, impair mucociliary clearance, and increase oxidative stress, ultimately exacerbating chronic respiratory conditions like COPD and asthma [92]. In addition to direct colonization, chronic oral infections contribute to systemic inflammation by elevating biomarkers such as C-reactive protein (CRP), reflecting a persistent host immune response that can heighten inflammatory activity within the lungs and worsen respiratory outcomes [92]. The risk is particularly high in vulnerable populations, including nursing home residents and hospitalized patients, where aspiration of bacteria-laden oral secretions contributes significantly to the development of pneumonia, making nursing home-acquired pneumonia a major cause of morbidity and mortality [93].

Poor oral hygiene not only increases microbial load but also alters the oral microbiome, favoring pathogenic species that produce virulence factors capable of evading host immunity and disrupting epithelial barriers, thereby facilitating pulmonary infection [94]. Studies have demonstrated that maintaining good oral hygiene, including regular tooth brushing, the use of antiseptic mouth rinses, and professional dental cleanings, reduces the microbial burden in the oral cavity, thereby lowering the risk of aspiration-related respiratory infections [95]. This is especially critical in intensive care units (ICUs), where patients are highly susceptible to ventilator-associated pneumonia; here, comprehensive oral care protocols that include antimicrobial agents and mechanical debridement of biofilms have been shown to significantly decrease infection incidence and improve survival outcomes [96]. At the molecular level, oral pathogens can influence systemic immune regulation by stimulating Toll-like receptors (TLRs) on airway epithelial cells, leading to the activation of nuclear factor-kappa B (NF-κB) pathways and the upregulation of inflammatory mediators that perpetuate lung tissue damage [92,93]. Furthermore, the lipopolysaccharides (LPS) of Gram-negative oral bacteria, such as *P. gingivalis,* not only enhance neutrophil recruitment to the lungs but also impair their phagocytic efficiency, creating a paradoxical environment of hyperinflammation and reduced bacterial clearance, which worsens respiratory disease progression. These interconnected mechanisms underscore the critical role of oral health in respiratory disease pathogenesis and emphasize the importance of interdisciplinary healthcare approaches, where integrating dental care into systemic disease management can reduce inflammatory burden, prevent respiratory infections, and improve patient outcomes across high-risk populations.

Rheumatoid arthritis: Rheumatoid arthritis (RA) is a chronic autoimmune disease characterized by persistent joint inflammation and systemic complications, and increasing evidence highlights a close association between RA and periodontal disease. Among oral pathogens, *P. gingivalis* plays a particularly important role because it expresses the enzyme peptidylarginine deiminase (PAD), which catalyzes the citrullination of host proteins [97]. This modification leads to the formation of anti-citrullinated protein antibodies (ACPAs), a hallmark of RA strongly correlated with disease onset and severity. The production of ACPAs reflects a breakdown of immune tolerance in which the immune system begins to recognize modified self-proteins as foreign, triggering chronic inflammation and tissue damage in the joints [98].

This process can be explained by molecular mimicry, a mechanism whereby microbial antigens resemble host proteins so closely that the immune system cannot clearly distinguish between them [99]. In the case of *P. gingivalis*, citrullinated bacterial peptides may resemble human citrullinated proteins present in joint tissues, prompting the immune system to mount a response against both the pathogen and the body's own tissues. Over time, this cross-reactivity promotes the generation of autoantibodies, sustains synovial inflammation, and accelerates joint destruction. The role of molecular mimicry in RA is therefore crucial, as it provides a mechanistic link between periodontal infection and autoimmune pathology, suggesting that oral pathogens may act as triggers in genetically or immunologically susceptible individuals. Furthermore, periodontal disease itself generates a chronic pro-inflammatory environment characterized by elevated systemic levels of mediators such as TNF-α and IL-6, which not only worsen local oral inflammation but also contribute to the systemic inflammatory burden that drives RA progression. Clinical studies reinforce this dual relationship, showing that RA patients often present with more severe periodontitis and that periodontal treatment can improve RA symptoms by reducing systemic inflammation and antibody levels. These findings underscore the importance of considering oral health as a component of comprehensive RA management, as addressing periodontal disease may help mitigate systemic autoimmunity, reduce disease activity, and improve overall patient outcomes [100].

In addition, understanding the molecular mimicry processes involved opens new perspectives for therapeutic interventions aimed at disrupting the autoimmune responses initiated by oral pathogens, which could provide innovative strategies for preventing or slowing the progression of RA and possibly other autoimmune diseases with similar pathogenic pathways.

Neural diseases: Oral biofilm has gained increasing recognition for its role in the pathogenesis of neural diseases, particularly neurodegenerative disorders such as Alzheimer's disease (AD) and Parkinson's disease (PD), through mechanisms that primarily involve chronic inflammation and microbial invasion. Periodontal pathogens residing in oral biofilms can enter the bloodstream via inflamed or compromised periodontal tissues, as often occurs in chronic periodontitis, and once in systemic circulation, they stimulate immune responses that elevate pro-inflammatory cytokines, contributing to a state of persistent systemic inflammation [101]. This systemic inflammation is now regarded as a critical driver of neuroinflammation, a central feature in the onset and progression of both AD and PD, as inflammatory mediators can cross or weaken the blood–brain barrier and initiate or worsen pathological processes within the brain [101].

In AD, the periodontal pathogen *P. gingivalis* has been detected in brain tissues of affected individuals, strongly suggesting its ability to invade neural structures and penetrate the blood–brain barrier under conditions of systemic inflammation [101]. The presence of *P. gingivalis* is closely linked to amyloid-beta plaque formation, a neuropathological hallmark of AD, as its toxins and metabolic products stimulate amyloid aggregation while also triggering local inflammatory responses that amplify neuronal injury and neurodegeneration [101]. Furthermore, *P. gingivalis* produces gingipains, powerful proteolytic enzymes that have been identified in brain tissues, where they degrade essential neuronal proteins, activate microglial cells, and perpetuate cycles of inflammation and neuronal loss, thereby directly contributing to AD pathology [101].

In PD, the role of oral biofilm may extend beyond direct neural invasion to include modulation of the gut–brain axis, an increasingly recognized communication pathway between the gastrointestinal tract and the central nervous system. Periodontal pathogens have been shown to influence the composition of the gut microbiota, inducing dysbiosis, which can provoke chronic intestinal inflammation and alter immune signaling pathways [102]. This state of dysbiosis may contribute to the misfolding and aggregation of alpha-synuclein in enteric neurons, a process thought to initiate PD pathology, with the subsequent transmission of these pathological signals to the brain via the vagus nerve, a direct neural conduit between the gut and central nervous system [102]. Through this axis, inflammatory and microbial signals originating in the gut can reach the brain, thereby fueling the neuroinflammation and dopaminergic neuronal damage characteristic of PD [102].

Together, these mechanisms highlight the multifaceted role of oral biofilm in neurological disease: it can act directly by transporting pathogens and toxins into the brain, or indirectly by sustaining systemic inflammation and influencing gut–brain communication, both of which contribute to neurodegenerative processes. This growing body of evidence underscores the importance of oral health in systemic and neurological well-being, suggesting that maintaining oral hygiene and preventing periodontal disease may represent valuable strategies for reducing systemic inflammatory load, preserving blood–brain barrier integrity, and ultimately lowering the risk or slowing the progression of neurodegenerative diseases such as AD and PD [101,102].

Cancer development: The disruption of microbial homeostasis in oral biofilms has emerged as a significant contributor to carcinogenesis, particularly in head and neck cancers and in distant malignancies such as colorectal cancer (CRC). Under healthy conditions, oral microbial communities maintain immune balance and tissue homeostasis; however, environmental and systemic factors such as smoking, poor oral hygiene, chronic systemic diseases, and sustained inflammation can disrupt this equilibrium, enabling pathogenic bacteria, including *P. gingivalis*, *F. nucleatum*, and *Treponema denticola*, to dominate [103]. These dysbiotic pathogens promote cancer development through multiple mechanisms. *P. gingivalis*, for example, can subvert host immune defenses by impairing neutrophil activity, promoting immune evasion, and sustaining chronic low-grade inflammation, all of which create a microenvironment favorable to tumor initiation [103]. Additionally, it directly influences epithelial cell biology by inhibiting apoptosis, disrupting cell cycle regulation, and upregulating oncogenic mediators such as matrix metalloproteinases (MMPs) and interleukin-6 (IL-6), which are closely associated with tumor invasion, angiogenesis, and metastasis [103].

These effects are particularly relevant in head and neck squamous cell carcinoma (HNSCC), where dysbiosis leads to decreased microbial diversity and the enrichment of anaerobic and pathogenic taxa at tumor sites. Large-scale cohort studies and systematic reviews consistently report that patients with oral squamous cell carcinoma exhibit distinct microbiome signatures compared with healthy controls, confirming the association between dysbiosis, tumor presence, and disease progression [104,105].

Beyond the oral cavity, *F. nucleatum* has been strongly implicated in CRC, where it is frequently detected within tumor tissues and is associated with more aggressive and treatment-resistant phenotypes [106]. Mechanistically, *F. nucleatum* adheres to intestinal epithelial cells through the FadA adhesion molecule, activating the Wnt/β-catenin signaling pathway and inducing the expression of oncogenes, thereby driving uncontrolled cell proliferation [106]. In parallel, it shapes the tumor microenvironment by recruiting myeloid-derived suppressor cells (MDSCs) and impairing natural killer (NK) cell-mediated cytotoxicity, leading to immune evasion and tumor progression [106]. The translocation of *F. nucleatum* and other oral pathogens from the mouth to distal organs likely occurs through hematogenous dissemination or gastrointestinal colonization facilitated by swallowing, particularly in the context of systemic inflammation or compromised mucosal barriers [107]. These findings underscore the role of oral pathogens in carcinogenesis and suggest that strategies aimed at preserving microbial homeostasis, preventing dysbiosis, and targeting microbe–host interactions may represent promising approaches in the prevention and management of cancer.

2.4. Future Directions in Diagnosis, Therapy, and Regeneration

In recent years, significant progress has been made in identifying diagnostic markers within the oral cavity that reflect systemic health conditions. Among these advances, salivary diagnostics have gained considerable attention due to their non-invasive nature and easy sample collection. Saliva contains a wide range of biomarkers, including inflammatory cytokines such as interleukin-6 (IL-6) and tumor necrosis factor-alpha (TNF-α), matrix metalloproteinases, and acute-phase proteins like C-reactive protein (CRP). These molecules are increasingly being recognized for their potential to serve as early indicators of systemic diseases such as cardiovascular disease and type 2 diabetes, which have well-documented associations with chronic periodontal inflammation [108,109]. Salivary proteomics, the comprehensive study of salivary proteins, has opened new avenues for detecting novel biomarkers associated with periodontitis and other inflammatory conditions. These biomarkers may help diagnose oral diseases and provide insights into the onset and progression of systemic disorders. The development of standardized protocols and emerging analytical technologies has further improved the reliability and reproducibility of salivary biomarker assessments.

Moreover, microbial signature profiling, particularly through next-generation sequencing (NGS) and metagenomic analysis, has enabled a more refined understanding of the oral microbiome's role in systemic health. These tools can detect shifts in microbial composition and identify dysbiosis patterns that are linked to chronic diseases such as diabetes, cardiovascular conditions, and even certain cancers [110]. Unlike traditional culture-based methods, NGS offers a comprehensive view of microbial communities, including non-culturable organisms, thereby enhancing diagnostic accuracy.

An exciting development in this area is the integration of machine learning and artificial intelligence (AI) in analyzing complex microbial and biomarker datasets. AI algorithms can detect subtle patterns and correlations that may not be evident through conventional statistical approaches. By training models on large datasets, researchers can differentiate between health and disease states with high accuracy, facilitating earlier and more precise diagnosis [111].

The management of oral biofilms is undergoing a transformative shift from conventional mechanical debridement and broad-spectrum antimicrobial use toward more targeted and sophisticated strategies. Among the most promising innovations are biofilm-disrupting agents, which are designed to degrade the extracellular polymeric substances (EPS) that protect biofilm-embedded bacteria. Enzymes such as *dispersin B* specifically target and break down polysaccharides in the biofilm matrix, thereby weakening the biofilm structure and enhancing the efficacy of antimicrobial agents. Similarly, antimicrobial peptides (AMPs) are being engineered to penetrate biofilms and exert bactericidal effects while minimizing host toxicity [112]. Another cutting-edge approach involves quorum-sensing inhibitors (QSIs), which disrupt microbial communication systems responsible for coordinating virulence factor expression, biofilm maturation, and resistance behavior. By interfering with quorum-sensing pathways, QSIs can prevent the establishment and persistence of pathogenic biofilms without exerting selective pressure that leads to resistance, making them a sustainable option for long-term biofilm control [113,114].

In parallel, immunomodulatory therapies are being explored to recalibrate host responses to biofilm-associated infections. These therapies aim not just to eliminate pathogens but to restore balanced host–microbe interactions. For instance, Toll-like receptor (TLR) antagonists can reduce excessive immune activation triggered by biofilms, while biologics targeting key inflammatory pathways may help suppress chronic inflammation that contributes to systemic disease progression [115,116]. These approaches reflect an understanding that host response plays a critical role in biofilm persistence and associated systemic effects.

The field of regenerative dentistry has witnessed rapid advances, largely driven by the discovery and application of dental pulp stem cells (DPSCs). These stem cells, derived from the dental pulp of permanent or deciduous teeth, possess remarkable self-renewal capacity and multilineage differentiation potential, making them ideal candidates for tissue engineering in oral and maxillofacial regeneration inflammation [117]. DPSCs have shown the ability to differentiate into a variety of cell types, including odontoblasts, osteoblasts, adipocytes, and neural-like cells. As a result, they are being intensively investigated for use in regenerating the pulp-dentin complex, reconstructing the periodontal ligament, and even bioengineering entire teeth. Their immunomodulatory properties also enhance their therapeutic potential by promoting tissue healing and reducing inflammation [117,118]. Recent innovations have significantly strengthened the regenerative capacity of DPSCs. For instance, Liu et al. (2024) demonstrated that DPSCs, when treated with cannabidiol (CBD) and cultured into organoid-like microspheroids, exhibit enhanced osteogenic potential through the upregulation of *WNT6*, a key gene involved in bone and tissue regeneration [118]. This highlights how bioactive molecules and 3D culture conditions can synergistically improve stem cell-based therapies.

However, the emergence of gene editing technologies, particularly CRISPR-Cas9, has opened new possibilities for enhancing the therapeutic efficacy of stem cells. These tools allow precise modifications of the stem cell genome, such as correcting pathogenic mutations or upregulating genes that encode growth factors and regenerative signals. This strategy not only optimizes cell behavior but also tailors' treatment to individual genetic profiles, representing a step toward precision regenerative medicine [119]. Moreover, the integration of advanced scaffold technologies and 3D bioprinting is revolutionizing the structural design of regenerative constructs. Modern biomaterials used for scaffolds now offer improved biocompatibility, mechanical strength, and controlled biodegradability, which are essential for supporting cell attachment, proliferation, and differentiation. Bioprinting techniques further enable the creation of complex tissue architectures that mimic the native organization of dental and periodontal tissues [120,121]. These technological advances, combining DPSCs, gene editing, and 3D bioprinting, are rapidly bridging the gap between experimental research and clinical application. As a result, the prospect of the functional, patient-specific regeneration of dental tissues is becoming increasingly realistic. Continued interdisciplinary collaboration will be essential to ensure the safe, ethical, and effective translation of these therapies into clinical practice.

Persistent oral dysbiosis has been linked to chronic low-grade inflammation, which plays a key role in the pathogenesis of a variety of systemic conditions. The chronic presence of biofilm-associated pathogens stimulates innate immune receptors, resulting in sustained production of pro-inflammatory mediators that can enter systemic circulation and exacerbate extraoral diseases [122]. Recent studies highlight the role of microbial-derived metabolites and extracellular vesicles in mediating crosstalk between the oral cavity and distant immune tissues. These bioactive molecules can influence T-cell differentiation, notably promoting Th17 responses, a phenotype implicated in mucosal and systemic autoimmunity. Such findings suggest that the oral microbiome may act as a reservoir for immune-activating signals that contribute to chronic inflammation and immune dysregulation beyond the oral cavity [123,124]. The immunological effects of microbial ecosystems are not limited to their pro-inflammatory capacity. Dysbiosis can impair the development of immune tolerance, which is essential for preventing overactive immune responses. This is particularly relevant in autoimmune diseases, where microbial imbalances in the gut and oral cavity have been shown to disrupt regulatory T-cell function and antigen tolerance [125]. Moreover, the overuse or inappropriate use of antibiotics may further disrupt microbial balance, leading to resistance and impairing the beneficial functions of the microbiome [126]. Integrating cross-disciplinary insights from oral biology, immunology, and microbiome research provides a broad view of how biofilm-associated dysbiosis may initiate or exacerbate systemic disease. It also opens new therapeutic avenues, such as microbiome modulation, targeted immune therapies, and biofilm-specific interventions, aimed at both preventing and treating chronic inflammatory diseases with an oral–systemic connection.

2.5. Conclusions

The exploration of oral biofilms in this chapter reveals their profound influence, not only on oral health but also on a wide range of systemic diseases, emphasizing the critical intersection between dentistry and overall medical care. These complex microbial communities, when disrupted, can lead to significant health issues beyond the oral cavity. The association between oral biofilms and systemic conditions such as CVD, diabetes, RA, and neural disorders like AD underscores the importance of managing oral health as part of a comprehensive approach to overall well-being.

The mechanisms through which oral biofilms influence systemic health are multifaceted. Bacteremia, resulting from the dissemination of oral bacteria into the bloodstream, can lead to systemic infections and contribute to chronic inflammatory conditions. The inflammatory response triggered by these bacteria plays a pivotal role in linking oral infections to systemic diseases, with elevated levels of inflammatory markers like CRP serving as a bridge between periodontal disease and conditions such as atherosclerosis and neuroinflammation, which is implicated in the progression of Alzheimer's disease.

Moreover, the phenomenon of molecular mimicry, where oral pathogens share antigens similar to those of host tissues, can provoke autoimmune responses, potentially leading to conditions like rheumatoid arthritis. Additionally, the chronic inflammation associated with oral biofilms can disrupt metabolic processes, exacerbating conditions like diabetes and contributing to the development of atherosclerosis. Recent research also suggests that systemic inflammation and microbial translocation caused by oral biofilms may play a role in the pathogenesis of neurodegenerative diseases, further highlighting the importance of oral health in preventing these debilitating conditions. These connections emphasize the critical importance of maintaining oral health, not only to prevent oral diseases but also to mitigate the risk of systemic and neural conditions.

Future research should continue to explore the intricate links between oral and systemic health, particularly in relation to neural diseases, paving the way for integrated healthcare approaches that address the oral–systemic–neural health nexus. For clinicians, this underscores the need for a holistic approach to patient care, where the management of oral biofilms is recognized as an essential component of preventing and treating systemic and neural diseases. The insights gained from understanding the role of oral biofilms in systemic and neural health emphasize the need for ongoing research, education, and collaboration across medical and dental disciplines to improve patient outcomes.

References

1. Volponi, A.A.; Pang, Y.; Sharpe, P.T. Stem cell-based biological tooth repair and regeneration. *Trends Cell Biol.* **2010**, *20*, 715–722. [CrossRef]
2. Yu, T.; Klein, O.D. Molecular and cellular mechanisms of tooth development, homeostasis and repair. *Development* **2020**, *147*, dev184754. [CrossRef] [PubMed]
3. Birjandi, A.A.; Sharpe, P. Wnt Signalling in Regenerative Dentistry. *Front. Dent. Med.* **2021**, *2*, 725468. [CrossRef]
4. Gómez-Gil, D.; Camila Orjuela-Vásquez, M.; Pino-Duque, M.; Pino-Araujo, A.; Sánchez-Garzón, J. Historic Background and Current Perspectives in Dental Crown Formation [Internet]. In *Embryology Update*; IntechOpen: London, UK, 2023. [CrossRef]
5. Huang, L.; Lu, W.; Ning, Y.; Liu, J. Reverse effects of Streptococcus mutans physiological states on neutrophil extracellular traps formation as a strategy to escape neutrophil killing. *Front. Cell. Infect. Microbiol.* **2022**, *12*, 1023457. [CrossRef]
6. Hajishengallis, G. Immunomicrobial pathogenesis of periodontitis: Keystones, pathobionts, and host response. *Trends Immunol.* **2014**, *35*, 3–11. [CrossRef]
7. Kowalski, J.; Nowak, M.; Górski, B.; Górska, R. What Has Immunology Brought to Periodontal Disease in Recent Years? *Arch. Immunol. Ther. Exp.* **2022**, *70*, 26. [CrossRef]
8. Matsuoka, M.; Soria, S.A.; Pires, J.R.; Sant'Ana, A.C.P.; Freire, M. Natural and induced immune responses in oral cavity and saliva. *BMC Immunol.* **2025**, *26*, 34. [CrossRef] [PubMed]

9. Zhao, A.; Sun, J.; Liu, Y. Understanding bacterial biofilms: From definition to treatment strategies. *Front. Cell. Infect. Microbiol.* **2023**, *13*, 1137947. [CrossRef] [PubMed]
10. Van Roy, Z.; Kielian, T. Immune-based strategies for the treatment of biofilm infections. *Biofilm* **2025**, *9*, 100264. [CrossRef]
11. Rathee, M.; Sapra, A. Dental Caries. In *StatPearls [Internet]*; StatPearls Publishing: Treasure Island, FL, USA, 2024. Available online: https://www.ncbi.nlm.nih.gov/books/NBK551699/ (accessed on 21 June 2023).
12. Shao, Q.; Feng, D.; Yu, Z.; Chen, D.; Ji, Y.; Ye, Q.; Cheng, D. The role of microbial interactions in dental caries: Dental plaque microbiota analysis. *Microb. Pathog.* **2023**, *185*, 106390. [CrossRef]
13. Philip, N.; Suneja, B.; Walsh, L. Beyond Streptococcus mutans: Clinical implications of the evolving dental caries aetiological paradigms and its associated microbiome. *Br. Dent. J.* **2018**, *224*, 219–225. [CrossRef]
14. Chen, X.; Daliri, E.B.; Kim, N.; Kim, J.R.; Yoo, D.; Oh, D.H. Microbial Etiology and Prevention of Dental Caries: Exploiting Natural Products to Inhibit Cariogenic Biofilms. *Pathogens* **2020**, *9*, 569. [CrossRef]
15. van Loveren, C. Sugar Restriction for Caries Prevention: Amount and Frequency. Which Is More Important? *Caries Res.* **2019**, *53*, 168–175. [CrossRef]
16. Lagerweij, M.; van Loveren, C. Chapter 7: Sugar and Dental Caries. *Monogr. Oral. Sci.* **2020**, *28*, 68–76. [CrossRef]
17. Delgado-Angulo, E.K.; Bernabé, E. Influence of host-related risk indicators on dental caries in permanent dentition. *Acta Odontol. Latinoam.* **2006**, *19*, 85–92. [PubMed]
18. Lopes, P.C.; Carvalho, T.; Gomes, A.T.P.C.; Veiga, N.; Blanco, L.; Correia, M.J.; Mello-Moura, A.C.V. White spot lesions: Diagnosis and treatment—A systematic review. *BMC Oral Health* **2024**, *24*, 58. [CrossRef]
19. Roberts, W.E.; Mangum, J.E.; Schneider, P.M. Pathophysiology of Demineralization, Part II: Enamel White Spots, Cavitated Caries, and Bone Infection. *Curr. Osteoporos. Rep.* **2022**, *20*, 106–119. [CrossRef] [PubMed]
20. Denis, M.; Atlan, A.; Vennat, E.; Tirlet, G.; Attal, J.P. White defects on enamel: Diagnosis and anatomopathology: Two essential factors for proper treatment (part 1). *Int. Orthod.* **2013**, *11*, 139–165, (In English, French). [CrossRef]
21. Abdelaziz, M. Detection, Diagnosis, and Monitoring of Early Caries: The Future of Individualized Dental Care. *Diagnostics* **2023**, *13*, 3649. [CrossRef]
22. Ghodasra, R.; Brizuela, M. Dental Caries Diagnostic Testing. In *StatPearls [Internet]*; StatPearls Publishing: Treasure Island, FL, USA, 2024. [PubMed]
23. Nassar, Y.; Brizuela, M. The Role of Fluoride on Caries Prevention. In *StatPearls [Internet]*; StatPearls Publishing: Treasure Island, FL, USA, 2024. [PubMed]
24. Toumba, K.J.; Twetman, S.; Splieth, C.; Parnell, C.; van Loveren, C.; Lygidakis, N.A. Guidelines on the use of fluoride for caries prevention in children: An updated EAPD policy document. *Eur. Arch. Paediatr. Dent.* **2019**, *20*, 507–516. [CrossRef] [PubMed]
25. Wei, Y.; Dang, G.P.; Ren, Z.Y.; Wan, M.C.; Wang, C.Y.; Li, H.B.; Zhang, T.; Tay, F.R.; Niu, L.N. Recent advances in the pathogenesis and prevention strategies of dental calculus. *NPJ Biofilms Microbiomes.* **2024**, *10*, 56. [CrossRef]

26. Kalesinskas, P.; Kačergius, T.; Ambrozaitis, A.; Pečiulienė, V.; Ericson, D. Reducing dental plaque formation and caries development. A review of current methods and implications for novel pharmaceuticals. *Stomatologija* **2014**, *16*, 44–52. [PubMed]
27. Unterbrink, P.; Schulze Zur Wiesche, E.; Meyer, F.; Fandrich, P.; Amaechi, B.T.; Enax, J. Prevention of Dental Caries: A Review on the Improvements of Toothpaste Formulations from 1900 to 2023. *Dent. J.* **2024**, *12*, 64. [CrossRef]
28. Walsh, T.; Worthington, H.V.; Glenny, A.M.; Marinho, V.C.; Jeroncic, A. Fluoride toothpastes of different concentrations for preventing dental caries. *Cochrane Database Syst. Rev.* **2019**, *3*, CD007868. [CrossRef]
29. Abedi, M.; Ghasemi, Y.; Nemati, M.M. Nanotechnology in toothpaste: Fundamentals, trends, and safety. *Heliyon* **2024**, *10*, e24949. [CrossRef]
30. Limeback, H.; Enax, J.; Meyer, F. Improving Oral Health with Fluoride-Free Calcium-Phosphate-Based Biomimetic Toothpastes: An Update of the Clinical Evidence. *Biomimetics* **2023**, *8*, 331. [CrossRef]
31. O'Hagan-Wong, K.; Enax, J.; Meyer, F.; Ganss, B. The use of hydroxyapatite toothpaste to prevent dental caries. *Odontology* **2022**, *110*, 223–230. [CrossRef] [PubMed]
32. Selvaraj, K.; Bharath, N.; Natarajan, R.; Dinesh, S.; Murugesan, S.; Selvaraj, S. Comparative Evaluation of Antimicrobial Efficacy of Toothpastes Containing Probiotic and Neem as Primary Ingredient on Salivary Streptococcus mutans in Melmaruvathur Population: An In Vivo Study. *J. Pharm. Bioallied Sci.* **2020**, *12*, S595–S600. [CrossRef] [PubMed]
33. Meto, A.; Colombari, B.; Odorici, A.; Giva, L.B.; Pericolini, E.; Regina, A.L.; Blasi, E. Antibacterial Effects of MicroRepair®BIOMA-Based Toothpaste and Chewing Gum on Orthodontic Elastics Contaminated In Vitro with Saliva from Healthy Donors: A Pilot Study. *Appl. Sci.* **2020**, *10*, 6721. [CrossRef]
34. Dionysopoulos, D.; Papageorgiou, S.; Papadopoulos, C.; Davidopoulou, S.; Konstantinidis, A.; Tolidis, K. Effect of Whitening Toothpastes with Different Active Agents on the Abrasive Wear of Dentin Following Tooth Brushing Simulation. *J. Funct. Biomater.* **2023**, *14*, 268. [CrossRef]
35. Jamwal, N.; Rao, A.; Shenoy, R.; Pai, M.; Ks, A.; Br, A. Effect of whitening toothpaste on surface roughness and microhardness of human teeth: A systematic review and meta-analysis. *F1000Research* **2022**, *11*, 22. [CrossRef]
36. Tungare, S.; Paranjpe, A.G. Diet and Nutrition to Prevent Dental Problems. In *StatPearls [Internet]*; StatPearls Publishing: Treasure Island, FL, USA, 2024. Available online: https://www.ncbi.nlm.nih.gov/books/NBK534248/ (accessed on 10 July 2023).
37. Chhaliyil, P.; Fischer, K.F.; Schoel, B.; Chhalliyil, P. A Novel, Simple, Frequent Oral Cleaning Method Reduces Damaging Bacteria in the Dental Microbiota. *J. Int. Soc. Prev. Community Dent.* **2020**, *10*, 511–519. [CrossRef]
38. Ng, T.C.; Chu, C.H.; Yu, O.Y. A concise review of dental sealants in caries management. *Front. Oral Health* **2023**, *4*, 1180405. [CrossRef]
39. Cho, K.; Rajan, G.; Farrar, P.; Prentice, L.; Prusty, B.G. Dental resin composites: A review on materials to product realizations. *Compos. Part B Eng.* **2022**, *230*, 109495. [CrossRef]

40. Gasner, N.S.; Schure, R.S. Periodontal Disease. 2025 May 12. In: StatPearls [Internet]. Treasure Island (FL): StatPearls Publishing; 2025 Jan–. PMID: 32119477. Available online: https://www.ncbi.nlm.nih.gov/books/NBK554590/ (accessed on 3 June 2025). [PubMed]
41. Hajishengallis, G.; Chavakis, T.; Lambris, J.D. Current understanding of periodontal disease pathogenesis and targets for host-modulation therapy. *Periodontol 2000* **2020**, *84*, 14–34. [CrossRef] [PubMed]
42. Abdulkareem, A.A.; Al-Taweel, F.B.; Al-Sharqi, A.J.B.; Gul, S.S.; Sha, A.; Chapple, I.L.C. Current concepts in the pathogenesis of periodontitis: From symbiosis to dysbiosis. *J. Oral Microbiol.* **2023**, *15*, 2197779. [CrossRef] [PubMed]
43. Genco, R.J.; Borgnakke, W.S. Risk factors for periodontal disease. *Periodontol 2000* **2013**, *62*, 59–94. [CrossRef]
44. Jacobs, R.; Fontenele, R.C.; Lahoud, P.; Shujaat, S.; Bornstein, M.M. Radiographic diagnosis of periodontal diseases—Current evidence versus innovations. *Periodontol 2000* **2024**. [CrossRef]
45. Meto, A.; Halilaj, G. The Integration of Cone Beam Computed Tomography, Artificial Intelligence, Augmented Reality, and Virtual Reality in Dental Diagnostics, Surgical Planning, and Education: A Narrative Review. *Appl. Sci.* **2025**, *15*, 6308. [CrossRef]
46. Slots, J. Periodontitis: Facts, fallacies and the future. *Periodontol 2000* **2017**, *75*, 7–23. [CrossRef]
47. Radu, C.M.; Radu, C.C.; Arbănaşi, E.M.; Hogea, T.; Murvai, V.R.; Chiș, I.A.; Zaha, D.C. Exploring the Efficacy of Novel Therapeutic Strategies for Periodontitis: A Literature Review. *Life* **2024**, *14*, 468. [CrossRef] [PubMed]
48. Teshome, A.; Derese, K.; Andualem, G. The Prevalence and Determinant Factors of Oral Halitosis in Northwest Ethiopia: A Cross-Sectional Study. *Clin. Cosmet. Investig. Dent.* **2021**, *13*, 173–179. [CrossRef]
49. Izidoro, C.; Botelho, J.; Machado, V.; Reis, A.M.; Proença, L.; Alves, R.C.; Mendes, J.J. Revisiting Standard and Novel Therapeutic Approaches in Halitosis: A Review. *Int. J. Environ. Res. Public Health* **2022**, *19*, 11303. [CrossRef]
50. Grudziąż-Sękowska, J.; Iwanicka-Grzegorek, E. Aetiology, diagnosis and management of halitosis—A narrative review. *J. Educ. Health Sport* **2022**, *13*, 235–245. [CrossRef]
51. Kapoor, U.; Sharma, G.; Juneja, M.; Nagpal, A. Halitosis: Current concepts on etiology, diagnosis and management. *Eur. J. Dent.* **2016**, *10*, 292–300. [CrossRef]
52. Szalai, E.; Tajti, P.; Szabó, B.; Kói, T.; Hegyi, P.; Czumbel, L.M.; Varga, G.; Kerémi, B. Organoleptic and Halitometric Assessments Do Not Correlate Well in Intra-Oral Halitosis: A Systematic Review And Meta-Analysis. *J. Evid. Based Dent. Pract.* **2023**, *23*, 101862. [CrossRef]
53. Khounganian, R.M.; Alasmari, O.N.; Aldosari, M.M.; Alghanemi, N.M. Causes and Management of Halitosis: A Narrative Review. *Cureus* **2023**, *15*, e43742. [CrossRef] [PubMed]
54. Vila, T.; Sultan, A.S.; Montelongo-Jauregui, D.; Jabra-Rizk, M.A. Oral Candidiasis: A Disease of Opportunity. *J. Fungi* **2020**, *6*, 15. [CrossRef] [PubMed]
55. Jørgensen, M.R. Pathophysiological microenvironments in oral candidiasis. *APMIS* **2024**. [CrossRef]

56. Lu, S.-Y. Oral Candidosis: Pathophysiology and Best Practice for Diagnosis, Classification, and Successful Management. *J. Fungi* **2021**, *7*, 555. [CrossRef]
57. Telles, D.R.; Karki, N.; Marshall, M.W. Oral Fungal Infections: Diagnosis and Management. *Dent. Clin. N. Am.* **2017**, *61*, 319–349. [CrossRef]
58. Coronado-Castellote, L.; Jiménez-Soriano, Y. Clinical and microbiological diagnosis of oral candidiasis. *J. Clin. Exp. Dent.* **2013**, *5*, e279-86. [CrossRef]
59. Contaldo, M.; Di Stasio, D.; Romano, A.; Fiori, F.; Della Vella, F.; Rupe, C.; Lajolo, C.; Petruzzi, M.; Serpico, R.; Lucchese, A. Oral Candidiasis and Novel Therapeutic Strategies: Antifungals, Phytotherapy, Probiotics, and Photodynamic Therapy. *Curr. Drug Deliv.* **2023**, *20*, 441–456. [CrossRef]
60. Quindós, G.; Gil-Alonso, S.; Marcos-Arias, C.; Sevillano, E.; Mateo, E.; Jauregizar, N.; Eraso, E. Therapeutic tools for oral candidiasis: Current and new antifungal drugs. *Med. Oral. Patol. Oral Cir. Bucal.* **2019**, *24*, e172–e180. [CrossRef]
61. Lavanya, N.; Jayanthi, P.; Rao, U.K.; Ranganathan, K. Oral lichen planus: An update on pathogenesis and treatment. *J. Oral. Maxillofac. Pathol.* **2011**, *15*, 127–132. [CrossRef] [PubMed]
62. Elenbaas, A.; Enciso, R.; Al-Eryani, K. Oral Lichen Planus: A review of clinical features, etiologies, and treatments. *Dent. Rev.* **2022**, *2*, 100007. [CrossRef]
63. Boorghani, M.; Gholizadeh, N.; Taghavi Zenouz, A.; Vatankhah, M.; Mehdipour, M. Oral lichen planus: Clinical features, etiology, treatment and management; a review of literature. *J. Dent. Res. Dent. Clin. Dent. Prospect.* **2010**, *4*, 3–9. [CrossRef]
64. Rotaru, D.I.; Sofineti, D.; Bolboacă, S.D.; Bulboacă, A.E. Diagnostic Criteria of Oral Lichen Planus: A Narrative Review. *Acta Clin. Croat.* **2020**, *59*, 513–522. [CrossRef]
65. Andabak-Rogulj, A.; Vindiš, E.; Aleksijević, L.H.; Škrinjar, I.; Juras, D.V.; Aščić, A.; Brzak, B.L. Different Treatment Modalities of Oral Lichen Planus-A Narrative Review. *Dent. J.* **2023**, *11*, 26. [CrossRef]
66. Raj, G.; Raj, M. Oral Lichen Planus. In *StatPearls [Internet]*; StatPearls Publishing: Treasure Island, FL, USA, 2024. Available online: https://www.ncbi.nlm.nih.gov/books/NBK578201/ (accessed on 6 February 2023).
67. Schwarz, F.; Derks, J.; Monje, A.; Wang, H.L. Peri-implantitis. *J. Clin. Periodontol.* **2018**, *45*, S246–S266. [CrossRef] [PubMed]
68. Berglundh, T.; Mombelli, A.; Schwarz, F.; Derks, J. Etiology, pathogenesis and treatment of peri-implantitis: A European perspective. *Periodontol 2000* **2024**. [CrossRef]
69. Ng, E.; Tay, J.R.H.; Mattheos, N.; Bostanci, N.; Belibasakis, G.N.; Seneviratne, C.J. A Mapping Review of the Pathogenesis of Peri-Implantitis: The Biofilm-Mediated Inflammation and Bone Dysregulation (BIND) Hypothesis. *Cells* **2024**, *13*, 315. [CrossRef]
70. Romandini, M.; Lima, C.; Pedrinaci, I.; Araoz, A.; Costanza Soldini, M.; Sanz, M. Clinical signs, symptoms, perceptions, and impact on quality of life in patients suffering from peri-implant diseases: A university-representative cross-sectional study. *Clin. Oral Implants Res.* **2021**, *32*, 100–111. [CrossRef]
71. Sahrmann, P.; Kühl, S.; Dagassan-Berndt, D.; Bornstein, M.M.; Zitzmann, N.U. Radiographic assessment of the peri-implant site. *Periodontol 2000* **2024**. [CrossRef]

72. Meto, A.; Conserva, E.; Liccardi, F.; Colombari, B.; Consolo, U.; Blasi, E. Differential Efficacy of Two Dental Implant Decontamination Techniques in Reducing Microbial Biofilm and Re-Growth onto Titanium Disks In Vitro. *Appl. Sci.* **2019**, *9*, 3191. [CrossRef]
73. Kormas, I.; Pedercini, C.; Pedercini, A.; Raptopoulos, M.; Alassy, H.; Wolff, L.F. Peri-Implant Diseases: Diagnosis, Clinical, Histological, Microbiological Characteristics and Treatment Strategies. A Narrative Review. *Antibiotics* **2020**, *9*, 835. [CrossRef]
74. Perussolo, J.; Donos, N. Maintenance of peri-implant health in general dental practice. *Br. Dent. J.* **2024**, *236*, 781–789. [CrossRef] [PubMed]
75. Li, X.; Kolltveit, K.M.; Tronstad, L.; Olsen, I. Systemic diseases caused by oral infection. *Clin. Microbiol. Rev.* **2000**, *13*, 547–558. [CrossRef] [PubMed]
76. Nomura, R.; Matayoshi, S.; Otsugu, M.; Kitamura, T.; Teramoto, N.; Nakano, K. Contribution of Severe Dental Caries Induced by Streptococcus mutans to the Pathogenicity of Infective Endocarditis. *Infect. Immun.* **2020**, *88*, e00897-19. [CrossRef]
77. Pussinen, P.J.; Kopra, E.; Pietiäinen, M.; Lehto, M.; Zaric, S.; Paju, S.; Salminen, A. Periodontitis and cardiometabolic disorders: The role of lipopolysaccharide and endotoxemia. *Periodontol 2000* **2022**, *89*, 19–40. [CrossRef]
78. Chen, L.; Deng, H.; Cui, H.; Fang, J.; Zuo, Z.; Deng, J.; Li, Y.; Wang, X.; Zhao, L. Inflammatory responses and inflammation-associated diseases in organs. *Oncotarget* **2017**, *9*, 7204–7218. [CrossRef]
79. Mendoza, M.F.; Anzelmo, M.A.; Suan, N.M.; Cuccia, C.S.; Lavie, C.J. More than Just a Toothache: Inflammatory Mechanisms Linking Periodontal Disease to Cardiovascular Disease and the Protective Impact of Cardiorespiratory Fitness. *Biomedicines* **2025**, *13*, 1512. [CrossRef] [PubMed]
80. Zaman, M.S.; Alam, S.M.G.; Razzaque, M.S. Oral Hygiene and Cardiovascular Health. *Hygiene* **2025**, *5*, 14. [CrossRef]
81. Kleinstein, S.E.; Nelson, K.E.; Freire, M. Inflammatory Networks Linking Oral Microbiome with Systemic Health and Disease. *J. Dent. Res.* **2020**, *99*, 1131–1139. [CrossRef]
82. Galicia-Garcia, U.; Benito-Vicente, A.; Jebari, S.; Larrea-Sebal, A.; Siddiqi, H.; Uribe, K.B.; Ostolaza, H.; Martín, C. Pathophysiology of Type 2 Diabetes Mellitus. *Int. J. Mol. Sci.* **2020**, *21*, 6275. [CrossRef]
83. Mouliou, D.S. C-Reactive Protein: Pathophysiology, Diagnosis, False Test Results and a Novel Diagnostic Algorithm for Clinicians. *Diseases* **2023**, *11*, 132. [CrossRef]
84. Chung, Y.L.; Lee, J.J.; Chien, H.H.; Chang, M.C.; Jeng, J.H. Interplay between diabetes mellitus and periodontal/pulpal-periapical diseases. *J. Dent. Sci.* **2024**, *19*, 1338–1347. [CrossRef]
85. Aizenbud, I.; Wilensky, A.; Almoznino, G. Periodontal Disease and Its Association with Metabolic Syndrome-A Comprehensive Review. *Int. J. Mol. Sci.* **2023**, *24*, 13011. [CrossRef]
86. Tsikouras, P.; Oikonomou, E.; Nikolettos, K.; Andreou, S.; Kyriakou, D.; Damaskos, C.; Garmpis, N.; Monastiridou, V.; Nalmpanti, T.; Bothou, A.; et al. The Impact of Periodontal Disease on Preterm Birth and Preeclampsia. *J. Pers. Med.* **2024**, *14*, 345. [CrossRef]

87. Nannan, M.; Xiaoping, L.; Ying, J. Periodontal disease in pregnancy and adverse pregnancy outcomes: Progress in related mechanisms and management strategies. *Front. Med.* **2022**, *9*, 963956. [CrossRef] [PubMed]
88. Arbildo-Vega, H.I.; Padilla-Cáceres, T.; Caballero-Apaza, L.; Cruzado-Oliva, F.H.; Mamani-Cori, V.; Cervantes-Alagón, S.; Vásquez-Rodrigo, H.; Coronel-Zubiate, F.T.; Aguirre-Ipenza, R.; Meza-Málaga, J.M.; et al. Effect of Treating Periodontal Disease in Pregnant Women to Reduce the Risk of Preterm Birth and Low Birth Weight: An Umbrella Review. *Medicina* **2024**, *60*, 943. [CrossRef]
89. Meto, A.; Sula, A.; Peppoloni, S.; Meto, A.; Blasi, E. Leveraging Dental Stem Cells for Oral Health during Pregnancy: A Concise Review. *Dent. J.* **2024**, *12*, 127. [CrossRef]
90. Dong, J.; Li, W.; Wang, Q.; Chen, J.; Zu, Y.; Zhou, X.; Guo, Q. Relationships Between Oral. *Microecosystem and Respiratory Diseases. Front. Mol. Biosci.* **2022**, *8*, 718222. [CrossRef]
91. Imai, K.; Iinuma, T.; Sato, S. Relationship between the oral cavity and respiratory diseases: Aspiration of oral bacteria possibly contributes to the progression of lower airway inflammation. *Jpn. Dent. Sci. Rev.* **2021**, *57*, 224–230. [CrossRef] [PubMed]
92. Lin, P.; Liu, A.; Tsuchiya, Y.; Noritake, K.; Ohsugi, Y.; Toyoshima, K.; Tsukahara, Y.; Shiba, T.; Nitta, H.; Aoki, A.; et al. Association between periodontal disease and chronic obstructive pulmonary disease. *Jpn. Dent. Sci. Rev.* **2023**, *59*, 389–402. [CrossRef]
93. Ashford, J.R. Impaired oral health: A required companion of bacterial aspiration pneumonia. *Front. Rehabil. Sci.* **2024**, *5*, 1337920. [CrossRef] [PubMed]
94. Marusiak, M.J.; Paulden, M.; Ohinmaa, A. Professional oral health care prevents mouth-lung infection in long-term care homes: A systematic review. *Can. J. Dent. Hyg.* **2023**, *57*, 180–190.
95. Satheeshkumar, P.S.; Papatheodorou, S.; Sonis, S. Enhanced oral hygiene interventions as a risk mitigation strategy for the prevention of non-ventilator-associated pneumonia: A systematic review and meta-analysis. *Br. Dent. J.* **2020**, *228*, 615–622. [CrossRef]
96. Kelly, N.; Blackwood, B.; Credland, N.; Stayt, L.; Causey, C.; Winning, L.; McAuley, D.F.; Lundy, F.T.; El Karim, I. Oral health care in adult intensive care units: A national point prevalence study. *Nurs. Crit. Care* **2023**, *28*, 773–780. [CrossRef]
97. Messina, B.M.; Grippaudo, C.; Polizzi, A.; Blasi, A.; Isola, G. The Key Role of *Porphyromonas gingivalis* in the Pathogenesis of Periodontitis Linked with Systemic Diseases. *Appl. Sci.* **2025**, *15*, 6847. [CrossRef]
98. Krutyhołowa, A.; Strzelec, K.; Dziedzic, A.; Bereta, G.P.; Łazarz-Bartyzel, K.; Potempa, J.; Gawron, K. Host and bacterial factors linking periodontitis and rheumatoid arthritis. *Front. Immunol.* **2022**, *13*, 980805. [CrossRef]
99. English, J.; Patrick, S.; Stewart, L.D. The potential role of molecular mimicry by the anaerobic microbiota in the aetiology of autoimmune disease. *Anaerobe* **2023**, *80*, 102721. [CrossRef]
100. Suárez, L.J.; Garzón, H.; Arboleda, S.; Rodríguez, A. Oral Dysbiosis and Autoimmunity: From Local Periodontal Responses to an Imbalanced Systemic Immunity. A Review. *Front. Immunol.* **2020**, *11*, 591255. [CrossRef] [PubMed]
101. Nicholson, J.S.; Landry, K.S. Oral Dysbiosis and Neurodegenerative Diseases: Correlations and Potential Causations. *Microorganisms* **2022**, *10*, 1326. [CrossRef]

102. Plachokova, A.S.; Gjaltema, J.; Hagens, E.R.C.; Hashemi, Z.; Knüppe, T.B.A.; Kootstra, T.J.M.; Visser, A.; Bloem, B.R. Periodontitis: A Plausible Modifiable Risk Factor for Neurodegenerative Diseases? A Comprehensive Review. *Int. J. Mol. Sci.* **2024**, *25*, 4504. [CrossRef]
103. Shahoumi, L.A.; Saleh, M.H.A.; Meghil, M.M. Virulence Factors of the Periodontal Pathogens: Tools to Evade the Host Immune Response and Promote Carcinogenesis. *Microorganisms* **2023**, *11*, 115. [CrossRef] [PubMed]
104. Benjamin, W.J.; Wang, K.; Zarins, K.; Bellile, E.; Blostein, F.; Argirion, I.; Taylor, J.M.G.; D'Silva, N.J.; Chinn, S.B.; Rifkin, S.; et al. Oral Microbiome Community Composition in Head and Neck Squamous Cell Carcinoma. *Cancers* **2023**, *15*, 2549. [CrossRef]
105. Yu, X.; Shi, Y.; Yuan, R.; Chen, Z.; Dong, Q.; Han, L.; Wang, L.; Zhou, J. Microbial dysbiosis in oral squamous cell carcinoma: A systematic review and meta-analysis. *Heliyon* **2023**, *9*, e13198. [CrossRef]
106. Brennan, C.A.; Garrett, W.S. Fusobacterium nucleatum—Symbiont, opportunist and oncobacterium. *Nat. Rev. Microbiol.* **2019**, *17*, 156–166. [CrossRef] [PubMed]
107. Kostic, A.D.; Chun, E.; Robertson, L.; Glickman, J.N.; Gallini, C.A.; Michaud, M.; Clancy, T.E.; Chung, D.C.; Lochhead, P.; Hold, G.L.; et al. Fusobacterium nucleatum potentiates intestinal tumorigenesis and modulates the tumor-immune microenvironment. *Cell Host Microbe* **2013**, *14*, 207–215. [CrossRef]
108. Corana, M.; Baima, G.; Iaderosa, G.; Franco, F.; Zhang, J.; Berta, G.N.; Romano, F.; Aimetti, M. Salivary Proteomics for Detecting Novel Biomarkers of Periodontitis: A Systematic Review. *J. Periodontal Res.* **2025**, *60*, 633–655. [CrossRef]
109. Constantin, V.; Luchian, I.; Goriuc, A.; Budala, D.G.; Bida, F.C.; Cojocaru, C.; Butnaru, O.-M.; Virvescu, D.I. Salivary Biomarkers Identification: Advances in Standard and Emerging Technologies. *Oral* **2025**, *5*, 26. [CrossRef]
110. Sáenz-Ravello, G.; Hernández, M.; Baeza, M.; Hernández-Ríos, P. The Role of Oral Biomarkers in the Assessment of Noncommunicable Diseases. *Diagnostics* **2024**, *15*, 78. [CrossRef]
111. Fonseca, D.C.; da Rocha Fernandes, G.; Waitzberg, D.L. Artificial intelligence and human microbiome: A brief narrative review. *Clin. Nutr. Open Sci.* **2025**, *59*, 134–142. [CrossRef]
112. Asma, S.T.; Imre, K.; Morar, A.; Herman, V.; Acaroz, U.; Mukhtar, H.; Arslan-Acaroz, D.; Shah, S.R.A.; Gerlach, R. An Overview of Biofilm Formation-Combating Strategies and Mechanisms of Action of Antibiofilm Agents. *Life* **2022**, *12*, 1110. [CrossRef]
113. Al-Madboly, L.A.; Aboulmagd, A.; El-Salam, M.A.; Kushkevych, I.; El-Morsi, R.M. Microbial enzymes as powerful natural anti-biofilm candidates. *Microb. Cell Fact.* **2024**, *23*, 343. [CrossRef]
114. Iaconis, A.; De Plano, L.M.; Caccamo, A.; Franco, D.; Conoci, S. Anti-Biofilm Strategies: A Focused Review on Innovative Approaches. *Microorganisms* **2024**, *12*, 639. [CrossRef]
115. Owen, A.M.; Fults, J.B.; Patil, N.K.; Hernandez, A.; Bohannon, J.K. TLR Agonists as Mediators of Trained Immunity: Mechanistic Insight and Immunotherapeutic Potential to Combat Infection. *Front. Immunol.* **2021**, *11*, 622614. [CrossRef] [PubMed]
116. Batoni, G.; Martinez-Pomares, L.; Esin, S. Editorial: Immune Response to Biofilms. *Front Immunol.* **2021**, *12*, 696356. [CrossRef] [PubMed]

117. Grawish, M.E. Human dental pulp stem/stromal cells in clinical practice. *World J. Stem Cells* **2024**, *16*, 54–57. [CrossRef]
118. Liu, F.; Wu, Q.; Liu, Q.; Chen, B.; Liu, X.; Pathak, J.L.; Watanabe, N.; Li, J. Dental pulp stem cells-derived cannabidiol-treated organoid-like microspheroids show robust osteogenic potential via upregulation of WNT6. *Commun. Biol.* **2024**, *7*, 972. [CrossRef]
119. Azeez, S.S.; Hamad, R.S.; Hamad, B.K.; Shekha, M.S.; Bergsten, P. Advances in CRISPR-Cas technology and its applications: Revolutionising precision medicine. *Front. Genome Ed.* **2024**, *6*, 1509924. [CrossRef]
120. Sousa, A.C.; Alvites, R.; Lopes, B.; Sousa, P.; Moreira, A.; Coelho, A.; Santos, J.D.; Atayde, L.; Alves, N.; Maurício, A.C. Three-Dimensional Printing/Bioprinting and Cellular Therapies for Regenerative Medicine: Current Advances. *J. Funct. Biomater.* **2025**, *16*, 28. [CrossRef]
121. Ma, Y.; Deng, B.; He, R.; Huang, P. Advancements of 3D bioprinting in regenerative medicine: Exploring cell sources for organ fabrication. *Heliyon.* **2024**, *10*, e24593. [CrossRef]
122. Rajasekaran, J.J.; Krishnamurthy, H.K.; Bosco, J.; Jayaraman, V.; Krishna, K.; Wang, T.; Bei, K. Oral Microbiome: A Review of Its Impact on Oral and Systemic Health. *Microorganisms* **2024**, *12*, 1797. [CrossRef]
123. Lu, S.; Wang, C.; Ma, J.; Wang, Y. Metabolic mediators: Microbial-derived metabolites as key regulators of anti-tumor immunity, immunotherapy, and chemotherapy. *Front. Immunol.* **2024**, *15*, 1456030. [CrossRef] [PubMed]
124. Lu, J.; Wang, Y.; Wu, J.; Duan, Y.; Zhang, H.; Du, H. Linking microbial communities to rheumatoid arthritis: Focus on gut, oral microbiome and their extracellular vesicles. *Front. Immunol.* **2025**, *16*, 1503474. [CrossRef] [PubMed]
125. Shao, T.; Hsu, R.; Rafizadeh, D.L.; Wang, L.; Bowlus, C.L.; Kumar, N.; Mishra, J.; Timilsina, S.; Ridgway, W.M.; Gershwin, M.E.; et al. The gut ecosystem and immune tolerance. *J. Autoimmun.* **2023**, *141*, 103114. [CrossRef]
126. Cusumano, G.; Flores, G.A.; Venanzoni, R.; Angelini, P. The Impact of Antibiotic Therapy on Intestinal Microbiota: Dysbiosis, Antibiotic Resistance, and Restoration Strategies. *Antibiotics* **2025**, *14*, 371. [CrossRef] [PubMed]

3. Pathogenic Microbial Influence on Pulp–Periodontal Pathologies

3.1. *Role of Oral Microbiome in Pulp–Periodontal Pathologies*

Following the discussion of dental biofilm in the preceding chapters, attention now turns to the oral microbiome and its crucial role in the development of pulp–periodontal pathologies. The human oral cavity hosts a highly diverse microbial community, comprising over 700 to 1000 species of bacteria, fungi, viruses, and protozoa, collectively referred to as the oral microbiome. This ecosystem plays a vital role in maintaining oral health by balancing beneficial (commensal) and harmful (pathogenic) microorganisms. However, this balance is delicate and can be disrupted in a process known as dysbiosis, which has profound implications in the context of pulp–periodontal pathologies [1,2].

Dysbiosis refers to a microbial imbalance that favors the proliferation of pathogenic species at the expense of commensals [3]. This shift results in the emergence of virulent microbial communities capable of evading immune surveillance, establishing resilient biofilms, and sustaining persistent inflammation across pulpal and periodontal tissues (Table 9). Keystone pathogens such as *Porphyromonas gingivalis*, *Treponema denticola*, and *Fusobacterium nucleatum* possess specialized virulence factors, such as proteolytic enzymes, fimbriae, and outer membrane vesicles, that enable them to penetrate host tissues, modulate immune responses, and disrupt epithelial integrity, thereby promoting disease progression [4].

Table 9. Key mechanisms linking dysbiosis to pulp–periodontal pathologies.

Pathogenic Mechanism	Description	Representative Microbes	Clinical Implications
Microbial Virulence Factors	Production of enzymes (e.g., gingipains), adhesins, and toxins by keystone pathogens like *P. gingivalis*, *T. denticola*, enabling tissue invasion and immune evasion [1–3].	*P. gingivalis*, *T. denticola*, *F. nucleatum*	Enhanced tissue destruction, apical periodontitis progression, and increased risk of endodontic–periodontal communication [1,3,4].
Biofilm Formation	Formation of structured microbial communities resistant to antimicrobials and host defenses; uses quorum sensing to coordinate virulence [2–4].	*E. faecalis*, *F. nucleatum*, *C. albicans*	Leads to persistent infections, treatment failure, and reinfection following endodontic therapy [3,4].
Immune Response Modulation	Disruption of normal immune signaling, degradation of complement proteins, and chronic inflammation due to altered cytokine responses [1–3].	*P. gingivalis*, *F. alocis*	Chronic inflammation, periodontal pocket formation, and exacerbation of pulpal–periodontal lesions [1–4].

Source: Table by author.

Biofilm formation is a central pathogenic mechanism in pulp–periodontal diseases. Within these structured microbial communities, pathogens are encased in a self-produced matrix that protects them from antimicrobial agents and host immune defenses. This biofilm mode of growth enhances microbial survival in both root canals and periodontal pockets. Furthermore, quorum-sensing mechanisms within biofilms allow for the coordinated regulation of virulence genes and adaptive responses to environmental stress, sustaining chronic inflammation and tissue destruction associated with apical periodontitis, periapical lesions, and combined endodontic–periodontal infections [5].

The host immune response plays a central but often paradoxical role. Although activated in response to microbial invasion, it frequently becomes dysregulated [6]. *P. gingivalis*, for example, can manipulate complement and Toll-like receptor (TLR) signaling to degrade C3 and C5 complement proteins, disrupt cytokine cascades, and impair neutrophil recruitment [7]. These immune-modulatory tactics promote chronic inflammation and impair lesion resolution [8]. Persistent infections also drive the release of inflammatory mediators, including cytokines such as IL-1β and TNF-α, which stimulate osteoclast activity and increase vascular permeability, thereby accelerating bone resorption and pulpal breakdown. Elevated prostaglandin E_2 (PGE_2) levels exacerbate pain and osteoclastogenesis via RANKL signaling, while matrix metalloproteinases (MMP-2, MMP-8, MMP-9) degrade collagen, dentin, and extracellular matrix components, further undermining periodontal support and pulpal structure (Table 10). Such mediators are particularly elevated in lesions of apical periodontitis and chronic periodontitis. In chronic pulp–periodontal infections, immune tolerance may emerge as a compensatory host mechanism to limit tissue damage [9]. Regulatory T cells (Tregs) secrete IL-10 and TGF-β, dampening pro-inflammatory responses but inadvertently facilitating pathogen persistence. At the same time, pathogens like *Filifactor alocis* exploit these regulatory environments and deploy additional immune-evasive strategies, such as upregulating antioxidant pathways or resisting neutrophil-mediated killing, further complicating eradication [5].

Table 10. Host immune mediators in pulp–periodontal pathology.

Mediator	Source	Function	Clinical Implication
IL-1β	Macrophages, dendritic cells	Potent proinflammatory cytokine that activates osteoclast differentiation and amplifies inflammatory signaling in infected tissues [5,6,9].	Promotes alveolar bone resorption and pulpal necrosis during chronic infection [5,9].
TNF-α	Neutrophils, macrophages	Induces cytokine cascades, increases vascular permeability, and sustains leukocyte recruitment at infection sites [6,7,9].	Contributes to chronic lesion formation, periapical inflammation, and tissue destruction [7,9].

Table 10. *Cont.*

Mediator	Source	Function	Clinical Implication
PGE_2	Fibroblasts, macrophages	Mediator of vasodilation, nociception, and osteoclast activation; enhances inflammatory pain responses [5,6,9].	Associated with symptomatic inflammation, tissue degradation, and bone loss in endodontic-periodontal lesions [6,9].
MMP-8, MMP-9	Neutrophils	Proteolytic enzymes that degrade type I collagen and extracellular matrix components, facilitating lesion expansion [5,7,8].	Lead to periapical and periodontal connective tissue breakdown and impaired healing [7,8].
IL-10, TGF-β	Tregs, dendritic cells	Anti-inflammatory cytokines that suppress excessive immune activation and promote immune tolerance [6,8,9].	Enable chronic infection persistence by limiting bacterial clearance and favoring immune evasion [8,9].

Source: Table by author.

Recognizing the multifactorial nature of pulp–periodontal pathologies, the European Society of Endodontology has emphasized the importance of integrated diagnostic and therapeutic approaches. Their guidelines emphasize the importance of comprehensively understanding microbial etiology, host–pathogen interactions, and anatomical communication between pulp and periodontal tissues to develop effective, evidence-based treatment strategies [10]. Elevated levels of IL-1β and MMP-8, for instance, are being evaluated as biomarkers in point-of-care diagnostic tools to assess periodontal disease activity, while adjunctive therapies such as Non-Steroidal Anti-Inflammatory Drugs (NSAIDs), MMP inhibitors, and biologics targeting pro-inflammatory cytokines (e.g., IL-1 receptor antagonists) show promise alongside conventional antimicrobial regimens.

Recent advances in next-generation sequencing (NGS) technologies have revolutionized our understanding of microbial shifts in pulp–periodontal pathologies. Using 16S rRNA gene sequencing, studies have revealed that diseased sites harbor distinct microbial signatures compared to healthy controls. There is notable enrichment of anaerobic Gram-negative bacteria such as Prevotella, Fusobacterium, and Dialister, alongside opportunistic fungi like Candida albicans, particularly in chronic or refractory cases [11,12]. These findings confirm the polymicrobial nature of endo-periodontal lesions and the frequent overlap between endodontic and periodontal microbial reservoirs.

Further NGS-based analyses by Arias-Moliz et al. (2024) have identified specific keystone taxa in post-treatment endodontic infections, such as *E. faecalis* and *F. alocis* [5]. These organisms exhibit notable resilience to intracanal medicaments and are strongly associated with persistent infections due to their robust biofilm-forming capacity and antibiotic resistance. Their identification reinforces the role of dysbiosis as a critical driver of treatment failure and underscores the need for microbiome-informed therapeutic strategies.

3.2. Anatomy and Pathophysiology of Dental Pulp and Periodontal Tissues

The dental pulp is a specialized connective tissue located at the core of the tooth, residing within the pulp chamber and extending into the root canals. This tissue is essential to the tooth's vitality as it contains an abundant supply of blood vessels, sensory and autonomic nerves, and various cellular components, including odontoblasts, fibroblasts, and immune cells. Odontoblasts, which line the periphery of the pulp chamber, are responsible for producing dentin, the calcified tissue that constitutes the bulk of the tooth structure (Figure 8a). This process, known as dentinogenesis, continues throughout life and enables the tooth to respond to physiological wear, decay, and injury by forming reparative dentin. Beyond its formative role, the dental pulp fulfills a vital sensory function: it responds to external stimuli such as temperature changes, chemical insults, and mechanical forces by transmitting pain signals to the central nervous system. This nociceptive response is a crucial defense mechanism, alerting the host to potential threats to the tooth's structural integrity [13,14].

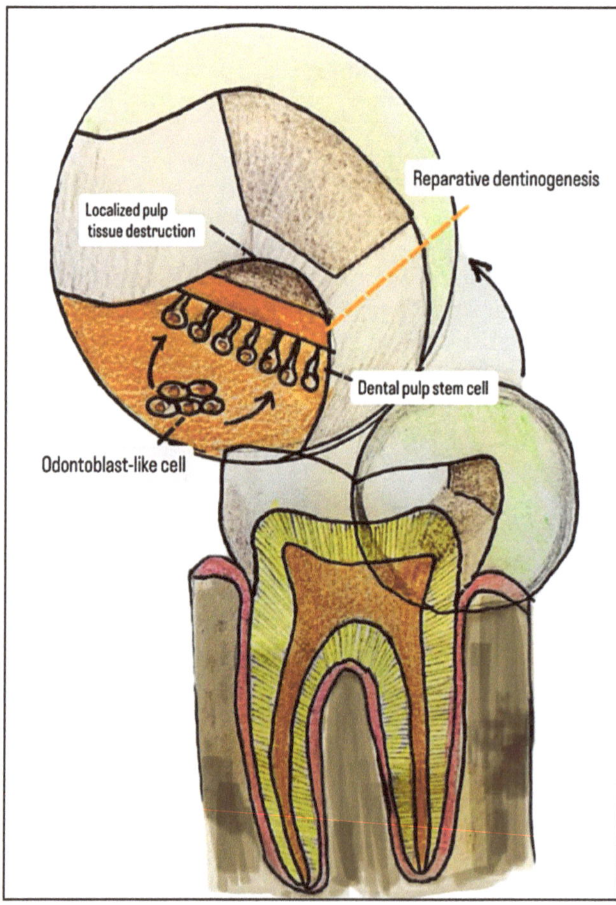

(a)

Figure 8. *Cont.*

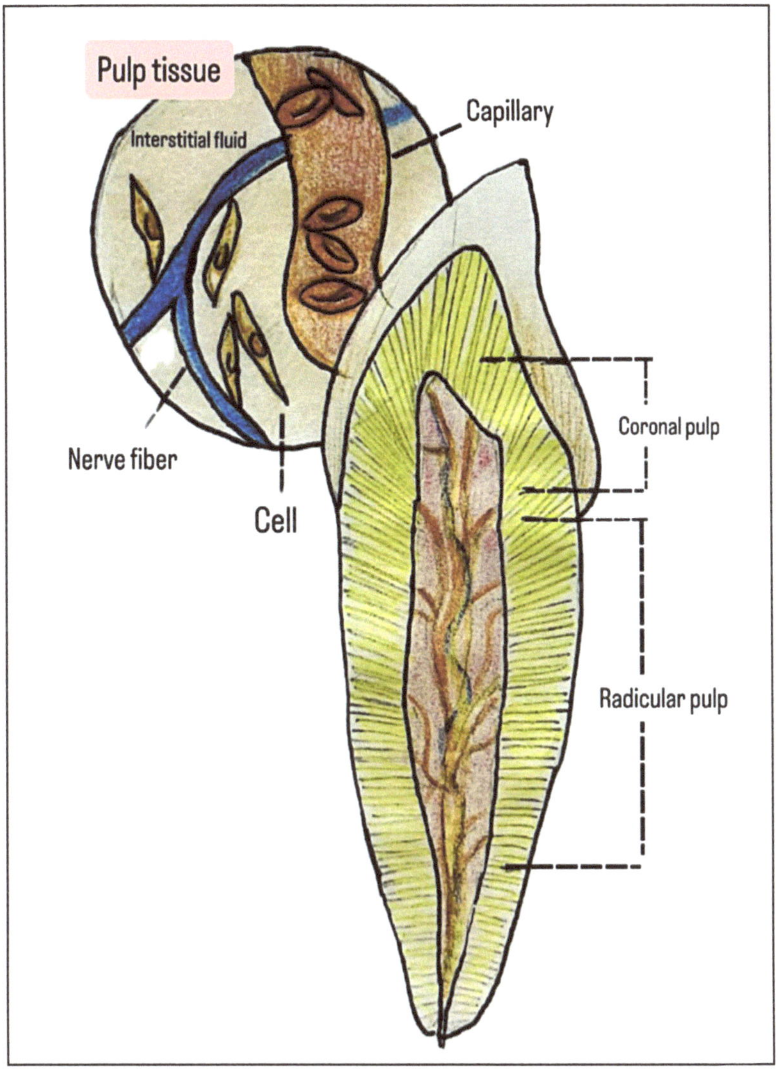

(**b**)

Figure 8. *Cont.*

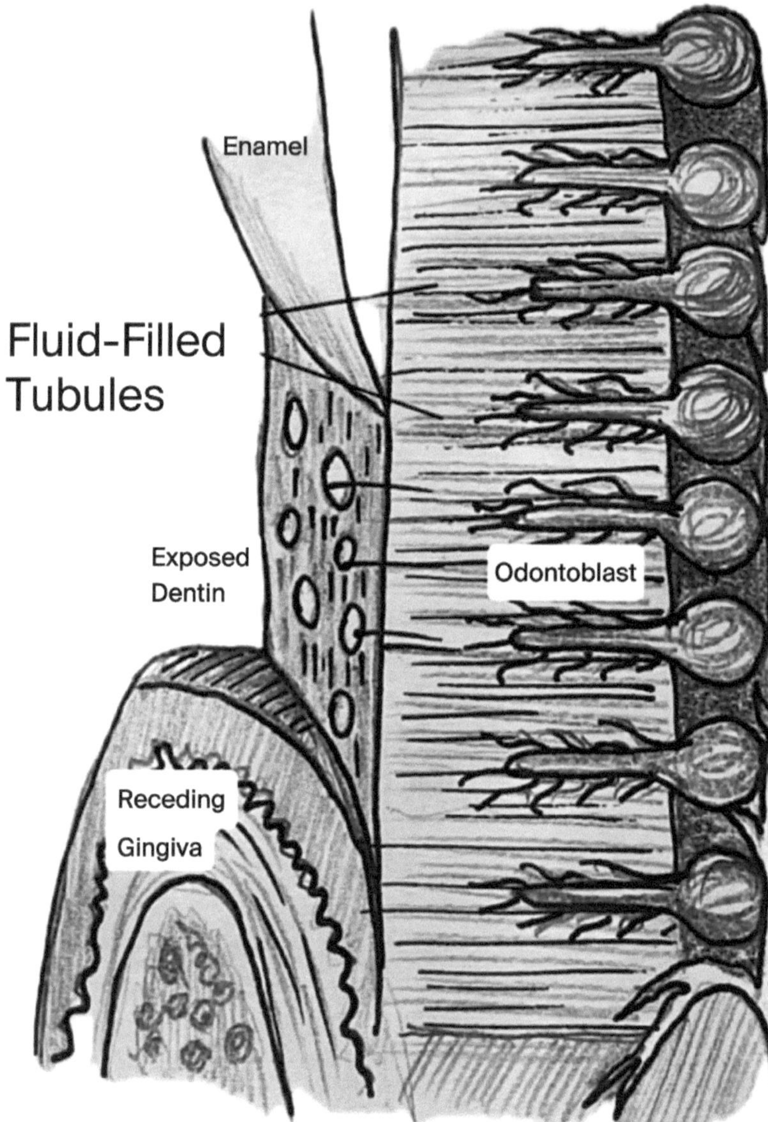

(c)

Figure 8. (**a**) Schematic illustration of reparative dentinogenesis following localized pulp tissue destruction. Injury to the pulp stimulates the recruitment of dental pulp stem cells to the damaged site, where they differentiate into odontoblast-like cells. These newly formed cells contribute to the deposition of reparative dentin, creating a protective barrier that helps restore the structural and functional integrity of the pulp–dentin complex. (**b**) Anatomical organization of dental pulp and its microstructure. The diagram shows the coronal and radicular pulp within the tooth, highlighting their continuity. The magnified view illustrates the pulp tissue, including capillaries, interstitial fluid, nerve fibers, and resident cells, emphasizing the highly vascularized and innervated nature of the pulp that supports tooth vitality and sensory function. (**c**) Schematic representation of dentin hypersensitivity associated with gingival recession. The illustration shows exposed dentin at the cervical region following gingival recession, revealing open fluid-filled dentinal tubules that communicate directly with the odontoblast processes in the pulp. Fluid movement within these tubules can trigger sensory nerve responses, explaining the pain experienced in exposed dentin areas. Credit: © Nensi Kallfani, used with permission.

Anatomically, the pulp is divided into two major regions: the coronal pulp, which occupies the crown of the tooth and extends into the pulp horns toward the cusps, and the radicular pulp, which descends into the root canals and tapers near the apex (Figure 8b). The pulp communicates with the surrounding periodontal tissues primarily through the apical foramen, a small opening at the root tip that allows the passage of neurovascular bundles. Additionally, the root canal system frequently contains accessory and lateral canals, particularly in the apical third or furcation areas, which may complicate both diagnosis and treatment if left unidentified. The intricate arrangement of these anatomical pathways underscores the central importance of thorough knowledge of pulp morphology for successful endodontic therapy [15,16].

The root canal system is encased by dentin and surrounded externally by cementum, a mineralized tissue that anchors the tooth to the periodontal ligament (PDL). The PDL is a specialized fibrous connective tissue that suspends the tooth within the alveolar socket, serving both as a shock absorber during mastication and as a source of proprioceptive feedback. The apical foramen itself is a critical site in endodontics because it often represents the focal point of periapical pathology. Proper understanding of the anatomical continuity among dentin, cementum, the PDL, and alveolar bone is vital, as these components work as a dynamic unit to maintain tooth stability and function [13].

A clinical illustration of this complexity is provided in Figure 9, showing tooth #4.5 before and after endodontic treatment. The pre-treatment radiograph reveals a periapical abscess, while the post-treatment image demonstrates a clearly visualized network of micro-canals within the root canal system, emphasizing the significance of addressing even the finer microstructures for optimal disinfection and sealing. This case exemplifies how comprehensive endodontic treatment that extends beyond the main canal into micro-canals can profoundly affect both the immediate therapeutic outcome and the long-term success of the procedure.

The structure of the dental root varies considerably depending on the type and position of the tooth. Maxillary molars, for example, often exhibit more complex root canal anatomies, such as a second mesiobuccal canal, whose presence is a common source of treatment failure when overlooked. The external root surface is lined with cementum, which integrates with PDL fibers to secure the tooth to the alveolar bone. This periodontal attachment apparatus is highly dynamic, adapting to functional stresses like occlusal loading while allowing a degree of physiologic tooth mobility. Such adaptive remodeling highlights the intricate interplay between anatomical form and biomechanical function in the pulp–periodontal complex [13,17].

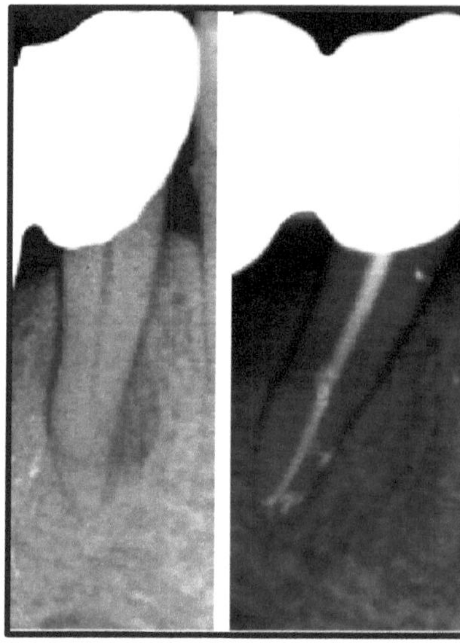

Figure 9. A clinical case, the tooth #4.5 before treatment (**left**) and after treatment (**right**), where the micro-canals within the root canal are shown. Credit: © Alessandra Odorici, used with permission.

A key microscopic feature of dentin is the presence of dentinal tubules, minute channels that extend radially from the pulp chamber to the dentino-enamel or dentino-cemental junction. These tubules enable the exchange of fluids and nutrients between the pulp and dentin, but also present a potential conduit for bacterial invasion when the protective layers of enamel or cementum are breached (Figure 8c).

Once pathogens penetrate these tubules, they may provoke pulpal inflammation (pulpitis), and if unchecked, the infection can progress through the apical foramen or accessory canals, eventually inducing periapical lesions characterized by bone resorption and chronic inflammatory changes at the root apex [15,16].

Pathophysiologic alterations of the dental pulp arise from diverse etiologies, including carious lesions, traumatic injury, and iatrogenic factors such as deep restorative procedures. These insults can lead to pulpitis, an inflammatory reaction that may progress from a reversible state to irreversible pulpitis or ultimately pulp necrosis if untreated. Pulpal necrosis frequently results in periapical abscess formation and may facilitate the dissemination of infection into adjacent periodontal tissues. Similarly, periodontal disease, such as periodontitis, involves chronic inflammation and destruction of the PDL, cementum, and alveolar bone, which can culminate in tooth mobility and loss. In advanced stages, periodontal pathogens can breach cementum and infiltrate the PDL space, occasionally gaining access to the pulp via apical or lateral canals, thereby creating endo-periodontal lesions that are notoriously complex to diagnose and manage [18,19].

The anatomical features and microbial pathogenesis of pulp and periodontal tissues are deeply interconnected. The apical foramen serves as the principal anatomical communication between these tissues, acting as a bidirectional pathway for the spread of bacteria, inflammatory mediators, and necrotic debris. Such communication allows primary endodontic or primary periodontal lesions to evolve into true combined endo-periodontal lesions when infections are left unresolved [20, 21]. Besides the apical foramen, accessory and lateral canals, especially in the apical third and furcation regions, offer additional routes for microbial invasion, promoting early translocation of bacteria even in the absence of overt clinical signs, particularly in the presence of deep periodontal pockets or pulpal necrosis [22,23].

Dentinal tubules further contribute to this microbial pathway. These microscopic channels, exposed through caries, abrasion, erosion, or periodontal attachment loss, allow bacteria to penetrate deeper into dentin and pulp tissues. Research has demonstrated that oral pathogens can colonize dentinal tubules, persist in viable form, and withstand conventional disinfection protocols, thereby contributing to persistent or recurrent infections [24,25]. The combined complexity of these anatomical pathways and the microbial challenges they present underscores the importance of a precise diagnostic approach. Successful therapy depends on recognizing how these structures influence microbial spread and the efficacy of mechanical and chemical debridement, as well as the effectiveness of sealing during endodontic and periodontal treatment.

Accessory Canals: Anatomical Pathways with Clinical Consequences

Accessory canals are critical anatomical structures that significantly influence the complexity, diagnosis, and prognosis of endo-periodontal lesions (Figure 10).

These narrow lateral branches of the root canal system are most commonly located in the apical third, furcation zones, or along lateral root surfaces, establishing direct communication pathways between the dental pulp and the periodontal ligament. Their prevalence has been reported in up to 30% of molars, particularly in the furcation region, which underscores their potential role in the propagation of disease and in treatment failure [22,23].

These canals permit bidirectional microbial migration, allowing bacteria, toxins, and inflammatory mediators to move between the pulp and periodontal tissues. When infection originates in the pulp, microorganisms can disseminate through accessory canals into the periodontium, often mimicking the clinical and radiographic features of primary periodontal disease. Conversely, in cases of advanced periodontitis, bacterial invasion into the pulp via the same canals may result in pulpal necrosis even in the absence of direct carious exposure or trauma. This dynamic interplay highlights the role of accessory canals in the pathogenesis of combined endodontic–periodontal lesions [20,26,27].

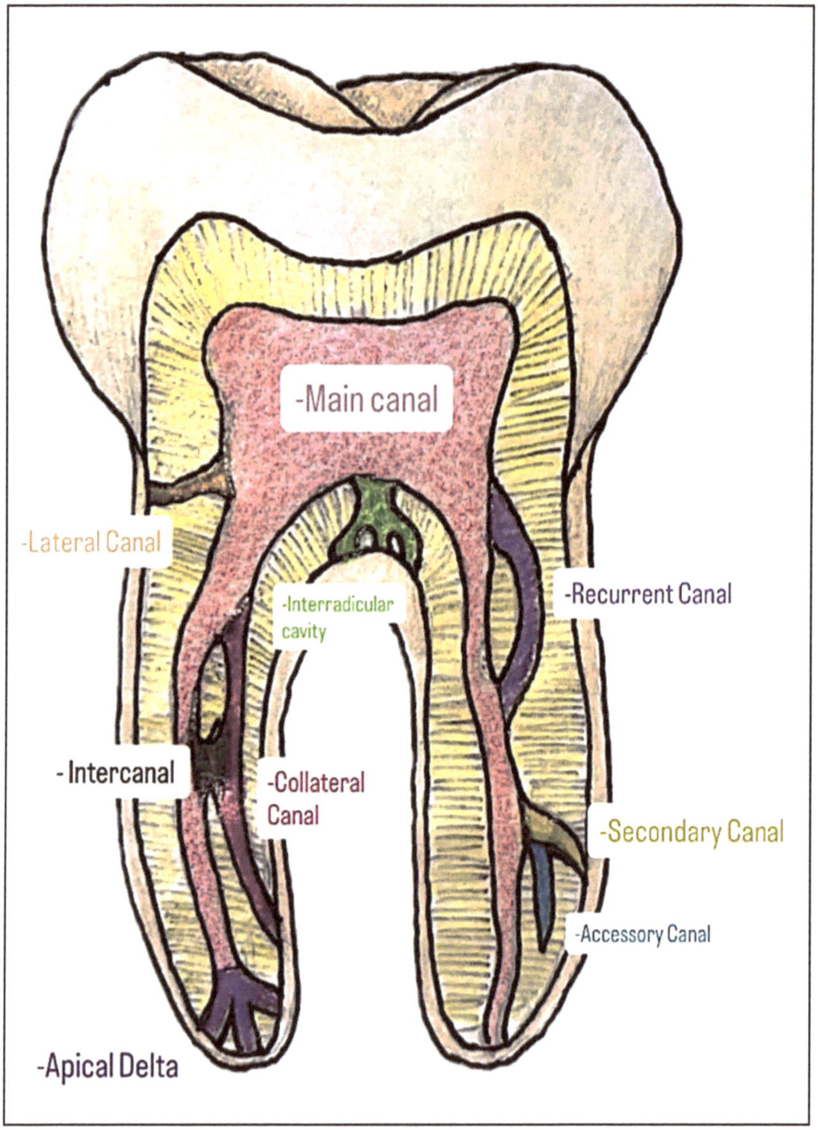

Figure 10. Anatomical complexity of the root canal system. The diagram illustrates the main canal and its intricate network of collateral pathways, including lateral canals, secondary and accessory canals, recurrent canals, intercannals, and apical deltas, as well as the interradicular cavity. These anatomical variations highlight the challenges in achieving complete debridement and disinfection during endodontic treatment. Credit: © Nensi Kallfani, used with permission.

The detection of accessory canals presents considerable diagnostic challenges. Their minute size, variable morphology, and frequent occurrence in anatomically complex regions, such as the furcation area, make them difficult to visualize on conventional periapical radiographs. As a result, lesions associated with these canals may be overlooked, leading to incomplete or ineffective treatment. In recent years, cone-beam computed tomography (CBCT) has emerged as an essential tool in endodontic diagnostics. CBCT imaging provides three-dimensional visualization of the canal anatomy, enabling the identification of accessory canals that might otherwise remain undetected and allowing clinicians to adjust their treatment strategies to address these complexities [28,29].

From a therapeutic view, lesions involving accessory canals necessitate a comprehensive endodontic–periodontal treatment approach. Root canal therapy must be meticulously performed, employing enhanced disinfection techniques, intracanal medicaments, and in some cases, surgical debridement or regenerative periodontal procedures. Adjunctive treatments such as scaling and root planing may also be required to address associated periodontal destruction. Studies have demonstrated that the combination of appropriate endodontic therapy and periodontal intervention improves clinical attachment levels and reduces lesion recurrence in cases involving accessory canal communication [30,31].

3.3. Evolution of Classification Systems for Pulp–Periodontal Pathologies

The classification of pulp–periodontal lesions has evolved from simplistic models to more sophisticated frameworks that consider the multifaceted nature of these pathologies [32,33]. Initially, classifications were based on clinical observations and the apparent origin of the disease:

- Early 20th Century: The earliest attempts at classification were rudimentary, focusing primarily on the obvious clinical presentation. Clinicians differentiated between pulpitis and periodontitis without recognizing the intricate interconnections between the pulp and periodontal tissues.
- Mid-20th Century: As dental pathology advanced, particularly with the advent of radiographic imaging, the concept of "endo-perio" lesions began to take shape. The understanding that an infection in the pulp could lead to periodontal destruction (and vice versa) led to a more nuanced classification system, which began to acknowledge primary and secondary disease processes.
- Late 20th Century: The traditional classification, which is still widely taught, emerged. This model introduced the categorization of lesions based on their primary origin, whether the disease started in the pulp or the periodontal tissues, and acknowledged the existence of combined lesions where both systems are involved. This period also saw the introduction of terms like "retrograde periodontitis" and "primary endodontic lesions with secondary periodontal involvement".
- 21st Century: With advances in molecular biology, imaging technologies such as CBCT, and a deeper understanding of the root canal system's anatomy (including lateral canals and accessory canals), more refined classification systems have been developed. These include etiology-based classifications and those considering specific root defects like cemental tears.

Modern Classification of Pulp–Periodontal Pathologies

1. Traditional Classification

The traditional classification system categorizes pulp–periodontal pathologies based on the origin of the disease, which is crucial for determining the treatment approach [34,35]:

- Primary endodontic lesions: These lesions originate in the dental pulp, typically due to deep caries, trauma, or a cracked tooth. The infection spreads to the periodontal tissues through anatomical pathways such as the apical foramen, lateral canals, or accessory canals. Clinically, these lesions are often identified by symptoms like pain, swelling, and a history of pulpitis, with radiographs showing periapical radiolucencies.
- Primary periodontal lesions: These begin in the periodontal tissues, often due to plaque-induced periodontitis. Over time, the infection may extend to the pulp, particularly if the periodontal pocket deepens to reach the root apex, potentially causing pulp necrosis. These lesions typically present with generalized periodontal symptoms like deep pockets, gingival recession, and bone loss.
- Combined lesions: In cases where both the pulp and periodontal tissues are independently diseased, they can converge, creating complex lesions that involve both systems. These cases are challenging because they require integrated treatment plans addressing both the endodontic and periodontal aspects simultaneously.

2. Al-Fouzan's Classification

Recognizing the limitations of the traditional classification, Al-Fouzan proposed a more refined system that incorporates the presence or absence of root damage, such as fractures or cemental tears [36]:

- Endodontic–periodontal lesions with root damage: This classification considers lesions that occur due to structural defects in the root, such as fractures, resorption, or cemental tears. These defects can cause localized periodontal destruction, with or without pulp involvement, making diagnosis and treatment more complex. For instance, a cemental tear may allow bacteria to penetrate the periodontal ligament and, in some cases, reach the pulp, necessitating both periodontal and endodontic interventions.
- Endodontic–periodontal lesions without root damage: These lesions occur when infection spreads from the pulp to the periodontium or vice versa without any structural damage to the root. The primary focus is often on removing the infectious source through endodontic therapy, with periodontal management being a secondary consideration.

3. Etiology-Based Classification

An etiology-based classification of pulp–periodontal pathologies underscores the clinical importance of determining the primary source of infection before initiating treatment. It is important to identify whether the lesion originates in the pulp or in the periodontal apparatus to establish an accurate diagnosis, select the correct sequence of therapy, and predict prognosis [37].

- Lesions of endodontic origin: Typically arise from pulpal necrosis caused by caries, trauma, or restorative insults. Once the pulp becomes necrotic, bacteria and their byproducts can migrate through the apical foramen, lateral canals, or accessory canals, eventually involving the surrounding periodontal tissues. Clinically, these lesions often present with acute or chronic periapical inflammation that may mimic or exacerbate periodontal disease. The cornerstone of management is thorough endodontic therapy, principally root canal treatment aimed at eliminating the intraradicular infection, after which adjunctive periodontal procedures, if needed, address any residual periodontal breakdown. These lesions begin with pulp necrosis, where bacteria spread through the apical foramen, lateral canals, or accessory canals into the periodontal tissues. Treatment focuses primarily on endodontic therapy, such as root canal treatment, to eliminate the source of infection, followed by any necessary periodontal care.

- Lesions of periodontal origin: By contrast, these lesions begin within the periodontium, most commonly due to chronic periodontitis. Progressive attachment loss and formation of deep periodontal pockets allow bacteria and their toxins to reach the root surface and gain access to the pulpal tissues through apical or lateral canals. In advanced cases, this secondary pulpal involvement can lead to partial or total pulp necrosis. For such lesions, the primary line of treatment is periodontal therapy, including meticulous scaling and root-planing, control of the periodontal biofilm, and, where indicated, surgical periodontal intervention. Endodontic treatment is performed only if pulpal compromise is confirmed. These start in the periodontium, often due to chronic periodontitis. The infection can migrate to the pulp through deep periodontal pockets or accessory canals, potentially leading to pulp necrosis. Periodontal therapy, including scaling, root planing, and possibly surgical intervention, is the primary treatment, with endodontic therapy as a secondary measure if the pulp is compromised.

4. Cemental Tear Classification

Cemental tears, a specific type of root defect, can lead to endodontic–periodontal lesions. Lee and colleagues proposed a classification system that focuses on these defects [38]:

- Cemental tear with pulp involvement: When a cemental tear occurs, it can create a pathway for bacteria to infect both the periodontal ligament and the dental pulp, leading to complex lesions. Treatment typically involves periodontal surgery to address the tear and root canal therapy if the pulp is affected.
- Cemental tear without pulp involvement: In cases where the tear affects only the periodontal tissues, treatment focuses on managing the localized periodontal damage, such as through surgical repair of the tear and thorough debridement of the affected area.

To offer a clearer grasp of the various classification systems for pulp–periodontal pathologies, the following table (Table 11) outlines the key characteristics, clinical implications, and treatment considerations for each classification type.

Each system, whether traditional, etiology-based, or focused on specific root defects like cemental tears, provides a framework for addressing the multifaceted nature of pulp–periodontal pathologies and improving patient outcomes.

Table 11. Pulp–periodontal pathology classifications.

Classification Types	Subcategories	Characteristics	Clinical Implications	Treatment Considerations
Traditional Classification [32–35]	**Primary Endodontic Lesions**	Originates within the dental pulp and secondarily affects the periodontium through accessory canals or apical foramina [32,34].	Deep carious lesions, trauma, sinus tract formation, and periapical radiolucency [33,35].	Root canal therapy is the primary approach; monitor for secondary periodontal effects [34,35].
	Primary Periodontal Lesions	Originates in periodontal tissues with possible secondary pulpal involvement due to apical spread of infection [32,33].	Generalized periodontal destruction, deep periodontal pockets, possible mobility [33,34].	Primary focus on periodontal therapy; endodontic treatment may be required if pulpal necrosis occurs [34,35].
	Combined Lesions	Independent endodontic and periodontal disease processes that converge and interact [32,34].	Complex presentations with extensive bone loss and dual tissue involvement [34,35].	Multidisciplinary management combining endodontic and periodontal therapy for optimal healing [34,35].
Al-Fouzan's Classification [36]	**Endodontic–Periodontal Lesions with Root Damage**	Involves root fractures, internal/external resorption, or cemental tears compromising root integrity [36,37].	Isolated periodontal pockets, possible pulp necrosis, or periapical radiolucency [37].	Repair root defects, perform endodontic therapy, and coordinate with periodontal management [36,37].
	Endodontic–Periodontal Lesions Without Root Damage	Infection spreads via natural anatomical pathways (dentinal tubules, lateral canals) without structural root damage [36].	Localized radiolucency, pocket formation, or communication between pulp and periodontium [37].	Prioritize endodontic treatment; follow with periodontal maintenance as needed [36,37].
Etiology-Based Classification	**Lesions of Endodontic Origin**	Infection originates from necrotic pulp and spreads to the periodontium through the apical foramen or lateral canals [36,37].	Presence of periapical radiolucency, sinus tracts, tenderness on percussion [36,37].	Root canal therapy as first-line treatment; adjunct periodontal care may follow [36,37].

Table 11. *Cont.*

Classification Types	Subcategories	Characteristics	Clinical Implications	Treatment Considerations
	Lesions of Periodontal Origin	Infection begins in the periodontium and advances toward the pulp apex, potentially causing pulpal necrosis [36,37].	Periodontal pockets reaching the apex, generalized bone loss, tooth mobility [36,37].	Periodontal therapy to arrest disease progression; endodontic therapy if pulp involvement occurs [36,37].
Cemental Tear Classification [38]	**Cemental Tear with Pulp Involvement**	Separation of cementum leading to both periodontal and pulpal involvement; may occur following trauma or aging [38].	Localized deep pockets, inflammation, possible pulpitis or necrosis [38].	Combined approach: surgical removal or repair of cemental fragment and root canal therapy [38].
	Cemental Tear without Pulp Involvement	Tear affects only periodontal structures, with intact pulp vitality [38].	Localized periodontal breakdown, mobility without pulpal symptoms [38].	Periodontal treatment focused on debridement and stabilization of the affected site [38].

Source: Table by author.

3.4. Pathogens in Pulp–Periodontal Lesions

Pulp–periodontal lesions often involve a variety of pathogenic microorganisms that play a critical role in the initiation and progression of these conditions. These pathogens can originate from either the pulp or the periodontal tissues and can contribute to the disease process through direct tissue invasion, biofilm formation, and immune modulation. While *Porphyromonas gingivalis* and *Treponema denticola* have long been recognized as central players in pulp–periodontal pathogenesis, emerging evidence underscores the critical role of other pathogens in these complex infections. Among these, *Enterococcus faecalis*, *Fusobacterium nucleatum*, and *Prevotella intermedia* exhibit distinct virulence strategies that contribute significantly to disease progression, particularly in persistent or refractory lesions. Main pathogens implicated in pulp–periodontal lesions include the following:

E. faecalis is frequently isolated from post-treatment root canal infections and is notorious for its ability to withstand harsh conditions, including high pH environments and antimicrobial agents. This Gram-positive facultative anaerobe forms robust biofilms within the root canal system, contributing to reinfection and treatment failure. Its virulence arsenal includes aggregation substances, cytolysin, and extracellular superoxide production, enabling it to disrupt host tissues and evade immune clearance. Moreover, its ability to penetrate dentinal tubules and resist intracanal medicaments makes it a formidable pathogen in endodontic–periodontal lesions [39].

F. nucleatum plays a pivotal role in the pathogenesis of periodontal diseases and is a key bridging organism in the formation of complex biofilms in the oral cavity. This spindle-shaped, Gram-negative anaerobe plays a bridging role in oral biofilm maturation. *F. nucleatum* acts as a structural keystone by co-aggregating with both early and late colonizers, facilitating polymicrobial synergy. It expresses adhesins (e.g., FadA), which bind to epithelial cells and allow tissue invasion. Additionally, *F. nucleatum* triggers pro-inflammatory cytokines such as IL-6 and IL-8, contributing to local immune dysregulation and bone resorption. This bacterium is capable of integrating with other pathogenic species, such as *P. gingivalis* and *T. denticola*, enhancing their pathogenic potential within the biofilm. In pulp–periodontal lesions, *F. nucleatum* can facilitate the spread of infection from periodontal tissues into the pulp, or vice versa, contributing to the complexity and severity of the lesion [40].

A key member of the orange complex, *P. intermedia* is a Gram-negative anaerobe implicated in both periodontal pockets and infected root canals. It produces proteolytic enzymes and hemolysins that degrade host proteins and facilitate iron acquisition. This species also contributes to epithelial barrier disruption and exhibits synergistic interactions with *P. gingivalis*, enhancing biofilm virulence. Notably, *P. intermedia* has been linked to acute inflammatory exacerbations and suppurative lesions in endodontic–periodontal cases [41].

P. gingivalis is a keystone pathogen in the development of chronic periodontitis and plays a significant role in pulp–periodontal lesions when periodontal infection extends to the dental pulp. This anaerobic bacterium is highly adept at evading the host immune system and can induce a chronic inflammatory response that leads to the destruction of periodontal and pulpal tissues. Its presence in pulp–periodontal lesions is often associated with severe inflammation and rapid disease progression [42].

Candida species, particularly *C. albicans*, are increasingly recognized as contributors to complex endodontic and periodontal infections. These fungi can form biofilms in the root canal system, often in conjunction with bacterial pathogens like *E. faecalis*. The biofilms created by these dual-species communities are highly resistant to conventional antimicrobial treatments, making them particularly challenging to manage in pulp–periodontal lesions. The presence of *Candida* can exacerbate the infection and increase the likelihood of treatment failure [39].

T. denticola is a spirochete commonly found in advanced periodontal disease. Its motility and invasiveness enable it to penetrate deep into periodontal tissues and even into the root canal system. In pulp–periodontal lesions, *T. denticola* often works synergistically with other pathogens like *P. gingivalis* to enhance tissue destruction and evade immune responses. This bacterium is associated with the progression of both endodontic and periodontal infections, contributing to the complexity of treatment [40].

The pathogens involved in pulp–periodontal lesions employ various mechanisms to establish infection and contribute to disease progression:

Biofilm formation: Many of the pathogens involved in pulp–periodontal lesions, such as *E. faecalis*, *F. nucleatum*, and *P. gingivalis*, are proficient at forming biofilms. These biofilms serve as protective environments where pathogens can survive antimicrobial treatments and resist host immune responses. The biofilm matrix also facilitates close interactions between different microbial species, leading to the enhanced virulence and persistence of infection [43,44].

Quorum sensing: Pathogens within biofilms communicate through quorum sensing, a process that allows them to coordinate their behavior, including the regulation of virulence factors and resistance mechanisms. This communication enhances the ability of the microbial community to adapt to the hostile environment of the root canal and periodontal pocket, making treatment more challenging [43].

Immune evasion and modulation: Pathogens like *P. gingivalis* are adept at modulating the host immune response, promoting a chronic inflammatory state that leads to tissue destruction. This immune modulation not only allows the pathogens to persist but also exacerbates the damage to both the pulp and periodontal tissues, contributing to the progression of the lesion [42].

The complex interplay of these pathogens in pulp–periodontal lesions necessitates a multifaceted treatment approach. Traditional antimicrobial therapies may be insufficient due to the protective nature of biofilms and the resistance mechanisms employed by these pathogens. Therefore, effective treatment often requires a combination of mechanical debridement, the use of advanced antimicrobial agents, and sometimes surgical intervention to remove infected tissues. Gaining insight into the particular pathogens involved and their pathogenic mechanisms is crucial for tailoring treatment strategies that effectively address the root causes of pulp–periodontal lesions [39,45].

3.5. Clinical Manifestations of Pulp–Periodontal Pathologies

Pulp–periodontal pathologies encompass a wide range of dental conditions that demand precise diagnosis and careful management.

(a) Pulpal Pathologies

Pulpal diseases are primarily characterized by inflammation of the dental pulp, which can progress to necrosis if untreated. The clinical manifestations of pulpal pathologies are often acute and associated with significant pain, commonly referred to as odontogenic pain, such as the following:

Acute pulpitis: One of the most common conditions affecting the dental pulp is acute pulpitis, which is marked by intense, sharp pain frequently triggered by exposure to thermal stimuli like hot or cold foods and drinks. The pain is usually localized but can radiate to adjacent teeth or the jaw. Histologically, acute pulpitis is marked by a significant influx of inflammatory cells, including neutrophils and lymphocytes, into the pulp tissue, leading to tissue destruction and increased pressure within the pulp chamber, which exacerbates the pain [46].

Pulpal necrosis: When pulpitis progresses untreated, the pulp tissue may become necrotic, leading to the tooth becoming non-vital. Pulpal necrosis is often asymptomatic until the infection extends to the periapical tissues, resulting in conditions like apical periodontitis [10]. At this stage, the tooth typically does not respond to thermal stimuli but may be sensitive to pressure or biting [47].

Chronic apical Periodontitis: This condition is typically asymptomatic or causes only mild discomfort. It is characterized by the presence of a periapical radiolucency, indicating bone loss around the root apex, and may be associated with a sinus tract. The affected tooth usually shows signs of non-vitality, which is confirmed through clinical tests [48]. If left untreated, apical periodontitis can progress to more severe conditions such as periapical abscesses or cysts.

Acute apical abscess: This severe condition is characterized by spontaneous, intense pain, significant swelling, and tenderness to percussion and palpation; pus discharge, systemic symptoms such as fever, and lymphadenopathy are common.

The affected tooth is typically non-vital, and the abscess may spread to surrounding tissues, necessitating prompt treatment [48].

Periapical cyst: Often asymptomatic, periapical cysts are characterized by a well-defined radiolucent area at the apex of a non-vital tooth. While smaller cysts may go unnoticed, larger ones can cause swelling or displacement of adjacent teeth, making them more apparent during clinical examinations or radiographic evaluations [10].

(b) Periodontal Pathologies

Periodontal diseases are primarily inflammatory conditions that affect the supporting structures of the teeth, including the gingiva, periodontal ligament, cementum, and alveolar bone, such as the following:

Gingivitis: The earliest form of periodontal disease, gingivitis, is characterized by inflamed, swollen, and bleeding gums, particularly during brushing or flossing. This condition is reversible with proper oral hygiene, but if left untreated, it can progress to more severe forms of periodontal disease [49]. However, if left untreated, gingivitis can progress to periodontitis.

Chronic periodontitis: As gingivitis advances to chronic periodontitis, the inflammation extends deeper into the periodontal tissues, leading to the destruction of the periodontal ligament and alveolar bone. Symptoms include deep periodontal pockets, gum recession, tooth mobility, and, in severe cases, tooth loss. Chronic periodontitis is often linked to systemic conditions like diabetes, which can exacerbate the disease [50].

Periodontal–endodontic abscess: This condition is marked by severe pain, significant swelling, and the presence of a deep periodontal pocket with pus discharge. The tooth may exhibit increased mobility, and systemic involvement, such as fever, may be present. Depending on the extent of the infection, the tooth can be either vital or non-vital, making diagnosis and treatment more complex [51].

(c) Combined Pulp–Periodontal Lesions

When both the pulp and periodontal tissues are involved, the clinical manifestations can be particularly complex, reflecting the interplay between the two tissues as follows:

Primary endodontic lesions with secondary periodontal involvement: These lesions typically present with symptoms of pulpitis or necrosis, such as severe toothache, which may be accompanied by periodontal symptoms like deep pockets or gum swelling as the infection spreads from the pulp to the periodontal tissues through anatomical pathways such as the apical foramen or lateral canals. The primary source of infection is the pulp, and treatment usually involves root canal therapy followed by periodontal care [10].

Primary periodontal lesions with secondary endodontic involvement: In these cases, the initial pathology begins in the periodontal tissues, leading to periodontal symptoms such as gum recession, tooth mobility, and pocket formation. As the disease progresses, it can extend to the pulp, causing pulpal necrosis. These lesions are often more challenging to diagnose and treat because the primary focus of the disease is periodontal, with secondary pulpal involvement [51].

True combined lesions: True combined lesions occur when both pulp and periodontal tissues are independently diseased, and the conditions merge to form a single, complex lesion. Clinically, these lesions present with a combination of symptoms from both pulpitis and periodontitis, such as severe pain, swelling, deep periodontal pockets, and possible abscess formation. These lesions require a multidisciplinary approach to treatment, addressing both the endodontic and periodontal aspects of the disease [10].

3.6. Diagnostic Techniques for Identifying Pulp–Pathogenic Microbes

The accurate identification of pulp–pathogenic microbes is essential for diagnosing and managing pulp–periodontal pathologies effectively. These infections, often caused by a variety of bacteria, fungi, and viruses, require precise diagnostic techniques to ensure appropriate treatment. Over the years, advancements in microbiological diagnostics have significantly enhanced our ability to detect and identify these pathogens, employing both traditional and modern molecular techniques. Below are mentioned various diagnostic methods used to identify pulp–pathogenic microbes, their applications, and their significance in clinical practice.

1. Traditional microbiological methods: Historically, the identification of pathogenic microbes in dental infections relied heavily on traditional microbiological techniques, including culture-based methods and biochemical tests.

Culture-based techniques: Foundational methods in microbiological diagnostics include culture-based techniques, which are particularly essential for isolating and identifying microorganisms from infected pulp tissue or root canal samples. These methods involve cultivating microbes on selective or differential media that support the growth of specific types of bacteria or fungi. Once the microorganisms are cultured, they can be analyzed based on their growth patterns, colony morphology, and biochemical reactions. These characteristics are crucial for accurately identifying specific pathogens involved in the infection. Although culture-based techniques can be time-consuming and are sometimes limited by the difficulty in cultivating certain fastidious oral pathogens, they remain the gold standard in microbial identification. This is largely due to their ability to produce pure isolates, which are essential for subsequent testing, such as antibiotic susceptibility assays or further molecular analysis. The precision and reliability of culture-based methods make them indispensable in clinical microbiology, despite the advancements in faster molecular diagnostic techniques [52].

ELISA: A well-established technique in microbiological diagnostics, the ELISA is used to detect the presence of specific antigens or antibodies within a sample. This method operates by utilizing enzymes attached to antibodies or antigens, which, upon binding to their target molecule, produce a detectable signal, usually a color change, that can be measured quantitatively. ELISA is particularly valuable in the context of pulp infections, where it can be employed to identify specific bacterial proteins or toxins indirectly by assessing the immune response of the host. This approach allows clinicians to detect pathogens even when they are not directly present in large numbers or are difficult to culture by identifying the immune system's response to these pathogens. The ability of ELISA to detect minute quantities of antigens or antibodies makes it a sensitive and specific tool in the diagnostic process. Moreover, ELISA can be adapted to high-throughput screening, making it suitable for processing multiple samples simultaneously. However, it is important to note that while ELISA is highly effective in detecting established infections, its ability to identify pathogens at the very early stages of infection may be limited, as the immune response might not yet be fully developed [53].

Western blot: A widely utilized technique in molecular biology, Western blotting is employed for detecting specific proteins within a sample, providing detailed insights into the presence of pathogens by analyzing their unique protein profiles. The process involves separating proteins based on their size using gel electrophoresis, followed by their transfer onto a membrane, typically made of nitrocellulose or PVDF. The membrane is then probed with antibodies specific to the target protein, which are usually linked to an enzyme that generates a detectable signal, such as a colorimetric or chemiluminescent reaction. This technique allows for the identification of proteins that are characteristic of particular pathogens, making it a powerful tool in confirming the presence of infectious agents in cases of pulp infections. Western blotting is often used in conjunction with other diagnostic methods, such as ELISA or PCR, to verify the identity of pathogens that may be involved in complex or chronic infections. Despite its robustness and specificity, Western blotting can be labor-intensive and requires a high level of technical expertise, making it less suitable for rapid diagnostics but invaluable in research and confirmatory testing [54].

2. Molecular diagnostic techniques: In recent years, molecular techniques have revolutionized the field of microbial diagnostics, allowing for more rapid, accurate, and comprehensive identification of pathogens without the need for culture.

PCR: An advanced molecular technique, the PCR is renowned for its high sensitivity in detecting and amplifying specific DNA sequences, even from minute amounts of microbial DNA present in a sample. This method revolutionized microbiological diagnostics by enabling the identification of pathogens that are difficult to culture or grow slowly, which is often the case in chronic pulp infections. The PCR process involves repeated cycles of heating and cooling, which allows the targeted DNA segment to be duplicated exponentially. As a result, even a single copy of DNA can be amplified into millions of copies, making it detectable and analyzable. This capability is particularly useful for diagnosing infections caused by elusive pathogens that may be present in very low quantities or that cannot be easily grown in laboratory conditions. Additionally, PCR's speed and precision allow for rapid diagnosis, which is crucial for timely intervention in dental infections. Despite its significant advantages, PCR requires specialized equipment and technical expertise, which can limit its availability in some clinical settings. However, its ability to provide accurate and early identification of pathogens makes it an indispensable tool in the management of complex infections, including those found in endodontic practice [55].

NGS: Rapidly becoming a pivotal technology in the field of microbiology, NGS offers unparalleled capabilities for identifying a wide array of pathogens within a single assay. Unlike traditional methods that target specific pathogens, NGS allows for the comprehensive sequencing of entire microbial communities directly from clinical samples. This broad-spectrum approach is particularly valuable in understanding the microbial diversity within infected pulp tissues, where multiple pathogens may coexist, or in cases where novel or unexpected pathogens are suspected. By sequencing the entire DNA or RNA content of a sample, NGS can provide a detailed snapshot of the microbial environment, including bacteria, viruses, fungi, and other microorganisms. This depth of analysis not only aids in identifying the causative agents of infection but also enhances our understanding of the complex interactions within microbial communities that may influence disease progression and treatment outcomes. NGS is especially useful in challenging diagnostic scenarios, such as chronic or refractory pulp infections, where traditional culture methods may fail to detect all the pathogens involved. However, the implementation of NGS in routine clinical practice is still limited by its high cost, the need for sophisticated bioinformatics tools, and the expertise required to interpret the vast amounts of data generated. Despite these challenges, NGS represents a significant advancement in the diagnostic toolkit for endodontic and periodontal infections, providing insights that are crucial for developing targeted and effective treatment strategies [56].

MALDI-TOF MS: An advanced and rapid technique, MALDI-TOF MS is increasingly employed in clinical microbiology for the identification of bacterial and fungal species. This method works by analyzing the protein profiles of microorganisms, generating unique mass spectrometry fingerprints that can be used to identify pathogens with high precision. MALDI-TOF MS has gained popularity due to its remarkable speed and accuracy, allowing for the simultaneous identification of a wide range of pathogens in a matter of minutes. The process begins with the ionization of proteins extracted from microbial cells, followed by their separation based on the mass-to-charge ratio. The resulting spectra are then compared against extensive databases of known microbial profiles to determine the identity of the organism. One of the key advantages of MALDI-TOF MS is its ability to identify microorganisms directly from clinical samples with minimal preparation, making it an efficient tool in routine diagnostics. Moreover, it has proven particularly useful in identifying pathogens that are difficult to culture or require long incubation periods, such as certain fungi or anaerobic bacteria. While the initial setup costs for MALDI-TOF MS can be high, the technique offers long-term benefits through reduced reagent costs, quicker turnaround times, and enhanced diagnostic accuracy. This makes it a valuable addition to the arsenal of tools available for diagnosing infections, including those involving the dental pulp and periodontal tissues [57].

FISH: A powerful molecular technique, FISH uses fluorescently labeled probes to bind to specific DNA sequences within microbial cells, enabling the direct visualization and identification of pathogens in their natural environment. This technique is particularly valuable for detecting and identifying bacteria within biofilms, which are complex communities of microorganisms that often play a significant role in chronic pulp infections. FISH not only identifies the presence of specific pathogens but also provides critical spatial information about their location and organization within the infected tissue. This spatial context is essential for understanding the dynamics of microbial communities and how they interact with the host's tissues and immune response. By visualizing where pathogens are located in relation to one another and to the surrounding host cells, FISH helps clinicians and researchers gain insights into the mechanisms of infection and persistence within biofilms. This information can guide more targeted and effective treatment strategies, especially in cases where traditional culture methods may fail to capture the full complexity of the infection. Although FISH requires specialized equipment and expertise, its ability to provide both qualitative and quantitative data about microbial populations makes it an invaluable tool in the study and management of biofilm-associated infections [58].

3. Advanced imaging and biofilm analysis: Since pulp infections often involve biofilms, a complex community of microbes encased in a self-produced matrix, advanced imaging techniques are crucial for elucidating the role these biofilms play in disease progression.

CLSM: A cutting-edge imaging technique, CLSM, is extensively used to explore the intricate structure and composition of biofilms in pulp infections. CLSM utilizes laser light to scan specimens point-by-point, enabling the creation of high-resolution,

3D images that provide a detailed view of biofilm architecture. This capability allows researchers to observe the spatial organization and interactions between different microbial species within the biofilm, offering valuable insights into how these microorganisms coexist, communicate, and respond to environmental stimuli or antimicrobial treatments. One of the significant advantages of CLSM is its ability to generate precise 3D reconstructions without the need for extensive sample preparation, which preserves the natural state of the biofilm. This non-destructive imaging method facilitates the examination of biofilm thickness, density, and the distribution of specific pathogens within the infected pulp tissues. Additionally, CLSM can be combined with various fluorescent probes and dyes, enabling the simultaneous visualization of multiple microbial species and the extracellular matrix components that support biofilm stability. This multiplexing capability is essential for understanding the complex interactions and synergistic relationships that contribute to the resilience and pathogenicity of biofilms. When integrated with advanced image analysis software, CLSM provides quantitative data on biofilm parameters such as biomass, porosity, and the spatial distribution of microorganisms. These detailed metrics are crucial for assessing the effectiveness of antimicrobial treatments and for developing targeted therapeutic strategies. For instance, CLSM can be used to monitor changes in biofilm structure and microbial viability in response to different disinfectants or antibiotics, thereby informing more effective clinical interventions. Moreover, CLSM's high-resolution imaging is invaluable for studying the dynamic processes within biofilms, such as microbial growth, gene expression, and metabolic activity. By visualizing these processes in real-time, researchers can gain a deeper understanding of the mechanisms that drive biofilm formation, maintenance, and resistance to treatment. This comprehensive knowledge is essential for advancing endodontic practices and improving clinical outcomes for patients with chronic pulp infections. Despite its numerous benefits, the application of CLSM requires specialized equipment and technical expertise, which may limit its accessibility in some research and clinical settings. Additionally, the interpretation of CLSM data can be complex, necessitating advanced training in image analysis and bioinformatics. Nevertheless, the unparalleled insights provided by CLSM make it an indispensable tool in the study and management of biofilm-associated pulp infections, contributing significantly to the development of more effective diagnostic and therapeutic approaches [59].

Image analysis programs: Indispensable tools for processing and interpreting the extensive data generated by CLSM and other advanced imaging techniques are image analysis programs. These software applications are designed to handle the complex, multi-dimensional datasets that result from the high-resolution imaging of biofilms, enabling researchers to extract meaningful quantitative information from the visual data. By analyzing parameters such as biofilm thickness, density, and cell viability, image analysis programs provide crucial insights into the structural and functional characteristics of biofilms, which are often implicated in chronic pulp infections. These programs allow for the precise measurement of biofilm architecture, including the spatial distribution of microbial species and the extracellular matrix. This detailed quantification is essential for understanding the pathogenic potential of biofilms, as factors like increased thickness and density can correlate with greater resistance to antimicrobial treatments. Additionally, image analysis software can track changes in biofilm properties over time, providing valuable data on how biofilms develop, persist, and respond to therapeutic interventions. One of the key advantages of using image analysis programs in conjunction with CLSM is the ability to automate and standardize the analysis process, reducing human error and improving reproducibility. These tools often include a range of customizable features that allow researchers to tailor the analysis to specific experimental needs, such as differentiating between live and dead cells, assessing metabolic activity, or identifying particular microbial species within a mixed community. Moreover, advanced image analysis programs can integrate with bioinformatics tools to perform more complex analyses, such as correlating biofilm structure with gene expression profiles or metabolic pathways. This integration enhances our understanding of the molecular mechanisms underlying biofilm formation and resistance, offering new avenues for targeted treatment strategies. Despite the powerful capabilities of these tools, their effective use requires a certain level of technical expertise, particularly in terms of setting appropriate parameters and interpreting the results. Additionally, the complexity of the data and the sophistication of the analysis software can present challenges for users, particularly those without a strong background in computational biology or bioinformatics [59].

4. Metagenomics and transcriptomics in precision diagnostics: In addition to conventional 16S rRNA-based sequencing, advanced molecular diagnostic tools such as shotgun metagenomics and metatranscriptomics have emerged as transformative approaches for characterizing the microbial and functional complexity of pulp–periodontal lesions. Shotgun metagenomics allows for the comprehensive detection of all microbial genomes, encompassing bacteria, fungi, viruses, and archaea, while simultaneously identifying antimicrobial resistance genes, virulence factors, and metabolic pathways implicated in disease progression [5].

Metatranscriptomics: By contrast, it focuses on the active expression of microbial genes by analyzing messenger RNA transcripts. This technique offers valuable insight into which microbial genes are being expressed in situ, thereby distinguishing viable, metabolically active pathogens from dormant or dead cells. Such resolution enhances both diagnostic precision and the capacity to design targeted therapeutic strategies [60].

These molecular tools are especially useful in complex or refractory pulp–periodontal infections, where traditional methods often fail to detect low-abundance or non-culturable organisms embedded within resilient polymicrobial biofilms. Moreover, transcriptomic analyses have uncovered functionally significant genes involved in biofilm maturation, immune evasion, and antibiotic resistance mechanisms that contribute to chronicity and treatment failure [61].

Importantly, these high-throughput molecular strategies support the development of precision-guided therapies by aligning specific microbial functions, rather than mere presence, with clinical pathology. This function-based diagnostic paradigm enables clinicians to move beyond empirical treatment toward interventions tailored to the active microbial profile of each lesion [62].

Recent investigations employing metagenomic and metatranscriptomic analyses have also revealed previously uncharacterized microbial species, patterns of functional redundancy within microbial consortia, and significant shifts in microbial community composition following therapy, underscoring the clinical relevance of these tools in modern endodontics and periodontology [5,61].

5. Integrated approaches in clinical practice: In clinical settings, the integration of traditional and modern diagnostic techniques is often necessary to achieve accurate and comprehensive identification of pulp–pathogenic microbes. For instance, PCR and NGS can be used for rapid screening and identification of pathogens, while culture-based methods and MALDI-TOF MS provide additional confirmation and allow for antimicrobial susceptibility testing. Similarly, FISH and CLSM can be employed to study the microbial ecology of biofilms within the pulp and root canals, aiding in the development of targeted treatment strategies. The use of these advanced diagnostic techniques not only improves the accuracy of pathogen identification but also enhances our understanding of the microbial dynamics in pulp–periodontal pathologies. This, in turn, leads to more effective treatments and better clinical outcomes for patients.

Microbiome-Based Therapeutic Strategies for Pulp–Periodontal Diseases

With increasing recognition of microbial dysbiosis as a driving factor in pulp–periodontal diseases, there is a growing emphasis on therapeutic approaches that restore microbial balance rather than indiscriminately eradicating all microbes. Microbiome-based therapeutics, including probiotics, prebiotics, and bacteriophage therapy, represent an emerging frontier aimed at re-establishing ecological homeostasis and suppressing pathogenic consortia in a targeted, host-friendly manner.

Probiotics, defined as live microorganisms that confer health benefits to the host when administered in adequate amounts, have demonstrated promising anti-inflammatory, antimicrobial, and immunomodulatory effects in the context of periodontal therapy. Specific strains from the genera *Lactobacillus* and *Bifidobacterium* can inhibit keystone pathogens such as *P. gingivalis* and *Fusobacterium nucleatum* by mechanisms including competitive exclusion, bacteriocin production, co-aggregation interference, and immune modulation [63–66]. Clinical studies have shown that adjunctive probiotic therapy can reduce periodontal pocket depth, decrease inflammatory cytokine levels, and promote beneficial microbial colonization. Although their application in endodontics remains in the early stages, in vitro evidence suggests that probiotics may impair root canal biofilms and enhance periapical healing, positioning them as potential future adjuncts to intracanal disinfection.

Prebiotics, non-digestible dietary compounds that selectively promote the growth and metabolic activity of beneficial bacteria, also hold potential in modulating the oral microbiota. Ingredients such as inulin and fructooligosaccharides have been shown to support the colonization and persistence of probiotic species in the oral cavity, potentially amplifying their therapeutic effects. While prebiotics have been explored primarily in periodontal settings, their incorporation into endodontic irrigants, scaffolds, or medicaments represents a novel and largely untapped therapeutic strategy that warrants further investigation [67].

Another frontier in microbiome-targeted therapy is bacteriophage therapy, which involves the use of viruses that specifically infect and lyse pathogenic bacteria. Bacteriophage therapy, the use of viruses that selectively infect and lyse bacteria, is another cutting-edge approach gaining momentum in dental applications. Unlike broad-spectrum antimicrobials, bacteriophages offer precision targeting, disrupting pathogenic species while sparing commensals and reducing the risk of dysbiosis. Experimental studies have shown that lytic phages targeting *E. faecalis* or *P. gingivalis* can significantly disrupt biofilms, suppress virulence gene expression, and enhance host immune clearance [68–70]. The incorporation of phage formulations into endodontic irrigants, root canal sealers, or subgingival delivery systems is being actively explored as a strategy to manage persistent infections, especially in cases of refractory apical periodontitis and chronic periodontitis.

Together, these microbiome-modulating approaches represent a paradigm shift from pathogen eradication to ecological reprogramming of the oral microbiome. They are aligned with the emerging concept of precision microbiome engineering; wherein microbial consortia are reshaped to promote health-associated community structures and host–microbe symbiosis. Ongoing innovations include probiotic-infused pastes, phage-embedded hydrogel scaffolds, and prebiotic-enhanced regenerative materials for clinical use in both endodontic and periodontal therapies. Although many of these strategies remain experimental, they hold significant promise for minimizing antibiotic use, reducing treatment failure, and promoting long-term microbial resilience. As translational research continues to bridge bench and bedside, microbiome-based therapeutics may become integral to personalized, biologically informed dental care.

3.7. Endodontic Treatment with Emphasis on Irrigants for Intracanal Disinfection

Endodontic treatment, or root canal therapy, is a meticulous dental procedure aimed at eradicating infection from within the tooth's root canal system. This process involves the removal of infected or necrotic pulp tissue, followed by the thorough cleaning, shaping, and sealing of the root canals to prevent reinfection. The success of this procedure is highly dependent on the clinician's attention to detail during each step, particularly during the disinfection phase, where the selection and use of irrigants are crucial.

1. Preoperative assessment: Before the initiation of endodontic treatment, a comprehensive preoperative assessment is critical. This process includes taking a detailed medical and dental history, performing a clinical examination, and obtaining diagnostic radiographs, such as periapical X-rays or CBCT scans. The purpose of this assessment is to evaluate the extent of the infection, understand the complexity of the root canal system, and identify any periapical pathology that might influence the treatment plan [71].

2. Anesthesia and isolation: Once the preoperative assessment is complete, local anesthesia is administered to ensure patient comfort throughout the procedure. Following anesthesia, the tooth is isolated using a rubber dam. The use of a rubber dam is essential to prevent contamination of the operative field with saliva and to protect the patient from ingesting or inhaling the irrigants or other materials used during the procedure [72].

3. Access cavity preparation: An access cavity is prepared through the occlusal surface for posterior teeth or the lingual surface for anterior teeth using high-speed burs. This cavity provides direct access to the pulp chamber and root canal system. The design and size of the access cavity are dictated by the tooth's anatomy, ensuring that all canals, especially in multi-rooted teeth, are located. Proper access is essential for effective canal cleaning and shaping [73].

4. Pulp tissue removal and initial canal exploration: After gaining access to the pulp chamber, the coronal pulp tissue is removed using a sharp spoon excavator or an endodontic file. The root canals are then explored with small, flexible K-files to determine their patency and establish the initial working length. The working length is typically determined using an electronic apex locator in conjunction with

radiographs. Accurate determination of the working length is crucial for ensuring that the entire root canal system is cleaned and shaped properly [74].

5. Cleaning and shaping of the root canal system: The cleaning and shaping of the root canal system are critical steps in endodontic treatment. This process involves both mechanical instrumentation and chemical disinfection to remove infected tissue, debris, and bacteria from the canals while shaping them to facilitate effective irrigation and obturation.

Mechanical instrumentation: Rotary or reciprocating endodontic files are commonly used for canal preparation. These instruments are used sequentially to gradually enlarge the canals while maintaining their original curvature. The goal is to create a continuously tapering funnel shape that narrows as it approaches the apex. Special attention is given to avoiding procedural errors such as the ledging, zipping, or transportation of the canal [75].

Apical enlargement: The apical third of the canal is prepared using smaller files to ensure complete cleaning and to facilitate the penetration of irrigants. Some clinicians choose to perform additional apical enlargement, using larger files in the apical region to ensure thorough debridement. This is particularly important in cases with apical periodontitis, where the periapical tissues are inflamed or infected [73].

6. Intracanal irrigation for disinfection: Irrigation is an essential component of root canal therapy, aiding in the removal of debris, bacterial biofilm, and organic tissue that cannot be fully eliminated by mechanical instrumentation alone (Figure 11). The choice of irrigants and the method of irrigation significantly impact the success of the disinfection process.

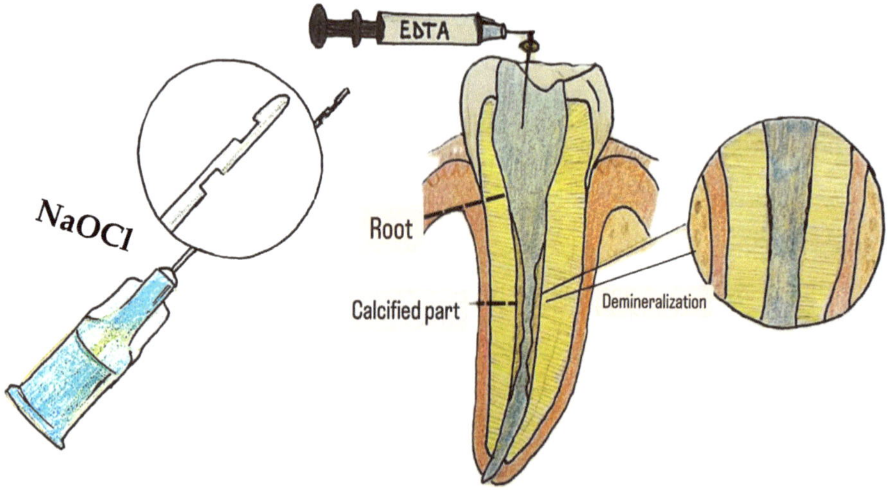

Figure 11. **Left:** Illustration of a side-vented irrigation needle delivering NaOCl solution into the root canal. The side-vent design promotes safer and more controlled irrigant flow, reducing the risk of extrusion beyond the apex. **Right:** Application of EDTA solution for managing calcified canals. The image shows EDTA-induced demineralization of the calcified dentin within the root canal, facilitating canal negotiation and preparation while preserving surrounding tooth structure. Credit: © Nensi Kallfani, used with permission.

Primary irrigant—NaOCl: The most widely used irrigant, due to its potent antimicrobial properties and ability to dissolve organic tissue, is NaOCl. Concentrations typically range from 0.5% to 6%, depending on the clinical situation and the clinician's preference. NaOCl is effective against a broad spectrum of microorganisms, including bacteria, fungi, and viruses, and is essential for cleaning the canal system thoroughly [76].

Chelating agents—EDTA: Often used in conjunction with NaOCl, EDTA is effective in removing the smear layer, a debris layer that forms on canal walls during instrumentation. The smear layer can harbor bacteria and block the penetration of irrigants into the dentinal tubules, so its removal is critical for effective disinfection. Typically, 17% EDTA is used towards the end of the cleaning process to ensure the canals are free of debris and ready for obturation [77].

Supplemental irrigants—CHX: Due to its broad-spectrum antimicrobial activity and its ability to bind to dentin for sustained antibacterial action, CHX is sometimes used as a final rinse. However, CHX is not a tissue solvent, so it is not used as the primary irrigant. It is particularly useful in cases of persistent infections or where NaOCl is contraindicated [75].

Activation of irrigants: To enhance the effectiveness of irrigation, various methods of irrigant activation can be employed. Ultrasonic activation is one of the most effective techniques, where ultrasonic energy is used to agitate the irrigant within the canal. This agitation increases the penetration of the irrigant into the complex anatomy of the root canal system, including lateral canals and dentinal tubules, thereby improving disinfection [77].

7. Drying the canals: After the cleaning, shaping, and irrigation process, the canals must be thoroughly dried before obturation. Sterile paper points are used to absorb any residual irrigant and moisture from the canals. Proper drying is essential to ensure that the root canal sealer adheres effectively during the obturation process [78].

8. Obturation of the root canal system: The obturation phase involves filling the cleaned and shaped canal system with a biocompatible material to seal the canal and prevent reinfection.

Gutta-percha: The most commonly used material for obturating, or filling, root canals in endodontic therapy is gutta-percha. As a thermoplastic material, gutta-percha offers flexibility and adaptability, which are essential for effectively sealing the complex anatomy of root canal systems. This material is primarily composed of the latex produced from the sap of the Palaquium gutta tree, combined with zinc oxide, waxes, and other agents to enhance its properties. Gutta-percha is available in several forms, most commonly as standard cones, which are tapered to fit the shape of the prepared canal, and in thermoplasticized versions, which allow for more advanced techniques such as injection or carrier-based systems. The process of obturation with gutta-percha typically involves first coating the material with a root canal sealer. The sealer, which can be made from a variety of substances including calcium hydroxide, epoxy resins, or bioceramics, acts as a binding agent, filling the microscopic spaces between the gutta-percha and the canal walls. This is crucial for preventing microbial leakage and ensuring the long-term success of the root canal treatment. Once coated with sealer, the gutta-percha is inserted into the prepared canal. To ensure the material fully occupies the canal space, techniques such as lateral or vertical compaction are employed. Lateral compaction involves inserting a master cone of gutta-percha into the canal and then using spreaders to compact additional gutta-percha cones laterally into the space. Vertical compaction, on the other hand, involves heating the gutta-percha and compacting it vertically within the canal, often in conjunction with the use of heat carriers or pluggers to achieve a dense, homogenous fill. These techniques, when performed correctly, help to create a tight seal that is vital for the success of endodontic therapy, as it prevents the reinfection of the canal system by bacteria. The effectiveness of gutta-percha as an obturation material has been well documented in the literature, with studies such as Ricucci et al. (2023) demonstrating its reliability in achieving successful long-term outcomes when used in conjunction with appropriate sealing techniques and materials [79].

Root canal sealers: The choice of sealer directly impacts the ability to prevent microbial infiltration and reinfection of the canal. Modern advancements in sealer technology, particularly with calcium silicate-based sealers, have significantly improved the outcomes of root canal therapy. These sealers are not only effective in sealing the canal space but also offer excellent biocompatibility, making them a preferred choice in contemporary endodontics. Calcium silicate-based sealers have unique properties that enhance their performance. Upon application, these sealers can penetrate the dentinal tubules, creating a physical and chemical bond with the tooth structure. One of the key advantages of these sealers is their ability to interact with the moisture present in the root canal environment. This interaction leads to the formation of hydroxyapatite, a mineral that is a natural component of tooth structure. The formation of hydroxyapatite at the sealer–tooth interface further strengthens the seal, reducing the risk of microleakage and promoting the healing of periapical tissues. Moreover, the biocompatibility of calcium silicate-based sealers is a significant advantage, as it minimizes the risk of adverse reactions and supports the healing process. These sealers are known to be bioactive, meaning they can induce a favorable biological response, such as the regeneration of bone and periodontal tissues around the root apex. This bioactivity is particularly beneficial in cases where there is periapical pathology, as the sealer can contribute to the resolution of inflammation and the regeneration of lost tissues [78].

9. Postoperative care and follow-up: After obturation, a temporary or permanent restoration is placed to seal the access cavity and restore the tooth's function. Postoperative instructions include advising the patient on what to expect in terms of discomfort and the importance of maintaining oral hygiene. The patient is scheduled for follow-up appointments to monitor healing and assess the success of the treatment. Radiographic evaluations are typically performed at follow-up visits to ensure that the periapical tissues are healing and that there are no signs of reinfection [71].

3.8. Treatment Strategies for Pulp–Periodontal Pathologies

The success of endodontic treatment fundamentally relies on a methodical approach to each phase of the procedure, with particular emphasis on root canal system disinfection. Utilizing effective irrigants and incorporating advanced techniques such as ultrasonic activation are critical for ensuring thorough debridement and microbial eradication, both of which are essential for the long-term success of the procedure. By rigorously following these protocols, clinicians can significantly enhance the chances of achieving favorable outcomes in endodontic therapy. Additionally, the effective management of pulp–periodontal pathologies requires an integrated approach that combines various treatment modalities, ranging from non-surgical interventions to advanced surgical and regenerative techniques.

1. Non-surgical treatment approaches: Non-surgical treatments are typically the first line of management for pulp–periodontal pathologies, especially when the disease is detected early. These approaches focus on minimizing tissue damage and promoting natural healing processes.

MINST: Recognized for its effectiveness in managing periodontal disease with minimal tissue disruption, MINST has gained significant attention. This technique involves the careful removal of plaque, calculus, and biofilm using advanced instruments such as ultrasonic scalers and fine curettes. Clinical studies have demonstrated that MINST can achieve outcomes comparable to more invasive procedures, with the added benefits of reduced patient discomfort and faster recovery times. This makes MINST particularly valuable in the management of early to moderate periodontitis, where preserving the structural integrity of periodontal tissues is paramount [80].

Ozone therapy: Emerging as a promising adjunctive treatment, ozone therapy is valued for its potent antimicrobial properties and its ability to promote tissue regeneration. Ozone can be applied directly to periodontal pockets, where it reduces microbial load and enhances oxygenation, thereby supporting the healing of both pulp and periodontal tissues. Studies have shown its efficacy in reducing bacterial counts and accelerating the resolution of periodontal infections, especially in cases that are resistant to conventional therapies [81].

Laser-assisted periodontal and pulp therapy: The integration of laser technology, particularly diode lasers, into periodontal and pulp therapy marks a significant advancement in dental care. In periodontal therapy, lasers offer the precise targeting of infected tissues while preserving healthy surrounding structures. This precision not only effectively reduces bacterial load but also promotes tissue regeneration and minimizes postoperative discomfort. When combined with traditional methods like scaling and root planing, laser therapy significantly enhances treatment outcomes, particularly by reducing periodontal pocket depth and improving clinical attachment levels [82,83]. Then, in pulp therapy, lasers provide a minimally invasive treatment option for conditions such as pulpitis and pulp–periodontal lesions. Lasers can decontaminate the root canal system with high efficacy by eliminating bacteria, reducing the need for extensive mechanical cleaning. Additionally, lasers promote tissue regeneration and accelerate healing within the pulp chamber, which is crucial for preserving tooth vitality. This use of lasers in pulp therapy not only enhances treatment outcomes but also minimizes patient discomfort and supports quicker recovery, making it a valuable tool in modern endodontic and periodontal procedures.

PDT: An innovative approach, PDT, involves the application of a photosensitizing agent followed by exposure to a specific wavelength of light. This process generates reactive oxygen species that effectively destroy microbial cells within biofilms, which are notoriously difficult to eradicate using conventional treatments alone. PDT has shown considerable promise in managing biofilm-associated infections in pulp–periodontal pathologies, particularly when used in conjunction with traditional antimicrobial therapies. This combination offers a robust strategy for controlling complex infections and promoting healing in both pulp and periodontal tissues [84].

2. Surgical treatment approaches: When non-surgical therapies are insufficient to manage pulp–periodontal pathologies, surgical interventions become necessary. These approaches are particularly effective in advanced cases where there is significant tissue destruction.

Periodontal flap surgery: A common procedure for accessing and cleaning the root surfaces and bone affected by deep periodontal pockets is periodontal flap surgery. The surgery involves lifting the gingival tissue to allow for thorough debridement and root planing, which are essential for removing calculus and infected tissue from areas not accessible by non-surgical methods. This procedure is often combined with regenerative techniques, such as bone grafting and GTR, to restore lost bone and periodontal structures, thereby improving the long-term stability of the affected teeth [85].

Regenerative periodontal surgery: Advances in regenerative dentistry have led to the development of new techniques and materials designed to restore lost periodontal structures. Regenerative periodontal surgery often involves using bone grafts, GTR membranes, and biologics-like growth factors to stimulate the natural regrowth of bone and periodontal ligaments. These techniques are particularly beneficial in severe periodontitis cases where significant bone loss has occurred. By promoting the regeneration of these tissues, regenerative periodontal surgery can significantly improve the prognosis of teeth that would otherwise be at risk of extraction [86].

3. Endodontic treatment strategies: Effective endodontic treatment is crucial for managing the pulpal component of pulp–periodontal pathologies. This involves both primary treatment strategies and retreatment options for cases where initial therapies have failed.

RCT: As previously discussed, it is important to reiterate that the primary goal of RCT is to remove infected pulp tissue, thoroughly disinfect the root canal system, and seal it to prevent reinfection. Recent studies highlight the critical importance of precise apical management in minimizing bacterial extrusion and promoting periapical healing. For example, the selection of an appropriate file size and the use of advanced irrigation techniques are crucial for ensuring the thorough disinfection of the apical third of the canal. The proper management of this area is essential for long-term success in endodontic treatment, as inadequate cleaning or improper obturation at the apex can lead to treatment failure. Research indicates that apical underfilling, rather than overfilling, may increase the likelihood of unfavorable outcomes, further emphasizing the need for precise techniques in apical management [74,87,88].

Retreatment of failed root canals: When an initial RCT fails, retreatment is often necessary to address persistent or recurrent infections. Retreatment involves the removal of the previous root canal filling, re-cleaning and reshaping of the canal system, and placement of a new filling. The process can be complex, particularly in cases with intricate canal anatomy or significant apical pathology. However, retreatment is often the only option for resolving chronic pulp–periodontal lesions and preventing further deterioration of the affected tooth [71,72].

Apical management techniques: Proper management of the apical third of the root canal is critical for the success of endodontic treatment. Techniques such as apical enlargement and the use of advanced irrigation methods, including ultrasonic activation, have been shown to improve disinfection outcomes and promote better periapical healing. These techniques are particularly important in cases involving complex canal anatomies, such as C-shaped canals, where thorough cleaning and disinfection are more challenging [73,76].

3.9. Advanced Materials in Endodontic and Periodontal Therapy

The evolution of materials used in endodontic and periodontal therapies has significantly impacted the success rates of treatments for pulp–periodontal pathologies. The development and application of new materials are critical in achieving optimal clinical outcomes, particularly in complex cases involving both the dental pulp and periodontal structures. This text explores the various advanced materials referenced in the provided studies, detailing their properties, applications, and clinical benefits.

1. Calcium silicate-based cements: A cornerstone in endodontic and periodontal therapies has been established by calcium silicate-based cements, such as MTA and its derivatives, due to their excellent biocompatibility, sealing ability, and regenerative properties.

MTA: Widely used for root-end filling, pulp capping, and perforation repair, MTA has become a standard material in these procedures (Figure 12).

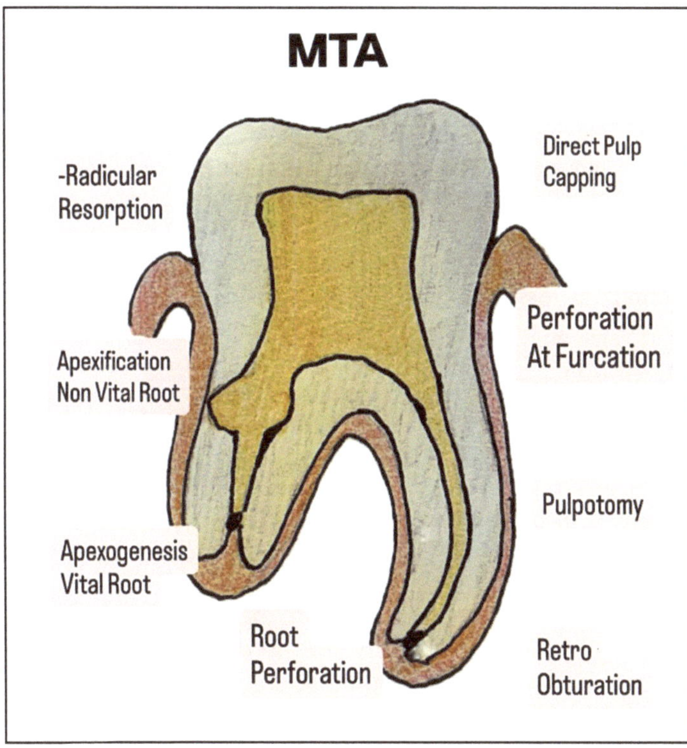

Figure 12. MTA in endodontics. The illustration highlights MTA's versatile use in managing diverse clinical scenarios, including direct pulp capping, pulpotomy, apexogenesis in vital roots, apexification in non-vital roots, repair of root and furcation perforations, retrograde obturation during apical surgery, and treatment of radicular resorption. Credit: © Nensi Kallfani, used with permission.

MTA is known for its capacity to stimulate hard tissue formation and create a durable seal that effectively blocks microbial infiltration, which is critical for the success of endodontic treatments. Its high pH and ability to form a mineralized barrier contribute significantly to its effectiveness. In the context of direct pulp capping, MTA has demonstrated long-term success, particularly in preserving pulp vitality and promoting the formation of a dentin bridge, which is essential for protecting the pulp and ensuring the longevity of the tooth. The regenerative properties of MTA also extend to its role in supporting the healing of periapical tissues, further underscoring its versatility and effectiveness in endodontic applications. Studies have consistently shown that MTA's ability to form a mineralized barrier and its alkaline environment contribute to its superior performance in clinical settings. Its application in endodontic procedures, such as root-end fillings and direct pulp capping, has been associated with high success rates, making it a material of choice for practitioners seeking reliable and predictable outcomes [79,89].

Premixed calcium silicate-based cements: These cements offer similar benefits to traditional MTA but with improved handling properties. For example, premixed cements such as Biodentine™ have been designed for easier application and reduced setting times while maintaining excellent biological properties. The use of these materials in root-end fillings has shown promising results in achieving a tight seal and promoting periapical healing, particularly when used with techniques that minimize nanoleakage [90].

2. Bioactive glasses: Bioactive glasses are used extensively in regenerative procedures due to their ability to bond with bone and promote tissue regeneration. These materials release ions that stimulate the cellular processes involved in bone formation and wound healing.

Bioactive glasses in bone grafting: The application of bioactive glasses in bone grafting procedures is particularly beneficial in cases of severe periodontal disease where significant bone loss has occurred. These materials not only provide a scaffold for new bone formation but also actively participate in the regenerative process by releasing silicate and calcium ions, which are critical for osteogenesis. Studies have demonstrated that bioactive glass can significantly improve the outcomes of bone grafting procedures by enhancing bone regeneration and ensuring the long-term stability of the grafted area [86].

3. Nanohydroxyapatite: A synthetic biomaterial that closely resembles the mineral component of bone and teeth, nanohydroxyapatite is increasingly used in endodontic and periodontal applications due to its biocompatibility and osteoconductive properties.

Applications in root canal therapy: Nanohydroxyapatite is used as a root canal sealer and in regenerative endodontics due to its ability to induce hard tissue formation. When applied in endodontic treatments, it helps in sealing the root canal system and promoting the healing of periapical tissues. Its nano-sized particles ensure deep penetration into the dentinal tubules, providing an effective barrier against bacterial infiltration [73].

Periodontal regeneration: In periodontal therapy, nanohydroxyapatite is used in combination with other regenerative materials to enhance bone regeneration in periodontal defects. It acts as a filler in bone grafts and helps in the re-establishment of the periodontal ligament and alveolar bone, making it an essential component in regenerative periodontal surgeries [86].

4. Sealing and filling materials: The effectiveness of endodontic and periodontal treatments heavily relies on the sealing and filling materials used to prevent microleakage and ensure long-term success.

Bioactive bioceramic root canal sealer: The choice of sealer is critical in root canal therapy to ensure the complete obturation of the canal system. Bioactive bioceramic sealers are particularly noted for their ability to release calcium ions, which stimulate the formation of hydroxyapatite, a crucial mineral for sealing dentinal tubules and preventing bacterial re-entry. This promotes a biologically favorable environment, supporting the regeneration of periapical tissues and contributing to the long-term success of root canal treatments. The superior biocompatibility and bioactivity of bioceramic sealers allow them to bond effectively with dentin, enhancing their sealing properties and actively participating in the healing process. Similarly, bioactive glass-based sealers offer promising results in endodontics. These sealers can be used without semisolid core materials, simplifying the obturation process while still providing a strong, durable seal [91,92].

Endodontic filling materials: The materials used for filling root canals, such as gutta-percha combined with advanced sealers, are essential for ensuring the complete obturation of the canal space. Newer materials like bioceramic-based fillers offer enhanced properties such as dimensional stability, bioactivity, and the ability to bond with the canal walls. These materials are particularly useful in retreatment cases where previous fillings have failed, providing a more reliable and durable solution [91].

5. Advanced irrigation systems: Effective irrigation is crucial in root canal therapy to ensure the complete removal of debris, bacteria, and biofilm from the canal system. Advanced irrigation systems and techniques have been developed to improve the efficacy of root canal disinfection.

Ultrasonic activation of irrigants: The use of ultrasonic devices to activate irrigants has been shown to enhance the cleaning efficacy of traditional irrigation solutions such as sodium hypochlorite. Ultrasonic activation allows the irrigant to penetrate more deeply into the root canal system, including lateral canals and isthmuses, where traditional irrigation methods may not reach. This technique has been shown to significantly improve the removal of biofilm and debris, leading to better clinical outcomes [75,77].

Irrigation needle design: The design of the irrigation needle plays a critical role in the effectiveness of the irrigation process. Recent studies have focused on optimizing needle design to improve the delivery and distribution of irrigants within the root canal system. Innovations in needle design have resulted in improved apical pressure and reduced extrusion of irrigants, minimizing the risk of postoperative complications and enhancing overall disinfection [76].

6. Biologic materials and growth factors: The use of biologic materials and growth factors has transformed regenerative endodontics and periodontics by promoting the natural healing and regeneration of dental and periodontal tissues.

Stem cell-based therapies: At the forefront of dental research, stem cell-based regenerative therapies offer the potential for the complete regeneration of dental tissues. These therapies involve the use of stem cells derived from various sources, including dental pulp and periodontal ligaments, which are capable of differentiating into the various cell types needed for tissue regeneration. The application of stem cells in combination with biocompatible scaffolds and growth factors has shown promising results in the regeneration of pulp tissue and the restoration of tooth vitality [86].

In the evolving field of dentistry, traditional endodontic procedures have long depended on a combination of mechanical instrumentation, chemical irrigants, and medicaments to achieve successful root canal treatments. These conventional methods, often utilizing synthetic agents with well-established efficacy, focus on thoroughly cleaning, shaping, and disinfecting the root canal system to eliminate infection and prevent reinfection. However, there is a growing interest in the integration of more biocompatible and natural alternatives within clinical practice, driven by the desire to enhance patient safety and outcomes. This shift has brought substances like propolis to the forefront of modern dental care, particularly in endodontic treatments. As we explore this transition in Chapter 4, we will delve into how propolis is being utilized to improve the outcomes of endodontic procedures.

3.10. Conclusions

The interplay between pathogenic microbes and the development of pulp–periodontal pathologies is a complex and significant aspect of oral health that requires a comprehensive understanding and strategic management. These pathologies, which represent the intersection of endodontic and periodontal diseases, are driven by a variety of pathogenic microorganisms that thrive within the unique environment of the oral cavity. The role of the oral microbiome, particularly in states of dysbiosis, is critical to the initiation and progression of these conditions. Specific pathogens such as *P. gingivalis*, *T. denticola*, and *E. faecalis* are recognized as key contributors to the pathogenesis of both pulpal and periodontal diseases, exacerbating tissue destruction and complicating treatment outcomes.

Advancements in molecular diagnostics and imaging technologies have significantly improved our ability to identify and understand the microbial diversity within pulp–periodontal lesions, allowing for more accurate diagnosis and targeted treatment strategies. The classification of these pathologies has evolved over time, reflecting an increased understanding of their multifactorial nature. Modern classification systems, which consider both the etiology and the presence of structural root defects, provide a more nuanced framework for clinical management.

Clinically, pulp–periodontal pathologies present with a wide range of symptoms, from acute pain associated with pulpal inflammation to the chronic progression of periodontal disease. The complexity of these conditions often necessitates a multidisciplinary approach that integrates both endodontic and periodontal therapies. Treatment strategies have advanced to include a combination of non-surgical and surgical interventions, with a growing emphasis on the use of novel and adjunctive therapies such as probiotics, advanced biomaterials, and enhanced irrigation techniques.

The ongoing development of advanced materials, including bioactive glasses and calcium silicate-based cements, along with the incorporation of biologic materials and growth factors, has further enhanced the potential for successful regenerative therapies. These innovations are critical for achieving long-term stability and healing in cases of severe pulp–periodontal pathologies.

Looking forward, continued research into the mechanisms of microbial pathogenicity, the refinement of diagnostic techniques, and the development of more effective therapeutic materials and approaches will be essential in improving outcomes for patients with pulp–periodontal diseases. The integration of these advancements into clinical practice holds the promise of not only more effective treatment but also the potential for the prevention of these complex and challenging conditions.

References

1. Di Stefano, M.; Polizzi, A.; Santonocito, S.; Romano, A.; Lombardi, T.; Isola, G. Impact of Oral Microbiome in Periodontal Health and Periodontitis: A Critical Review on Prevention and Treatment. *Int. J. Mol. Sci.* **2022**, *23*, 5142. [CrossRef] [PubMed]
2. Siddiqui, R.; Badran, Z.; Boghossian, A.; Alharbi, A.M.; Alfahemi, H.; Khan, N.A. The increasing importance of the oral microbiome in periodontal health and disease. *Future Sci. OA* **2023**, *9*, FSO856. [CrossRef] [PubMed]
3. Hajishengallis, G.; Lamont, R.J. Polymicrobial communities in periodontal disease: Their quasi-organismal nature and dialogue with the host. *Periodontol 2000* **2021**, *86*, 210–230. [CrossRef]
4. Wieczorkiewicz, K.; Jarząbek, A.; Bakinowska, E.; Kiełbowski, K.; Pawlik, A. Microbial Dynamics in Endodontic Pathology—From Bacterial Infection to Therapeutic Interventions—A Narrative Review. *Pathogens* **2025**, *14*, 12. [CrossRef]
5. Arias-Moliz, M.T.; Pérez-Carrasco, V.; Uroz-Torres, D.; Santana Ramos, J.D.; García-Salcedo, J.A.; Soriano, M. Identification of keystone taxa in root canals and periapical lesions of post-treatment endodontic infections: Next generation microbiome research. *Int. Endod. J.* **2024**, *57*, 933–942. [CrossRef]
6. Lamont, R.J.; Hajishengallis, G.; Koo, H. Social networking at the microbiome-host interface. *Infect. Immun.* **2023**, *91*, e0012423. [CrossRef]
7. Hajishengallis, G. New developments in neutrophil biology and periodontitis. *Periodontol 2000* **2020**, *82*, 78–92. [CrossRef]
8. Maekawa, T.; Krauss, J.L.; Abe, T.; Jotwani, R.; Triantafilou, M.; Triantafilou, K.; Hashim, A.; Hoch, S.; Curtis, M.A.; Nussbaum, G.; et al. Porphyromonas gingivalis manipulates complement and TLR signaling to uncouple bacterial clearance from inflammation and promote dysbiosis. *Cell Host Microbe* **2014**, *15*, 768–778. [CrossRef]
9. Hajishengallis, G. Immunomicrobial pathogenesis of periodontitis: Keystones, pathobionts, and host response. *Trends Immunol.* **2014**, *35*, 3–11. [CrossRef]
10. Duncan, H.F.; Kirkevang, L.L.; Peters, O.A.; El-Karim, I.; Krastl, G.; Del Fabbro, M.; Chong, B.S.; Galler, K.M.; Segura-Egea, J.J.; Kebschull, M. ESE Workshop Participants and Methodological Consultant. Treatment of pulpal and apical disease: The European Society of Endodontology (ESE) S3-level clinical practice guideline. *Int. Endod. J.* **2023**, *56*, 238–295. [CrossRef] [PubMed]
11. Sun, P.; Guo, Z.; Guo, D.; Wang, J.; Wu, T.; Li, T.; Liu, J.; Liu, X. The Microbiota Profile Analysis of Combined Periodontal-Endodontic Lesions Using 16S rRNA Next-Generation Sequencing. *J. Immunol. Res.* **2021**, *2021*, 2490064. [CrossRef]
12. Tak, E.J.; Park, O.J.; Lee, J.S.; Yoo, Y.J.; Perinpanayagam, H.; Jeong, Y.S.; Lee, J.Y.; Bae, J.W.; Kum, K.Y.; Han, S.H. Microbiota associated with caries and apical periodontitis: A next-generation sequencing study. *Int. Endod. J.* **2025**, *58*, 890–901. [CrossRef]
13. Evans, M. The endodontic-periodontal juncture: Where two worlds meet. An overview of endo-perio lesions. *Aust. Dent. J.* **2023**, *68*, S56–S65. [CrossRef]
14. Ghannam, M.G.; Alameddine, H.; Bordoni, B. Anatomy, Head and Neck, Pulp (Tooth). In *StatPearls [Internet]*; StatPearls Publishing: Treasure Island, FL, USA, 2024. [PubMed]
15. Sedani, S.; Kriplani, S.; Thakare, A.; Patel, A. The Hidden World Within: Microbial Dynamics in Root Canal Systems. *Cureus* **2024**, *16*, e60577. [CrossRef]

16. Karamifar, K.; Tondari, A.; Saghiri, M.A. Endodontic Periapical Lesion: An Overview on the Etiology, Diagnosis and Current Treatment Modalities. *Eur. Endod. J.* **2020**, *5*, 54–67. [CrossRef] [PubMed]
17. Plotino, G. *Minimally Invasive Approaches in Endodontic Practice*; Springer Nature Switzerland AG: Cham, Switzerland, 2021. [CrossRef]
18. Zhu, L.; Tang, Z.; Hu, R.; Gu, M.; Yang, Y. Ageing and Inflammation: What Happens in Periodontium? *Bioengineering* **2023**, *10*, 1274. [CrossRef] [PubMed]
19. Van Dyke, T.E.; Bartold, P.M.; Reynolds, E.C. The Nexus Between Periodontal Inflammation and Dysbiosis. *Front. Immunol.* **2020**, *11*, 511. [CrossRef] [PubMed]
20. Vertucci, F.J. Root canal anatomy of the human permanent teeth. *Oral Surg. Oral Med. Oral. Pathol.* **1984**, *58*, 589–599. [CrossRef]
21. Karabucak, B.; Setzer, F.C. Anatomy of the pulp–periodontal complex. *Dent. Clin. N. Am.* **2014**, *58*, 29–46. [CrossRef]
22. Mamat, R.; Nik Abdul Ghani, N.R. The complexity of the root canal anatomy and its influence on root canal debridement in the apical region: A review. *Cureus* **2023**, *15*, e49024. [CrossRef]
23. Chen, B.; Zhu, Y.; Lin, M.; Zhang, Y.; Li, Y.; Ouyang, X.; Ge, S.; Lin, J.; Pan, Y.; Xu, Y.; et al. Expert consensus on the diagnosis and therapy of endo-periodontal lesions. *Int. J. Oral Sci.* **2024**, *16*, 55. [CrossRef]
24. Ricucci, D.; Loghin, S.; Gonçalves, L.S.; Rôças, I.N.; Siqueira, J.F., Jr. Histobacteriologic conditions of the apical root canal system and periapical tissues in teeth associated with sinus tracts. *J. Endod.* **2018**, *44*, 405–413. [CrossRef]
25. Siqueira, J.F.; Rôças, I.N. Clinical implications and microbiology of bacterial persistence after treatment procedures. *J. Endod.* **2009**, *34*, 1291–1301. [CrossRef] [PubMed]
26. Durmazpınar, P.M.; Kanmaz, B.; Buduneli, N. Endo-Perio Lesions and Dentists' Treatment Approach: A Survey. *Med. Sci. Monit.* **2024**, *30*, e942544. [CrossRef] [PubMed]
27. Wong, I.; Ton, A.; Cassidy, A.J.; Fozzard, N.; Sharma, L.A.; Love, R.M.; Sharma, A. A retrospective study on the prognostic factors and success, survival, and failure outcomes of treated endodontic-periodontal lesions. *Clin. Exp. Dent. Res.* **2024**, *10*. [CrossRef]
28. Gulsahi, A.; Kulah, C.K.; Bakirarar, B.; Gulen, O.; Kamburoglu, K. Age estimation based on pulp/tooth volume ratio measured on cone-beam CT images. *Dentomaxillofac Radiol.* **2018**, *47*, 20170239. [CrossRef] [PubMed]
29. Meto, A.; Halilaj, G. The Integration of Cone Beam Computed Tomography, Artificial Intelligence, Augmented Reality, and Virtual Reality in Dental Diagnostics, Surgical Planning, and Education: A Narrative Review. *Appl. Sci.* **2025**, *15*, 6308. [CrossRef]
30. Al-Sibassi, A.; Niazi, S.A.; Clarke, P.; Adeyemi, A. Management of the endodontic-periodontal lesion. *Br. Dent. J.* **2025**, *238*, 536–544. [CrossRef]
31. Ichraq, O.; Mounsif, M.; Fennich, M.; El Yamani, A. A Multidisciplinary Approach in the Management of a Grade 3 Endo-Periodontal Lesion. *Cureus* **2025**, *17*, e85715. [CrossRef]
32. Armitage, G.C. Development of a classification system for periodontal diseases and conditions. *Ann. Periodontol.* **1999**, *4*, 1–6. [CrossRef]
33. Highfield, J. Diagnosis and classification of periodontal disease. *Aust. Dent. J.* **2009**, *54*, S11–S26. [CrossRef]

34. Shenoy, N.; Shenoy, A. Endo-perio lesions: Diagnosis and clinical considerations. *Indian J. Dent. Res.* **2010**, *21*, 579–585. [CrossRef]
35. Samir, P.V.; Mahapatra, N.; Dutta, B.; Bagchi, A.; Dhull, K.S.; Verma, R.K. A Correlation between Clinical Classification of Dental Pulp and Periapical Diseases with its Patho Physiology and Pain Pathway. *Int. J. Clin. Pediatr. Dent.* **2023**, *16*, 639–644. [CrossRef]
36. Al-Fouzan, K.S. A new classification of endodontic-periodontal lesions. *Int. J. Dent.* **2014**, *2014*, 919173. [CrossRef]
37. Tataryn, R.W.; Craig, J.R. Dental Evaluation: Endodontic and Periodontal. *Otolaryngol. Clin. N. Am.* **2024**, *57*, 1069–1082. [CrossRef] [PubMed]
38. Lee, A.H.C.; Neelakantan, P.; Dummer, P.M.H.; Zhang, C. Cemental tear: Literature review, proposed classification and recommendations for treatment. *Int. Endod. J.* **2021**, *54*, 2044–2073. [CrossRef]
39. Fiallos, N.d.M.; Ribeiro Aguiar, A.L.; da Silva, B.N.; Pergentino, M.L.M.; Rocha, M.F.G.; Sidrim, J.J.C.; Maia, D.C.B.d.S.C.; Cordeiro, R.d.A. The Potential of Phenothiazines against Endodontic Pathogens: A Focus on *Enterococcus-candida* Dual-Species Biofilm. *Antibiotics* **2022**, *11*, 1562. [CrossRef] [PubMed]
40. Sakanaka, A.; Kuboniwa, M.; Shimma, S.; Alghamdi, S.A.; Mayumi, S.; Lamont, R.J.; Fukusaki, E.; Amano, A. Fusobacterium nucleatum Metabolically Integrates Commensals and Pathogens in Oral Biofilms. *mSystems* **2022**, *7*, e0017022. [CrossRef]
41. Yekani, M.; Dastgir, M.; Fattahi, S.; Shahi, S.; Maleki Dizaj, S.; Memar, M.Y. Microbiological and molecular aspects of periodontitis pathogenesis: An infection-induced inflammatory condition. *Front. Cell. Infect. Microbiol.* **2025**, *15*, 1533658. [CrossRef] [PubMed]
42. Bezerra, B.; Monajemzadeh, S.; Silva, D.; Pirih, F.Q. Modulating the Immune Response in Periodontitis. *Front. Dent. Med.* **2022**, *3*, 879131. [CrossRef]
43. Erkihun, M.; Asmare, Z.; Endalamew, K.; Getie, B.; Kiros, T.; Berhan, A. Medical Scope of Biofilm and Quorum Sensing during Biofilm Formation: Systematic Review. *Bacteria* **2024**, *3*, 118–135. [CrossRef]
44. Luo, A.; Wang, F.; Sun, D.; Liu, X.; Xin, B. Formation, Development, and Cross-Species Interactions in Biofilms. *Front. Microbiol.* **2022**, *12*, 757327. [CrossRef]
45. Kozak, M.; Pawlik, A. The Role of the Oral Microbiome in the Development of Diseases. *Int. J. Mol. Sci.* **2023**, *24*, 5231. [CrossRef]
46. Dastpak, M.; Ghoddusi, J.; Jafarian, A.H.; Sarmad, M. Association between Clinical Symptoms and Histological Features of Molars with Acute Pulpitis. *Iran. Endod. J.* **2023**, *18*, 91–95. [CrossRef] [PubMed]
47. Renton, T. Dental (Odontogenic) Pain. *Rev. Pain.* **2011**, *5*, 2–7. [CrossRef] [PubMed]
48. Blake, A.; Tuttle, T.; McKinney, R. Apical Periodontitis. In *StatPearls [Internet]*; StatPearls Publishing: Treasure Island, FL, USA, 2024. Available online: https://www.ncbi.nlm.nih.gov/books/NBK589656/ (accessed on 17 July 2023).
49. Rathee, M.; Jain, P. Gingivitis. In *StatPearls [Internet]*; StatPearls Publishing: Treasure Island, FL, USA, 2024. Available online: https://www.ncbi.nlm.nih.gov/books/NBK557422/ (accessed on 27 March 2023).

50. Gasner, N.S.; Schure, R.S. Periodontal Disease. In *StatPearls [Internet]*; StatPearls Publishing: Treasure Island, FL, USA, 2024. Available online: https://www.ncbi.nlm.nih.gov/books/NBK554590/ (accessed on 10 April 2023).
51. Saad, W.; Almaslamani, M.; Saleh, A.R. Revascularization of a Permanent Tooth with Necrotic Pulp and Apical Periodontitis. *Clin. Cosmet. Investig. Dent.* **2024**, *16*, 227–235. [CrossRef]
52. Institute of Medicine (US) Committee on Emerging Microbial Threats to Health in the 21st Century; Smolinski, M.S.; Hamburg, M.A.; Lederberg, J. (Eds.) *Microbial Threats to Health: Emergence, Detection, and Response*; National Academies Press (US): Washington, DC, USA, 2003; Appendix C, Pathogen Discovery, Detection, and Diagnostics. Available online: https://www.ncbi.nlm.nih.gov/books/NBK221492/ (accessed on 11 June 2025).
53. Alhajj, M.; Zubair, M.; Farhana, A. Enzyme Linked Immunosorbent Assay. In *StatPearls [Internet]*; StatPearls Publishing: Treasure Island, FL, USA, 2024. Available online: https://www.ncbi.nlm.nih.gov/books/NBK555922/ (accessed on 23 April 2023).
54. Mahmood, T.; Yang, P.C. Western blot: Technique, theory, and trouble shooting. *N. Am. J. Med. Sci.* **2012**, *4*, 429–434. [CrossRef] [PubMed]
55. Whitfield, N.N.; Wolk, D.M. Identification of Pathogens by Nonculturing Molecular Techniques. In *The Prokaryotes*; Rosenberg, E., DeLong, E.F., Lory, S., Stackebrandt, E., Thompson, F., Eds.; Springer: Berlin/Heidelberg, Germany, 2013. [CrossRef]
56. Nafea, A.M.; Wang, Y.; Wang, D.; Salama, A.M.; Aziz, M.A.; Xu, S.; Tong, Y. Application of next-generation sequencing to identify different pathogens. *Front. Microbiol.* **2024**, *14*, 1329330. [CrossRef]
57. van Belkum, A.; Welker, M.; Pincus, D.; Charrier, J.P.; Girard, V. Matrix-Assisted Laser Desorption Ionization Time-of-Flight Mass Spectrometry in Clinical Microbiology: What Are the Current Issues? *Ann. Lab. Med.* **2017**, *37*, 475–483. [CrossRef]
58. Shakoori, A.R. Fluorescence In Situ Hybridization (FISH) and Its Applications. *Chromosome Struct. Aberrations* **2017**, 343–367. [CrossRef]
59. Mhade, S.; Kaushik, K.S. Tools of the Trade: Image Analysis Programs for Confocal Laser-Scanning Microscopy Studies of Biofilms and Considerations for Their Use by Experimental Researchers. *ACS Omega* **2023**, *8*, 20163–20177. [CrossRef]
60. Franzosa, E.A.; Morgan, X.C.; Segata, N.; Waldron, L.; Reyes, J.; Earl, A.M.; Giannoukos, G.; Boylan, M.R.; Ciulla, D.; Gevers, D.; et al. Relating the metatranscriptome and metagenome of the human gut. *Proc. Natl. Acad. Sci. USA* **2014**, *111*, E2329–E2338. [CrossRef]
61. Do, T.; Devine, D.; Marsh, P.D. Oral biofilms: Molecular analysis, challenges, and future prospects in dental diagnostics. *Clin Cosmet Investig Dent.* **2013**, *5*, 11-9. [CrossRef] [PubMed]
62. Lamont, R.J.; Hajishengallis, G. Polymicrobial synergy and dysbiosis in inflammatory disease. *Trends Mol. Med.* **2015**, *21*, 172–183. [CrossRef] [PubMed]
63. Allaker, R.P.; Stephen, A.S. Use of Probiotics and Oral Health. *Curr. Oral Health Rep.* **2017**, *4*, 309–318. [CrossRef] [PubMed]
64. Zhang, Y.; Ding, Y.; Guo, Q. Probiotic Species in the Management of Periodontal Diseases: An Overview. *Front. Cell. Infect. Microbiol.* **2022**, *12*, 806463. [CrossRef]

65. Retamal-Valdes, B.; Teughels, W.; Oliveira, L.M.; da Silva, R.N.; Fritoli, A.; Gomes, P.; Soares, G.M.S.; Temporão, N.; Furquim, C.P.; Duarte, P.M.; et al. Clinical, microbiological, and immunological effects of systemic probiotics in periodontal treatment: Study protocol for a randomized controlled trial. *Trials.* **2021**, *22*, 283. [CrossRef]
66. Sachelarie, L.; Scrobota, I.; Romanul, I.; Iurcov, R.; Potra Cicalau, G.I.; Todor, L. Probiotic Therapy as an Adjuvant in the Treatment of Periodontal Disease: An Innovative Approach. *Medicina* **2025**, *61*, 126. [CrossRef]
67. Vernon, J.J. Modulation of the Human Microbiome: Probiotics, Prebiotics, and Microbial Transplants. *Adv. Exp. Med. Biol.* **2025**, *1472*, 277–294. [CrossRef]
68. Luong, T.; Salabarria, A.C.; Roach, D.R. Phage Therapy in the Resistance Era: Where Do We Stand and Where Are We Going? *Clin. Ther.* **2020**, *42*, 1659–1680. [CrossRef]
69. Guo, X.; Wang, X.; Shi, J.; Ren, J.; Zeng, J.; Li, J.; Li, Y. A review and new perspective on oral bacteriophages: Manifestations in the ecology of oral diseases. *J. Oral Microbiol.* **2024**, *16*, 2344272. [CrossRef]
70. Kabwe, M.; Tucci, J.; Darby, I.; Dashper, S. Oral bacteriophages and their potential as adjunctive treatments for periodontitis: A narrative review. *J. Oral Microbiol.* **2025**, *17*, 2469890. [CrossRef] [PubMed]
71. Monteiro, T.M.; Cortes-Cid, V.O.; Marceliano-Alves, M.F.V.; Campello, A.F.; Bastos, L.F.; Lopes, R.T.; Siqueira, J.F., Jr.; Alves, F.R.F. Intracanal removal and apical extrusion of filling material after retreatment using rotary or reciprocating instruments: A new approach using human cadavers. *Int. Endod. J.* **2024**, *57*, 100–107. [CrossRef] [PubMed]
72. Gulabivala, K.; Ng, Y.L. Factors that affect the outcomes of root canal treatment and retreatment-A reframing of the principles. *Int. Endod. J.* **2023**, *56*, 82–115. [CrossRef]
73. Campos, G.O.; Dos Reis Prado, A.H.; de Assis Macedo, I.F.; da Costa Ferreira, I.; da Costa Ferreira, G.; Benetti, F.; da Cunha Peixoto, I.F.; Diniz Viana, A.C. Effect of Foraminal Enlargement on Periapical Healing in Necrotic Teeth: A Systematic Review. *Iran. Endod. J.* **2024**, *19*, 75–84. [CrossRef] [PubMed]
74. Ricucci, D. Apical limit of root canal instrumentation and obturation, part 1. Literature review. *Int. Endod. J.* **1998**, *31*, 384–393. [CrossRef]
75. Gazzaneo, I.; Amoroso-Silva, P.; Pacheco-Yanes, J.; Alves, F.R.F.; Marceliano-Alves, M.; Olivares, P.; Meto, A.; Mdala, I.; Siqueira, J.F., Jr.; Rôças, I.N. Disinfecting and Shaping Type I C-shaped Root Canals: A Correlative Micro-computed Tomographic and Molecular Microbiology Study. *J. Endod.* **2021**, *47*, 621–630. [CrossRef]
76. Baasch, A.; Campello, A.F.; Rodrigues, R.C.V.; Alves, F.R.F.; Voigt, D.D.; Mdala, I.; Perez, R.; Brasil, S.C.; Rôças, I.N.; Siqueira, J.F., Jr. Effects of the Irrigation Needle Design on Root Canal Disinfection and Cleaning. *J. Endod.* **2024**, *50*, 1463–1471. [CrossRef]
77. Loyola-Fonseca, S.C.; Campello, A.F.; Rodrigues, R.C.V.; Alves, F.R.F.; Brasil, S.C.; Vilela, C.L.S.; Gonçalves, L.S.; Provenzano, J.C.; Siqueira, J.F., Jr.; Rôças, I.N. Disinfection and Shaping of Vertucci Class II Root Canals after Preparation with Two Instrument Systems and Supplementary Ultrasonic Activation of Sodium Hypochlorite. *J. Endod.* **2023**, *49*, 1183–1190. [CrossRef]
78. Amoroso-Silva, P.; Brasil, S.C.; Pérez, A.R.; Tolentino, E.S.; Alves, F.R.F.; Siqueira, J.F., Jr.; Rôças, I.N. Influence of sealer type on treatment outcome of teeth with apical periodontitis: A systematic review. *Braz. Dent. J.* **2023**, *34*, 1–21. [CrossRef]

79. Ricucci, D.; Rôças, I.N.; Alves, F.R.F.; Cabello, P.H.; Siqueira, J.F., Jr. Outcome of Direct Pulp Capping Using Calcium Hydroxide: A Long-term Retrospective Study. *J. Endod.* **2023**, *49*, 45–54. [CrossRef]
80. Chung, W.C.; Huang, C.F.; Feng, S.W. Clinical Benefits of Minimally Invasive Non-Surgical Periodontal Therapy as an Alternative of Conventional Non-Surgical Periodontal Therapy-A Pilot Study. *Int. J. Environ. Res. Public Health* **2022**, *19*, 7456. [CrossRef]
81. El Meligy, O.A.; Elemam, N.M.; Talaat, I.M. Ozone Therapy in Medicine and Dentistry: A Review of the Literature. *Dent. J.* **2023**, *11*, 187. [CrossRef]
82. Jiang, Y.; Feng, J.; Du, J.; Fu, J.; Liu, Y.; Guo, L.; Liu, Y. Clinical and biochemical effect of laser as an adjunct to non-surgical treatment of chronic periodontitis. *Oral Dis.* **2022**, *28*, 1042–1057. [CrossRef]
83. Arias-Herrera, S.; Sánchez-Martos, R.; Alfaro-Ochoa, L. Introduction to Diode Laser Therapies in Dentistry [Internet]. Recent Advances and Future Perspectives in Periodontology [Working Title]. In *Frontiers in Periodontology—New Directions and Emerging Therapies*; IntechOpen: London, UK, 2024. [CrossRef]
84. Ribeiro, M.; Gomes, I.B.; Saavedra, M.J.; Simões, M. Photodynamic therapy and combinatory treatments for the control of biofilm-associated infections. *Lett. Appl. Microbiol.* **2022**, *75*, 548–564. [CrossRef]
85. Boehm, T.K.; Kim, C.S. Overview of Periodontal Surgical Procedures. In *StatPearls [Internet]*; StatPearls Publishing: Treasure Island, FL, USA, 2024. Available online: https://www.ncbi.nlm.nih.gov/books/NBK599507/ (accessed on 11 January 2024).
86. Thalakiriyawa, D.S.; Dissanayaka, W.L. Advances in Regenerative Dentistry Approaches: An Update. *Int. Dent. J.* **2024**, *74*, 25–34. [CrossRef] [PubMed]
87. Brignardello-Petersen, R. Apical underfilling, but not overfilling, in root canal treatment probably increases the odds of unfavorable outcomes. *J. Am. Dent. Assoc.* **2019**, *150*, e160. [CrossRef] [PubMed]
88. Cuellar, M.R.C.; Pereira, T.C.; de Vasconcelos, L.R.S.M.; Pedrinha, V.F.; Vivan, R.R.; Duarte, M.A.H.; de Andrade, F.B. Reducing Apical Bacterial Extrusion: The Impact of Reciproc File Size and Irrigation Technique. *Iran. Endod. J.* **2024**, *19*, 176–182.
89. Chaudhari, P.S.; Chandak, M.G.; Jaiswal, A.A.; Mankar, N.P.; Paul, P. A Breakthrough in the Era of Calcium Silicate-Based Cements: A Critical Review. *Cureus* **2022**, *14*, e28562. [CrossRef]
90. Enkhbileg, N.; Kim, J.W.; Chang, S.W.; Park, S.H.; Cho, K.M.; Lee, Y. A Study on Nanoleakage of Apical Retrograde Filling of Premixed Calcium Silicate-Based Cement Using a Lid Technique. *Materials* **2024**, *17*, 2366. [CrossRef] [PubMed]
91. Estivalet, M.S.; de Araújo, L.P.; Immich, F.; da Silva, A.F.; Ferreira, N.S.; da Rosa, W.L.O.; Piva, E. Bioactivity Potential of Bioceramic-Based Root Canal Sealers: A Scoping Review. *Life* **2022**, *12*, 1853. [CrossRef] [PubMed]
92. Washio, A.; Morotomi, T.; Yoshii, S.; Kitamura, C. Bioactive Glass-Based Endodontic Sealer as a Promising Root Canal Filling Material without Semisolid Core Materials. *Materials* **2019**, *12*, 3967. [CrossRef] [PubMed]

4. What Do We Know About Propolis in Modern Dentistry?

4.1. Propolis: A Lasting Link Between People and Bees

Often revered as nature's tireless architects, bees have long captivated the human imagination with their ability to build intricate hives, produce honey, and play a crucial role in pollination, activities that support the ecosystem (Figure 13). Among the myriad wonders of the hive, propolis stands out as a remarkable substance that exemplifies the ingenuity of these small yet mighty creatures. Propolis, a resinous compound, is meticulously made by bees (*Apis mellifera* L.) when they gather resin from tree buds, sap flows, and other botanical sources, blending it with beeswax and enzymes from their saliva. This compound is vital to the hive's structure, serving to fortify the hive, seal gaps, smooth surfaces, and protect the colony from external threats [1]. The name "propolis" is derived from the Greek words "pro", meaning "in front of", and "polis", meaning "city", reflecting its critical role in defending and maintaining the hive, much like a city's fortifications protect its inhabitants.

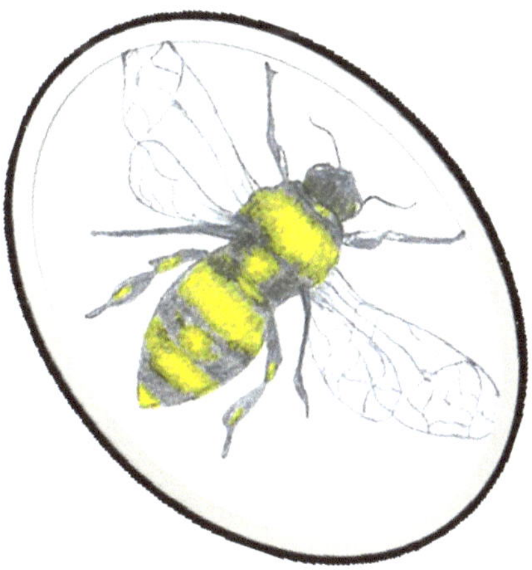

Bees, nature's golden architects, create delicate patterns of life and sweetness.

Figure 13. A bee illustration. Credit: © Nensi Kallfani, used with permission.

The use of propolis is not a modern phenomenon; its application dates back to ancient civilizations, where it was highly esteemed for its healing properties, particularly in treating wounds and infections. Archeological evidence suggests that humans have been practicing beekeeping for at least 8500 years, underscoring the deep-rooted and symbiotic relationship between humans and bees. This long-standing connection has provided humans with honey, beeswax, and propolis, each with significant therapeutic potential recognized and utilized for thousands of years [1].

In ancient Egypt, around 3000 BC, propolis played a crucial role in the mummification process. The Egyptians, aware of its antiseptic and preservative properties, used propolis to embalm mummies, preventing decay and ensuring their preservation for the afterlife. Additionally, propolis was employed in treating various skin conditions and wounds, showcasing its ability to promote healing and prevent infections. The significance of propolis was similarly acknowledged in ancient Greece and Rome. Hippocrates, often referred to as the "Father of Medicine," prescribed propolis for treating sores and ulcers, both externally and internally. Aristotle also documented the use of propolis as a natural remedy for infections and wounds, highlighting its versatile therapeutic properties. The Romans, who expanded upon Greek medical knowledge, used propolis extensively to reduce swelling, relieve pain, and treat a variety of ailments, embedding its use deeply into the medical traditions of the time [2,3].

Throughout the Middle Ages, propolis maintained its prominence as a medicinal substance across Europe. It was widely used in folk medicine to treat infections, wounds, and skin disorders, and its applications extended to oral health. The Renaissance period saw continued reliance on propolis, with European apothecaries and herbalists incorporating it into treatments for respiratory infections, skin ailments, and as an essential ingredient in balms and salves. By the 17th and 18th centuries, propolis was officially recognized in the London Pharmacopoeia as a valuable medicinal resource, solidifying its status as a legitimate therapeutic agent. In the 19th century, propolis became especially popular in Russia, where it earned the nickname "Russian penicillin" due to its potent antibacterial properties. Russian soldiers utilized propolis during World War II to treat wounds, benefiting from its ability to prevent infection and accelerate healing [4].

The 20th century marked a significant turning point in the understanding and application of propolis as scientific research began to uncover its complex chemical composition and therapeutic properties. Early studies identified a variety of bioactive compounds in propolis, including flavonoids, phenolic acids, and terpenoids, which are largely responsible for its antimicrobial, anti-inflammatory, and antioxidant effects. As research expanded globally, the diverse chemical composition of propolis, shaped by the botanical sources available to bees in different regions, became increasingly documented. This knowledge led to the incorporation of propolis into a wide range of commercial products, such as creams, ointments, lozenges, and mouthwashes, making its benefits accessible to a broader audience [5].

In the 21st century, the interest in propolis has continued to grow, driven by a broader trend towards natural and alternative medicines. Scientific studies have explored its potential applications in various fields, including dentistry, dermatology, and oncology. Propolis is now widely recognized in dental care for its ability to reduce plaque formation, treat gum diseases, and enhance overall oral health. Furthermore, ongoing research is investigating the potential of propolis in cancer treatment and immune system support, underscoring its relevance in modern medicine [6,7].

4.2. *Chemical Composition of Propolis*

Biochemical Composition of Propolis and Its Relevance to Oral Health

Propolis is a heterogeneous resinous mixture produced by honeybees from plant exudates, enriched with bees' own enzymes and waxes. Its composition is influenced by botanical source, geographical location, and seasonal variation, factors that in turn determine biological activities [8,9].

Typical major fractions include resins (50–70%), waxes (30–50%), essential oils (5–10%), pollen (~5%), and a wide variety of bioactive organic compounds. Among these, flavonoids, phenolic acids and their esters, and terpenoids play the most prominent roles in oral health, supported by essential fatty acids, amino acids, vitamins, and minerals. These components interact synergistically to inhibit oral pathogens, modulate inflammatory responses, and promote tissue regeneration [10,11].

Propolis is a complex and unique natural substance collected by bees from a variety of plant sources. Its composition is highly variable, depending on the geographical location and the specific plants available to the bees. This variability contributes to the diverse biological activities and medicinal properties attributed to propolis. The primary components of propolis include resins, waxes, essential oils, pollen, and a variety of organic compounds such as flavonoids and phenolic acids:

Resins (50–70%): Resins make up the bulk of propolis, accounting for 50% to 70% of its composition. These resins are primarily derived from the exudates of trees and other plants, which bees collect and then modify using their own enzymes. The primary components of these resins include flavonoids, phenolic acids, and their esters. These compounds are critical to the biological activity of propolis, contributing to its therapeutic properties.

Waxes (30–50%): Waxes comprise about 30% to 50% of propolis and serve as a binding agent, helping to hold the other components together. These waxes are primarily composed of long-chain fatty acids and alcohols, which contribute to the physical properties of propolis, such as its stickiness and ability to form protective barriers.

Essential oils (10%): Essential oils make up around 10% of propolis and provide it with its distinctive aroma. These oils are complex mixtures of volatile organic compounds, including terpenes and aromatic acids, which contribute to the antimicrobial and anti-inflammatory properties of propolis.

Pollen (5%): Pollen constitutes about 5% of propolis and is an essential component, providing various nutrients and contributing to the overall biological activity of propolis. Pollen in propolis is rich in proteins, vitamins, and minerals, which enhance its nutritional value.

Phenolic acids: Phenolic acids are another crucial component of propolis, known for their antioxidant and anti-inflammatory properties. These compounds, such as caffeic acid and ferulic acid, work synergistically with flavonoids to enhance the therapeutic effects of propolis. The concentration and types of phenolic acids in propolis vary depending on the botanical sources available to the bees, similar to flavonoids [12,13].

Other organic compounds: In addition, propolis contains various other organic compounds that contribute to its medicinal properties. These include vitamins, amino acids, and bioactive enzymes, which collectively enhance the health benefits of propolis.

Below is a detailed exploration of the chemical composition of propolis, highlighting its major components and their significance, starting with the following:

Flavonoids: A major component of propolis, flavonoids are a diverse group of phytonutrients (plant chemicals) found in many fruits, vegetables, and other plant products. These compounds are renowned for their potent biological activities, contributing to the wide range of medicinal properties attributed to propolis. The composition of flavonoids in propolis varies significantly depending on the geographical location, botanical sources available to bees, and environmental factors, making the study of these compounds both complex and fascinating. For example, propolis from temperate regions tends to be rich in flavonoids like galangin, pinocembrin, and chrysin, while propolis from tropical regions may contain different flavonoid profiles [14,15].

Propolis collected from various regions of Poland has been extensively studied, revealing a rich and varied flavonoid profile. These flavonoids are responsible for much of the biological activity associated with Polish propolis, including its antimicrobial, antioxidant, and anti-inflammatory properties. The diversity in the chemical composition of propolis from different regions underscores the influence of local flora on the flavonoid content, highlighting the importance of geographical factors in the therapeutic efficacy of propolis [14].

One of the significant advancements in understanding the role of flavonoids in propolis has been through the study of their biotransformation and metabolite activity in vivo. Research has shown that once ingested, flavonoids undergo various metabolic processes that enhance or modify their biological activity. This transformation is crucial for the bioavailability and efficacy of flavonoids, determining how these compounds exert their beneficial effects on the human body. For instance, certain flavonoid metabolites have been identified with enhanced anti-inflammatory and antioxidant properties, offering deeper insights into how propolis can be used effectively in therapeutic settings [15].

Historically, the identification and study of flavonoids in propolis dates back several decades. Early research, such as that conducted by Popravko and colleagues in 1969, laid the foundation for understanding the chemical diversity of flavonoids in propolis. Their work identified key flavonoid components that continue to be of interest in contemporary research due to their significant biological activities, including antimicrobial and anti-inflammatory effects. This pioneering research paved the way for further studies into the therapeutic potential of propolis flavonoids [12].

In more recent times, flavonoids found in propolis have gained attention for their potential in combating photoaging and psoriasis. These skin conditions, characterized by inflammation and oxidative stress, have shown positive responses to treatments incorporating propolis flavonoids. The antioxidant properties of these compounds are particularly beneficial in reducing the damage caused by ultraviolet (UV) radiation, a major factor in photoaging. Additionally, the anti-inflammatory effects of flavonoids help alleviate the symptoms of psoriasis, making them a promising component in skincare and dermatological applications [16].

The extraction, purification, and characterization of flavonoids from propolis have been subjects of intense study. Researchers have developed various methods to isolate and analyze these compounds, aiming to enhance their therapeutic potential. The biological properties of propolis flavonoids, including their antimicrobial, anti-inflammatory, and antioxidant effects, are closely linked to their chemical structure, which varies based on the source and method of extraction. This ongoing research is crucial for developing standardized propolis-based products with consistent efficacy and safety profiles [17].

Phenolic acids in propolis: Among the bioactive components of propolis, phenolic acids stand out for their substantial contributions to its antioxidant, antimicrobial, and anti-inflammatory effects. These organic compounds, whose concentrations vary depending on the geographical origin of the propolis, are essential in determining the therapeutic potential of this natural substance. Primarily derived from the plant resins that bees collect and metabolize, the phenolic acids in propolis are renowned for their potent antioxidant capabilities. These acids effectively neutralize free radicals, safeguarding cells from oxidative stress and contributing to the overall health benefits of propolis. This action is crucial in preventing various chronic diseases, including cardiovascular diseases and cancer. The antioxidant potential of phenolic acids is one of the primary reasons propolis has been historically and continues to be used in traditional medicine across different cultures [18].

One of the significant studies conducted on propolis samples from different regions of Anatolia demonstrated that the phenolic content varies significantly depending on the botanical sources available to bees in each region. This study utilized Principal Component Analysis (PCA) to cluster propolis samples based on their phenolic profiles, highlighting the diversity in composition and its implications for antioxidant and antimicrobial activities. The research underscores how regional factors influence the chemical makeup of propolis, particularly its phenolic acids, which are crucial for its biological efficacy [18].

Another critical study focused on the analysis of phenolic acids in propolis using High-Performance Liquid Chromatography (HPLC) techniques, providing detailed insights into the specific types of phenolic acids present in propolis samples. This study identified and quantified several key phenolic acids, including caffeic acid, p-coumaric acid, and ferulic acid, among others. These compounds are well-known for their health-promoting properties, including anti-inflammatory effects, which are essential in managing conditions such as arthritis and other inflammatory disorders. The HPLC analysis also highlighted the consistency and variability of phenolic acid content in propolis, depending on its geographical and botanical origins [19].

The antimicrobial activity of phenolic acids in propolis is another area of significant interest. These compounds have been shown to inhibit the growth of a wide range of pathogens, including bacteria, fungi, and viruses. This makes propolis a potent natural antimicrobial agent, capable of enhancing the body's defense mechanisms and preventing infections. The phenolic acids in propolis disrupt the cell membranes of pathogens, inhibit their enzyme activity, and interfere with their metabolic processes, leading to their eventual destruction. This antimicrobial property is particularly valuable in the development of natural health products and treatments aimed at combating antibiotic-resistant strains of bacteria [18].

Esters in propolis: Vital components with multifaceted biological activities, esters play a crucial role in the therapeutic potential of propolis. These compounds, formed through the reaction of an alcohol with an acid, are abundant in propolis and are particularly noted for their diverse biological activities, including anti-inflammatory, neuroprotective, hepatoprotective, and cardioprotective effects. One of the most well-studied esters in propolis is CAPE, which has garnered considerable attention for its wide range of health benefits. CAPE is a potent bioactive compound with a plethora of biological activities that make it a valuable component of propolis. It exerts strong antioxidant and anti-inflammatory effects by inhibiting the nuclear factor kappa B (NF-κB) pathway, a protein complex that plays a crucial role in regulating immune response, cytokine production, and cell survival. This inhibition reduces the production of pro-inflammatory cytokines and enzymes, thereby mitigating inflammation. CAPE also possesses antiviral and antibacterial properties, making it a versatile compound in the fight against various pathogens. Furthermore, it has demonstrated protective effects against cancer by inducing apoptosis in cancer cells and inhibiting tumor growth. Its ability to support immune function and protect against neurodegenerative diseases further underscores its significance as a therapeutic agent in both traditional and modern medicine [20]. The hepatoprotective properties of CAPE are another area of significant interest. Studies have shown that CAPE can protect liver cells from damage caused by toxins and oxidative stress, making it a promising candidate for the treatment of liver diseases. This protective effect is largely attributed to CAPE's ability to enhance the body's antioxidant defense mechanisms and reduce lipid peroxidation, a process that leads to cell membrane damage [20].

In addition to CAPE, propolis contains other esters that contribute to its therapeutic potential. Ferulic acid esters are another crucial group of esters in propolis, known for their potent antioxidant properties. These esters protect cells from oxidative stress, which is a major contributor to aging and various chronic diseases. Ferulic acid esters also exhibit anti-inflammatory and antimicrobial activities, contributing to the overall health benefits of propolis. Their ability to enhance skin health is particularly notable; they protect the skin from UV-induced damage, promote wound healing, and reduce signs of aging. Additionally, ferulic acid esters support cardiovascular health by mitigating oxidative damage to blood vessels, thereby reducing the risk of heart disease [21].

Chlorogenic acid esters are recognized for their powerful antioxidant and anti-inflammatory effects. These esters play a significant role in modulating glucose metabolism, making them beneficial for managing blood sugar levels and preventing diabetes-related complications. Chlorogenic acid esters also exhibit antimicrobial properties, enhancing the efficacy of propolis in fighting off infections. Moreover, these esters protect the liver from oxidative damage, reduce the risk of cardiovascular diseases, and contribute to overall metabolic health [22]. For instance, esters in propolis have been utilized in the functionalization of materials such as cellulose nanofiber/poly(vinyl alcohol) porous hydrogels. These hydrogels, enriched with Egyptian propolis extract, exhibit enhanced biological activities, including antimicrobial and wound-healing properties. This application highlights the versatility of esters in propolis, extending their use beyond traditional medicinal applications to advanced biomedical engineering and material sciences [22].

Cinnamic acid esters are widely studied for their antimicrobial and antioxidant activities. These esters inhibit the growth of various pathogens, including bacteria, fungi, and viruses, making them crucial components of propolis's antimicrobial efficacy. They also protect cells from oxidative damage, which can lead to inflammation and various chronic diseases. In addition to their antimicrobial properties, cinnamic acid esters support skin health by reducing inflammation and preventing infections, thereby promoting faster wound healing and healthier skin [23].

Benzoic acid benzyl ester is another important ester in propolis, known primarily for its antimicrobial properties. This ester is frequently used in various formulations for its preservative effects, helping to extend the shelf life of products while preventing microbial contamination. Its role in propolis contributes to the substance's overall ability to protect against infections and preserve its bioactive components [23].

Waxes in propolis, the role of long-chain fatty acids in structural integrity and biological activity: Waxes in propolis, which constitute 30% to 50% of its composition, are primarily made up of long-chain fatty acids (LCFAs) and their esters. These waxes play a critical role in providing the structural matrix that holds propolis together, contributing to its physical properties such as viscosity and adhesiveness. The

LCFAs found in propolis not only support its structural integrity but also contribute to various biological activities, making them essential components of this natural substance. Below is a detailed exploration of the key LCFAs found in propolis, highlighting their functions and associated health benefits.

Palmitic acid (C16:0) is a saturated fatty acid and one of the most common long-chain fatty acids found in propolis. It serves as a major component of cell membranes and is a precursor for the synthesis of other lipids, including triglycerides and phospholipids. It provides structural stability to cell membranes, which is crucial for maintaining cell integrity and function. It also supports energy storage and plays a vital role in the production of signaling molecules that regulate various biological processes. The presence of palmitic acid in propolis contributes to its overall stability and bioactivity, enhancing its effectiveness in various applications [24].

Stearic acid (C18:0) is another saturated fatty acid commonly found in propolis. It is involved in the formation of cell membranes and also serves as a significant energy source for cells. It is known for its neutral impact on cholesterol levels, distinguishing it from other saturated fats. It helps maintain the integrity of cell structures, which is essential for the proper functioning of various tissues, including skin and cardiovascular tissues. The inclusion of stearic acid in propolis supports its role in promoting skin health and protecting against oxidative damage [25].

Oleic acid (C18:1) is a monounsaturated fatty acid that plays a crucial role in maintaining the fluidity of cell membranes. It is involved in various metabolic processes, including the regulation of cholesterol levels. It supports cardiovascular health by reducing levels of low-density lipoprotein (LDL) cholesterol, often referred to as "bad" cholesterol, while increasing high-density lipoprotein (HDL) cholesterol, known as "good" cholesterol. It also exhibits anti-inflammatory and antioxidant properties, making it beneficial for reducing inflammation and protecting cells from oxidative stress. The presence of oleic acid in propolis enhances its cardiovascular protective effects and contributes to its overall health benefits [26].

Linoleic acid (C18:2) is a polyunsaturated fatty acid that is essential for human health. It serves as a precursor for the synthesis of other important fatty acids and signaling molecules, including prostaglandins, which are involved in inflammation and immune responses. It is crucial for maintaining healthy skin and cell membranes. It supports immune function and plays a significant role in modulating inflammatory responses. The presence of linoleic acid in propolis contributes to its anti-inflammatory and skin-protective properties, making it effective in promoting wound healing and reducing the signs of aging [27].

Arachidic acid (C20:0) is a saturated fatty acid that contributes to the structural integrity of cell membranes, particularly in nerve tissues where it plays a role in maintaining membrane stability and function. It supports the stability and function of cell membranes, which is especially important for the proper functioning of nerve cells. Its presence in propolis contributes to the substance's neuroprotective properties, aiding in the maintenance of nervous system health and the prevention of neurodegenerative conditions [28].

Essential oils and aromatic compounds in propolis: their roles and health benefits: Essential oils in propolis, comprising 5% to 10% of its composition, are volatile aromatic compounds that significantly contribute to the scent and biological activities of propolis. Among these, terpenes stand out as a major group of compounds responsible for the aromatic properties and diverse biological activities of propolis. Terpenes vary widely, ranging from simple monoterpenes to more complex triterpenes, each offering unique benefits, such as antimicrobial, anti-inflammatory, and antioxidant effects.

Monoterpenes, such as pinene and limonene, are the simplest form of terpenes, consisting of two isoprene units. These volatile compounds are responsible for the characteristic aroma of propolis and play a crucial role in its antimicrobial properties, making propolis effective against a variety of pathogens. Additionally, monoterpenes possess anti-inflammatory and antioxidant activities, contributing to the overall health benefits of propolis.

Sesquiterpenes, including β-caryophyllene and α-cubebene, consist of three isoprene units and are known for their more complex structures and diverse biological activities. β-caryophyllene, in particular, interacts with cannabinoid receptors, providing pain relief and strong anti-inflammatory effects. These sesquiterpenes enhance the antimicrobial efficacy of propolis, further supporting its use in treating infections and inflammatory conditions [29].

Diterpenes, such as lupeol and β-amyrin, are composed of four isoprene units and are typically found in plant resins. These compounds are less volatile than monoterpenes and sesquiterpenes but exhibit a wide range of biological activities, including anti-inflammatory, anticancer, and antimicrobial properties. Lupeol, for instance, is noted for its potential in treating skin disorders and cancer, highlighting the therapeutic value of diterpenes in propolis [30].

Triterpenes, such as the triterpenoid β-amyrin, consist of six isoprene units and are commonly found in plant resins and waxes. These compounds are renowned for their anti-inflammatory and hepatoprotective effects, making them effective in treating various inflammatory conditions and protecting liver health. The presence of triterpenes in propolis underscores its potential in managing chronic inflammatory diseases and supporting overall health.

Aromatic compounds are a significant and diverse class of components within propolis, and they play multiple essential roles that contribute to both its therapeutic efficacy and its distinctive sensory characteristics. Among these compounds, vanillin and eugenol are particularly notable. Vanillin, an aromatic aldehyde, is responsible for imparting a sweet, vanilla-like aroma to propolis, which not only enhances its sensory appeal but also contributes significantly to its biological activities. Vanillin possesses strong antimicrobial properties, which enable it to inhibit the growth of various pathogens, including bacteria and fungi. This antimicrobial activity is particularly valuable in the context of wound healing and infection prevention, where the control of microbial growth is crucial. Additionally, it exhibits antioxidant properties, which help protect cells from oxidative stress and contribute to the overall stability of propolis-based formulations [30].

Eugenol, another key aromatic compound found in propolis, is well-known for its potent antimicrobial and anti-inflammatory properties. This compound is commonly used in various medicinal and dental applications due to its ability to alleviate pain and reduce inflammation, making it a valuable component in treating oral infections and inflammatory skin conditions. The presence of eugenol in propolis enhances its effectiveness in managing wounds and infections, contributing to faster healing and reduced risk of secondary infections. Furthermore, eugenol's role in stabilizing propolis formulations ensures that these products maintain their efficacy over time, even under varying environmental conditions [29].

In addition to vanillin and eugenol, aromatic acids such as cinnamic acid and benzoic acid play crucial roles in the preservation and stability of propolis. Cinnamic acid, with its strong antimicrobial and anti-inflammatory properties, is particularly effective in preventing the growth of harmful microorganisms, thereby protecting wounds from infection and promoting healing. It also contributes to the structural stability of propolis, ensuring that its bioactive components remain intact and effective over time. Benzoic acid, another important aromatic acid in propolis, serves as a natural preservative. It helps extend the shelf life of propolis products by inhibiting microbial growth, which is essential for maintaining the quality and safety of these natural remedies. The combined action of these aromatic acids makes propolis a robust natural treatment for a variety of skin conditions, from minor cuts and abrasions to more serious infections [23].

The role of pollen in propolis: enhancing nutritional value and biological activities: Pollen, comprising 5% to 10% of propolis, plays a vital role in enhancing both the nutritional value and the biological activities of this remarkable natural substance. Pollen grains in propolis are rich in proteins and amino acids, essential nutrients that contribute to various biological functions. These compounds are critical for tissue repair, immune function, and enzyme activity, making them indispensable to the therapeutic properties of propolis.

Among the key proteins and amino acids found in propolis, leucine stands out for its crucial role in protein synthesis and muscle repair. As an essential amino acid, leucine is vital for initiating the process of protein synthesis in muscles, thereby supporting muscle growth and recovery. It also plays a significant role in regulating blood sugar levels by promoting insulin release. This dual action makes leucine particularly beneficial for athletes and individuals recovering from injury, as well as for maintaining stable blood sugar levels, which is crucial for overall metabolic health [24].

Tryptophan, another essential amino acid present in propolis, serves as a precursor to serotonin, a neurotransmitter that regulates mood, sleep, and appetite. Adequate levels of tryptophan can lead to improved mood and better sleep quality by increasing serotonin levels, which helps reduce anxiety and depression. Additionally, tryptophan's role in appetite control can be beneficial for weight management, contributing to overall mental and physical well-being [26].

Lysine is essential for the formation of collagen, a protein necessary for healthy skin, bones, and connective tissues. This amino acid also enhances calcium absorption, which is important for bone health, and supports immune function by promoting the production of antibodies. Lysine's involvement in collagen synthesis not only aids in faster wound healing and recovery from injuries but also helps maintain healthy skin and prevent bone disorders like osteoporosis [27].

Arginine is a semi-essential amino acid that plays a pivotal role in protein synthesis and the production of nitric oxide, a compound that helps relax blood vessels and improve blood flow. Arginine's ability to enhance blood circulation makes it beneficial for cardiovascular health, while its role in promoting the formation of new blood vessels supports wound healing. Additionally, arginine boosts immune function by stimulating the activity of white blood cells, enhancing the body's ability to fight infections [28].

Histidine is another important amino acid found in propolis, crucial for tissue growth and repair, the production of red and white blood cells, and the protection of nerve cells. Histidine also serves as a precursor to histamine, which plays a significant role in immune responses. By supporting the production of hemoglobin, histidine helps prevent anemia and contributes to overall neurological health by protecting nerve cells from damage [26,27].

The biological activity of propolis is significantly enhanced by the presence of pollen. Pollen contributes to the antimicrobial and anti-inflammatory properties of propolis, making it more effective in treating infections and inflammatory conditions. Furthermore, the immune-modulating effects of propolis are boosted by the proteins and amino acids found in pollen, which help strengthen the immune system and improve the body's ability to resist diseases and heal wounds [23].

Other chemical compounds in propolis: Vitamins, Minerals, and Sugars: Propolis is a complex natural substance that contains a wide array of chemical compounds, including vitamins, minerals, sugars, and organic acids, each contributing to its overall health benefits. These compounds work synergistically to enhance the biological activities of propolis, making it a powerful natural remedy with diverse therapeutic applications.

Vitamins in propolis: Propolis is rich in various vitamins that play crucial roles in numerous biochemical processes in the human body, including immune support, antioxidant protection, and metabolic functions. Among these, the B vitamins stand out as essential components. The B vitamin complex found in propolis includes B1 (thiamine), B2 (riboflavin), B3 (niacin), B5 (pantothenic acid), B6 (pyridoxine), B7 (biotin), B9 (folate), and B12 (cobalamin). These vitamins are vital for various metabolic processes and overall health.

Vitamin B1 (Thiamine) is crucial for energy production as it helps convert carbohydrates into energy and plays a role in nerve function. Adequate thiamine levels support optimal brain function and prevent complications such as beriberi [23]. Vitamin B2 (Riboflavin) is essential for energy production and the metabolism of fats, drugs, and steroids. It aids in the conversion of tryptophan to niacin and supports antioxidant activity, helping to maintain healthy skin, eyes, and nerve functions [24]. Vitamin B3 (Niacin) is involved in DNA repair and the production of stress- and sex-related hormones in the adrenal glands, which improves circulation and cholesterol levels, thereby reducing the risk of cardiovascular diseases and enhancing cognitive function [27]. Vitamin B5 (Pantothenic Acid) is vital for the synthesis of coenzyme A (CoA), which is important for fatty acid metabolism and energy production. It supports the health of skin, hair, eyes, liver, and the nervous system [28]. Vitamin B6 (Pyridoxine) is involved in amino acid metabolism, neurotransmitter synthesis, and the production of hemoglobin, supporting brain health, mood regulation, and immune function [27,28]. Vitamin B7 (Biotin) is essential for the metabolism of fats, carbohydrates, and proteins, supporting the health of hair, skin, and nails [24]. Vitamin B9 (Folate) is crucial for DNA synthesis, repair, and methylation, particularly important during periods of rapid growth such as pregnancy and infancy, helping to prevent neural tube defects in newborns [23]. Vitamin B12 (Cobalamin) is essential for red blood cell formation, neurological function, and DNA synthesis, helping to prevent anemia, support brain health, and maintain nerve function [26].

Vitamin C (Ascorbic Acid) is a powerful antioxidant that protects cells from damage by free radicals, aids in collagen synthesis, and supports the immune system. It enhances wound healing and helps prevent scurvy, a disease resulting from vitamin C deficiency [27]. Vitamin E (Tocopherol) acts as an antioxidant, protecting cell membranes from oxidative damage. It also plays a role in immune function, skin health, and the prevention of chronic diseases such as cardiovascular issues and cancer, while maintaining healthy skin and hair [24].

Minerals in propolis: Propolis is also rich in a variety of essential minerals that contribute to its health benefits and biological activities. These minerals play vital roles in numerous physiological processes and help support overall health [29,30].

Magnesium (Mg) is essential for over 300 enzymatic reactions in the body, including energy production, protein synthesis, and muscle and nerve function. Mg supports cardiovascular health, helps regulate blood pressure, and is crucial for bone health, as well as reducing symptoms of anxiety and improving sleep quality [28]. Calcium (Ca) is the most abundant mineral in the body, crucial for building and maintaining strong bones and teeth. It also plays a role in muscle contraction, blood clotting, and nerve transmission, helping to prevent osteoporosis and supporting heart and muscle functions [28]. Potassium (K) is vital for maintaining proper cell function, fluid balance, and nerve signaling. It helps regulate heart rhythm and muscle contractions, supporting cardiovascular health by lowering blood pressure and reducing the risk of stroke [23]. Sodium (Na) is essential for maintaining fluid balance, transmitting nerve impulses, and ensuring proper muscle function. However, it is important to balance sodium intake to prevent hypertension and associated cardiovascular diseases [27]. Copper (Cu) is involved in the formation of red blood cells, the absorption and utilization of iron, and the maintenance of healthy bones, blood vessels, nerves, and immune function, supporting cardiovascular health and connective tissue formation [24]. Zinc (Zn) is crucial for immune function, protein synthesis, wound healing, DNA synthesis, and cell division. It supports normal growth and development, particularly during pregnancy, childhood, and adolescence, and has antioxidant properties that protect against free radical damage [26]. Manganese (Mn) is involved in bone formation, blood clotting, and reducing inflammation, playing a role in carbohydrate, amino acid, and cholesterol metabolism [26]. Iron (Fe) is essential for the production of hemoglobin, which carries oxygen in the blood, and plays a role in energy metabolism and immune function, preventing anemia and enhancing immune response [23].

Sugars in propolis: Although propolis typically contains very low amounts of sugars, traces of certain sugars contribute to its overall composition and potential benefits.

Glucose is a simple sugar that serves as a primary energy source for cells, essential for metabolic processes and energy production. In small amounts, glucose provides a quick source of energy, supporting various cellular activities and maintaining proper cellular function. Fructose is a naturally occurring sugar found in many plants, metabolized primarily in the liver, where it is converted into glucose or stored as glycogen. It serves as an alternative energy source, supporting energy metabolism without causing significant spikes in blood sugar levels [27]. Sucrose is a disaccharide composed of glucose and fructose, providing a rapid release of energy. In trace amounts found in propolis, it supports quick metabolic boosts without significant health risks [23].

The following table (Table 12) offers a comprehensive overview of the key bioactive compounds in propolis, including flavonoids, phenolic acids, esters, long-chain fatty acids, terpenes, aromatic compounds, proteins, amino acids, vitamins, minerals, and sugars. Each compound's primary functions and associated health benefits are detailed, illustrating the broad therapeutic potential of propolis as a natural remedy.

Table 12. Comprehensive summary of bioactive compounds in propolis, their functions, and associated health benefits.

Compound Types	Specific Compounds	Functions	Health Benefits
Flavonoids [4–8,12–18,21–23]	**Galangin**	Antioxidant; scavenges free radicals, protecting cells from oxidative stress [12,15,17].	Anti-inflammatory, antimicrobial, and anticancer properties aiding systemic health maintenance [4,7,16].
	Apigenin	Strong anti-inflammatory and antioxidant; inhibits inflammatory enzyme cascades [15–17,21].	Reduces chronic disease risk (cancer, cardiovascular), exhibits neuroprotective effects [7,17].
	Pinocembrin	Antioxidant and anti-inflammatory; modulates immune responses, counters microbial infections [5,7,14,17].	Enhances neuroprotection, supports cardiovascular and immune health [15,16,18].
	Pinostrobin	Exhibits antimicrobial and anti-inflammatory activity; mitigates oxidative stress [5,13,15].	Reduces inflammation and infection risk; therapeutic potential in inflammatory conditions [14,18].
	Kaempferol	Strong antioxidant, reduces oxidative and inflammatory stress [7,14,17].	Lowers chronic disease risks, supports brain health, anti-aging effects [9,15,16].
	Chrysin	Anti-inflammatory, antioxidant; inhibits pro-oxidant enzymes [7,15,17,18].	Reduces anxiety, improves testosterone, anticancer properties [7,17].
	Quercetin	Stabilizes cell membranes, reduces histamine release; powerful antioxidant [7,13,14,17].	Supports cardiovascular and immune health, reduces allergy symptoms, anticancer potential [4,9,16].

Table 12. *Cont.*

Compound Types	Specific Compounds	Functions	Health Benefits
Phenolic Acids [5,7,13,14,17,19–23]	**Caffeic Acid**	Inhibits free radical formation, antioxidant and anti-inflammatory [19,20].	Protects cells from oxidative stress and inflammation; lowers chronic disease risk [7,20,21].
	p-Coumaric Acid	Antimicrobial and antioxidant activity [13,14,19].	Prevents microbial infections, supports immunity, enhances antioxidant defense [7,14].
	Ferulic Acid	Anti-inflammatory, antioxidant [5,7,19].	Protects cardiovascular health, reduces inflammation, anticancer potential [9,19,21].
	Gallic Acid	Strong antioxidant, antimicrobial [7,13,14].	Promotes wound healing, protects from oxidative damage, anticancer properties [7,9].
	Cinnamic Acid	Antimicrobial, antifungal, anti-inflammatory [5,13,14].	Inhibits microbial growth, supports immune health [7,13].
Esters [5,7,13,14,20–23]	**Caffeic Acid Phenethyl Ester (CAPE)**	Multifunctional: antioxidant, anti-inflammatory, antiviral, antibacterial, neuro- and cardioprotective [7,20,21].	Reduces inflammation, protects neurons, supports immunity, anticancer effects [20,21].
	Ferulic Acid Esters	Antioxidant, anti-inflammatory, antimicrobial [5,19].	Protects from oxidative stress, promotes wound healing and cardiovascular health [19,22].
	Chlorogenic Acid Esters	Modulate glucose metabolism; antimicrobial and antioxidant [7,19,21].	Improve glycemic control, protect liver, lower cardiovascular risk [7,19].
	Cinnamic Acid Esters	Antimicrobial, antioxidant [7,13,14].	Inhibits pathogens, protects cells from oxidative damage [7,14].

Table 12. *Cont.*

Compound Types	Specific Compounds	Functions	Health Benefits
	Benzoic Acid Benzyl Ester	Antimicrobial, preservative [5,13,14].	Extends product shelf life, prevents contamination [13].
Long-Chain Fatty Acids [7,23,25–28]	**Palmitic Acid (C16:0)**	Provides structural stability, lipid synthesis [25–27].	Supports membrane integrity, energy storage, signaling [25,27].
	Stearic Acid (C18:0)	Structural and energy function [25,27].	Maintains cell structure, neutral cholesterol effects [25,28].
	Oleic Acid (C18:1)	Regulates cholesterol, enhances membrane fluidity [25–27].	Improves cardiovascular health, anti-inflammatory action [25,27,28].
	Linoleic Acid (C18:2)	Precursor of essential fatty acids, modulates inflammation [25,26].	Supports immune and skin health, reduces inflammation [25,27].
	Arachidic Acid (C20:0)	Stabilizes neuronal membranes [25–27].	Supports neuroprotection and nerve function [27,28].
Terpenes [5,7,9,13,29,30]	**Monoterpenes (α-Pinene, Limonene)**	Volatile aromatic molecules with antimicrobial and antioxidant activity [7,13,29].	Reduce inflammation, act as antioxidants, antimicrobial [7,9,29].
	Sesquiterpenes (β-Caryophyllene, α-Cubebene)	Anti-inflammatory, antimicrobial, analgesic activity [7,9,30].	Pain relief, anti-inflammatory effects [29,30].
	Diterpenes (Lupeol, β-Amyrin)	Resin-based compounds with anti-inflammatory and anticancer actions [7,9,30].	Support anticancer therapy and wound healing [29,30].
	Triterpenes (β-Amyrin derivatives)	Found in resins and waxes; hepatoprotective, anti-inflammatory [7,9,30].	Protect liver, reduce oxidative stress [9,30].

Table 12. *Cont.*

Compound Types	Specific Compounds	Functions	Health Benefits
Aromatic Compounds [4,5,7,9,13,14]	**Cinnamic Acid**	Antimicrobial, anti-inflammatory [13,14].	Prevents infection, reduces inflammation [13,14].
	Benzoic Acid	Antimicrobial, preservative [5,13].	Prevents microbial contamination [5,13].
	Caffeic Acid	Antioxidant, anti-inflammatory [7,19,20].	Boosts immunity, reduces inflammation, protects from chronic diseases [7,20].
	Vanillin	Antimicrobial, antioxidant [13,14].	Protects from oxidative stress, infection [13,14].
	Benzyl Alcohol	Antimicrobial, preservative [5,13].	Enhances product stability, prevents contamination [5,13].
Proteins & Amino Acids [7,13,14,26,29]	**Leucine**	Initiates protein synthesis, regulates glucose [13,14].	Supports muscle repair, metabolic regulation [13,14].
	Tryptophan	Serotonin precursor; regulates mood, sleep, appetite [13,26].	Improves sleep and mood, reduces anxiety [13,26].
	Lysine	Essential for collagen formation, calcium absorption [13,14].	Supports tissue repair and immunity [13,14].
	Arginine	Nitric oxide precursor, promotes vasodilation [13,14,26].	Improves circulation and healing [13,14].
	Histidine	Supports cell growth, nerve protection [13,14].	Prevents anemia, protects neurons [13,14].
Vitamins, Minerals & Sugars [4–7,13,14,23,26,29]	**Vitamins B1–B12, C, E**	Antioxidant, metabolic, and immune regulatory functions [5,7,13,14].	Maintain nervous, cardiovascular, and immune health [7,13,14].
	Minerals (Mg, Ca, K, Na, Cu, Zn, Mn, Fe)	Enzyme cofactors, bone and nerve maintenance [5,7,23,26].	Support bone strength, metabolism, and immune function [5,7,23].
	Sugars (Glucose, Fructose, Sucrose)	Energy substrates for metabolism [5,7,13].	Provide immediate and sustained energy [5,13].

Source: Table by author.

4.3. Regional Variations in Propolis

Significant regional variations in both chemical composition and biological activities are evident in propolis. These differences are primarily influenced by the local flora from which the bees collect the resin, as well as by climate and geographical conditions. The diverse plant sources available in different regions lead to a wide range of propolis types, each with unique properties and health benefits.

In Europe, particularly in regions where poplar trees (*Populus* species) are prevalent, propolis is known as poplar-type propolis. This variety is rich in flavonoids and phenolic acids, including CAPE, which contribute to its strong antioxidant, antimicrobial, and anti-inflammatory properties. This type of propolis is widely used in health products and supplements due to its effectiveness in treating infections and protecting against oxidative stress [31].

Brazil is renowned for its green propolis, which is primarily derived from the resin of Baccharis dracunculifolia. This propolis is particularly rich in artepillin C and other prenylated phenylpropanoids, compounds known for their potent antimicrobial and anticancer activities. Green Brazilian propolis has gained popularity in traditional medicine, especially for its role in combating infections and reducing inflammation [32].

In Cuba and other Caribbean regions, red propolis is primarily sourced from the floral resin of Clusia rosea. This type of propolis is characterized by its high content of polyphenols, including isoflavonoids and prenylated benzophenones. Red Cuban propolis exhibits strong antioxidant, antimicrobial, and anti-inflammatory effects, making it beneficial in preventing and treating various chronic diseases [33].

Albanian propolis, collected from diverse regions across the country, including the southern and northern areas, showcases a mix of phenolic acids, flavonoids, and other bioactive compounds. Research has shown that this propolis is particularly effective against bacterial pathogens like *P. aeruginosa*, inhibiting biofilm formation and reducing virulence factors. These properties make Albanian propolis a valuable resource in the fight against infections [34].

Regional variations are also evident in propolis from New Zealand, which, although primarily resembling the poplar-type propolis, displays unique characteristics due to the specific flora of the region. Studies have identified distinct volatile organic compounds in New Zealand propolis, contributing to its strong antimicrobial and antioxidant properties, making it suitable for various health applications [33].

In the United States, propolis shows considerable regional variation in both its composition and antimicrobial activity, reflecting the diverse plant life from which bees collect resin. Research has demonstrated that US propolis is effective against a wide range of pathogens, including *Paenibacillus larvae* and *Ascosphaera apis*, which are responsible for significant diseases in bees. This variability underscores the importance of local flora in determining the bioactivity of propolis [35].

These regional differences in the composition and bioactivity of propolis underscore the need to understand the environmental factors, such as local flora, climate, and geography, that shape its properties. Insights into these variations allow researchers to optimize its therapeutic potential and adapt formulations to specific clinical needs. However, this same chemical diversity that enriches its bioactive profile poses a challenge for standardized use in dental care products. Variability in botanical sources, seasonal conditions, and extraction methods can alter the concentration of key compounds, leading to inconsistent clinical outcomes. To achieve reliable therapeutic effects, it is essential to implement harmonized extraction protocols and rigorous quality control standards that preserve the most effective bioactive constituents while minimizing variability from group to group [36,37].

4.4. *Propolis in Medicine and Dentistry*

Recognized for its extensive therapeutic properties, propolis, a natural substance, has become a valuable component in both medicine and dentistry. Its diverse biological activities, including antimicrobial, anti-inflammatory, antioxidant, immunomodulatory, and regenerative properties, have made propolis a key natural remedy in healthcare practices. This section explores the applications of propolis in medicine and dentistry, supported by recent scientific studies and clinical applications.

4.4.1. Propolis in Medicine

Propolis has been widely used in various medical fields due to its unique combination of therapeutic properties. Each of these properties contributes to its effectiveness in treating a broad range of health conditions.

Antimicrobial properties: Propolis exhibits strong antimicrobial activity against a broad spectrum of pathogens, including bacteria, fungi, and viruses. This antimicrobial action is primarily due to the presence of flavonoids, phenolic acids, and other bioactive compounds that disrupt microbial cell walls and membranes, thereby inhibiting their growth and proliferation. Propolis has been effectively used in treating infections, promoting wound healing, and serving as a natural preservative in various medical formulations [38].

Anti-inflammatory properties: The anti-inflammatory effects of propolis are attributed to its ability to inhibit the production of pro-inflammatory cytokines and enzymes, such as cyclooxygenase-2 (COX-2) and nitric oxide synthase (iNOS). These compounds contribute to the suppression of inflammatory responses in the body, making propolis effective in managing conditions such as arthritis, asthma, and inflammatory bowel disease. Its anti-inflammatory properties also play a crucial role in reducing pain and swelling associated with these conditions [39].

Antioxidant properties: Propolis is rich in flavonoids and phenolic acids, which are potent antioxidants. These compounds neutralize free radicals, reducing oxidative stress and protecting cells from damage. This antioxidant activity is particularly beneficial in preventing chronic diseases, slowing down the aging process, and protecting against environmental stressors. Propolis's ability to combat oxidative stress makes it a valuable supplement in various therapeutic regimes [40].

Immunomodulatory properties: Propolis modulates the immune system by enhancing the activity of immune cells, such as macrophages and lymphocytes, and boosting the production of antibodies. This immunomodulatory effect strengthens the body's defense mechanisms, helping it fight off infections more effectively and improving responses to vaccines. The immune-boosting properties of propolis have been utilized in both preventive and therapeutic contexts, making it a valuable natural adjunct in immune health [41].

Anticancer properties: Recent studies have shown that propolis possesses anticancer properties, primarily through its ability to induce apoptosis (programmed cell death) in cancer cells and inhibit their proliferation. Propolis compounds like CAPE have been identified as potent agents in reducing tumor growth and metastasis in various cancer models. These properties are being explored in clinical settings as complementary therapies in cancer treatment, offering potential benefits in managing cancer progression and improving patient outcomes [42,43].

4.4.2. Propolis in Dentistry

Propolis has found significant applications in dentistry, particularly in the prevention and treatment of dental caries, gingivitis, periodontitis, endodontic infections, and denture stomatitis. Its natural antimicrobial, anti-inflammatory, and regenerative properties make it an effective alternative or adjunct to conventional dental treatments (Figure 14).

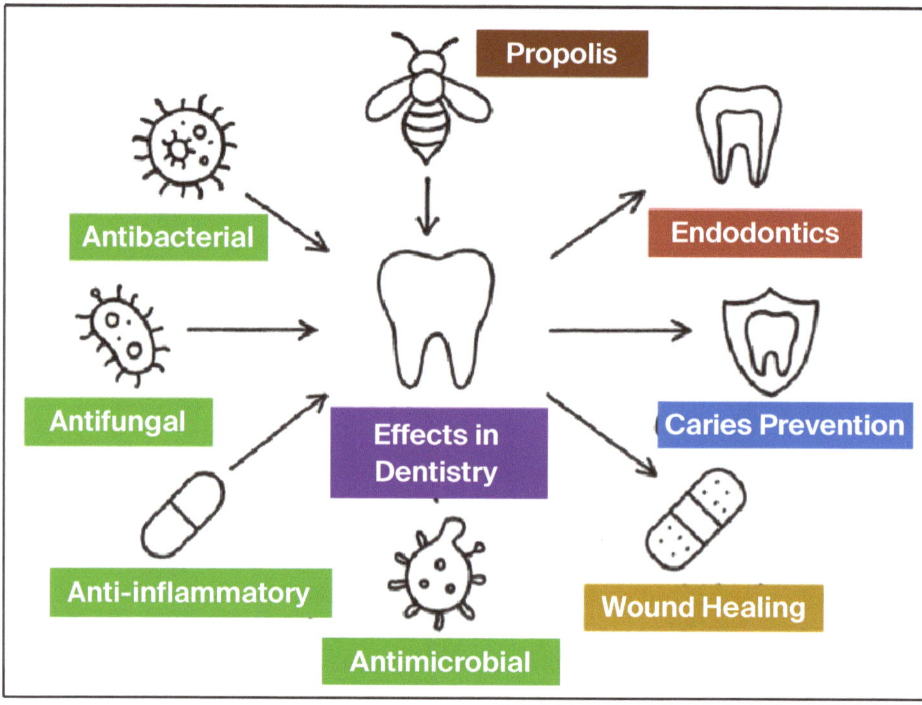

Figure 14. This flowchart visually illustrates the diverse effects of propolis in dentistry, highlighting its various applications and roles across different dental care practices. Source: Figure by author.

Mechanistic Overview of Antimicrobial Action

The antimicrobial activity of propolis is largely attributed to its rich content of flavonoids (e.g., pinocembrin, galangin, chrysin), phenolic acids and esters (e.g., caffeic acid phenethyl ester [CAPE]), and terpenoids. These compounds act synergistically to inhibit bacterial growth, impair biofilm formation, and disrupt microbial communication systems such as quorum sensing [10,11]. Propolis acts on multiple stages of biofilm development, inhibiting initial bacterial adhesion, preventing maturation, and facilitating detachment. Polyphenols penetrate the biofilm matrix, destabilizing extracellular polymeric substances (EPS) and making bacterial cells more susceptible to host defenses and antimicrobials. This effect has been confirmed in mixed-species biofilms containing *S. mutans*, *P. gingivalis*, and *F. nucleatum*, organisms central to cariogenesis and periodontitis [13].

Caries prevention: Propolis inhibits the growth of cariogenic bacteria, especially *S. mutans*, through the mechanisms that reduce biofilm formation and acid production. Flavonoids and CAPE inhibit *S. mutans* glucosyltransferases (GtfB, GtfC, GtfD), enzymes responsible for synthesizing extracellular glucans that form the structural backbone of dental plaque biofilms. By reducing extracellular polysaccharide production, propolis interferes with bacterial adhesion to enamel and decreases acidogenicity. Additionally, phenolic compounds alter bacterial membrane permeability, causing the leakage of intracellular constituents and metabolic disruption [11]. Moreover, propolis can enhance remineralization of enamel by supplying trace minerals such as calcium and phosphate. Regular incorporation into toothpastes and mouthwashes has been associated with reduced caries incidence [10,11].

Gingivitis and periodontitis treatment: The antimicrobial activity of propolis helps in controlling the oral pathogens responsible for gingivitis and periodontitis, while its anti-inflammatory properties reduce the swelling, redness, and pain associated with gum inflammation. Propolis also promotes the healing and regeneration of gum tissues, enhancing collagen production and tissue repair. These properties make it a valuable adjunct in periodontal therapy, where it is used in products like mouthwashes, gels, and ointments for targeted application on affected areas [10,11,13]. Terpenoids and phenolic acids in propolis exhibit potent activity against *P. gingivalis* by disrupting its outer membrane integrity and inhibiting cysteine proteases (gingipains), which are key virulence factors involved in connective tissue destruction. CAPE also downregulates inflammatory mediators induced by *P. gingivalis* lipopolysaccharide (LPS), thereby reducing periodontal tissue breakdown [11]. Beyond antimicrobial effects, propolis modulates the host inflammatory response. By suppressing NF-κB activation in gingival fibroblasts, flavonoids and CAPE reduce the secretion of IL-1β, TNF-α, and matrix metalloproteinases, attenuating soft tissue destruction and bone loss. When applied in gels or mouthrinses, propolis decreases plaque accumulation and gingival bleeding, improving periodontal parameters [10].

Endodontic treatment: In endodontics, propolis is recognized for its potential in root canal treatments due to its antimicrobial, anti-inflammatory, and regenerative properties [44,45]. Propolis can be used as an intracanal medicament to disinfect the root canal system, reducing microbial load and preventing reinfection. Figure 15a–c illustrates the ex vivo application of a 10% alcoholic propolis solution as an irrigant, showcasing its significant potential in endodontic treatment. SEM analysis demonstrates that this treatment not only effectively removes the smear layer but also seals the entrances of the dentinal tubules, thereby enhancing the integrity and cleanliness of the treated dentin surface.

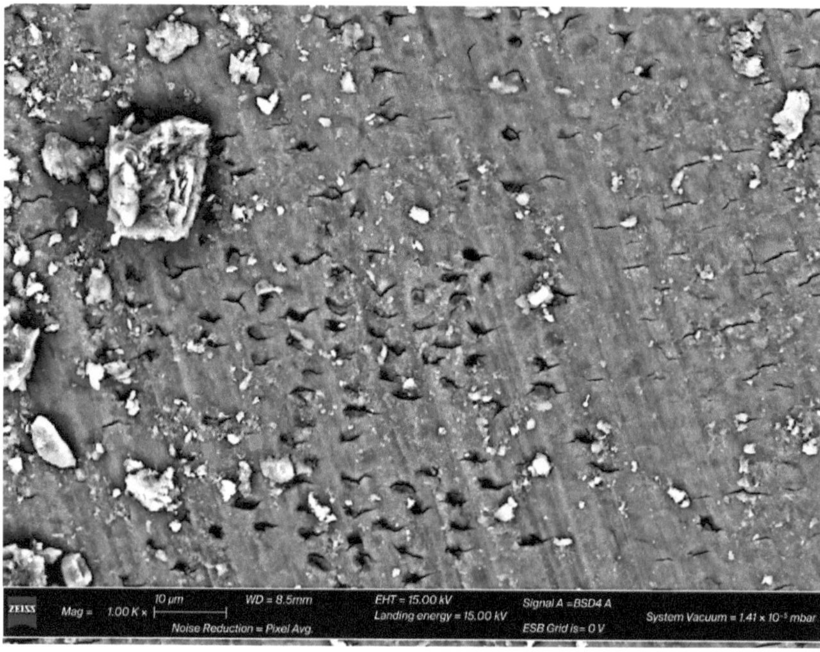

(**a**)

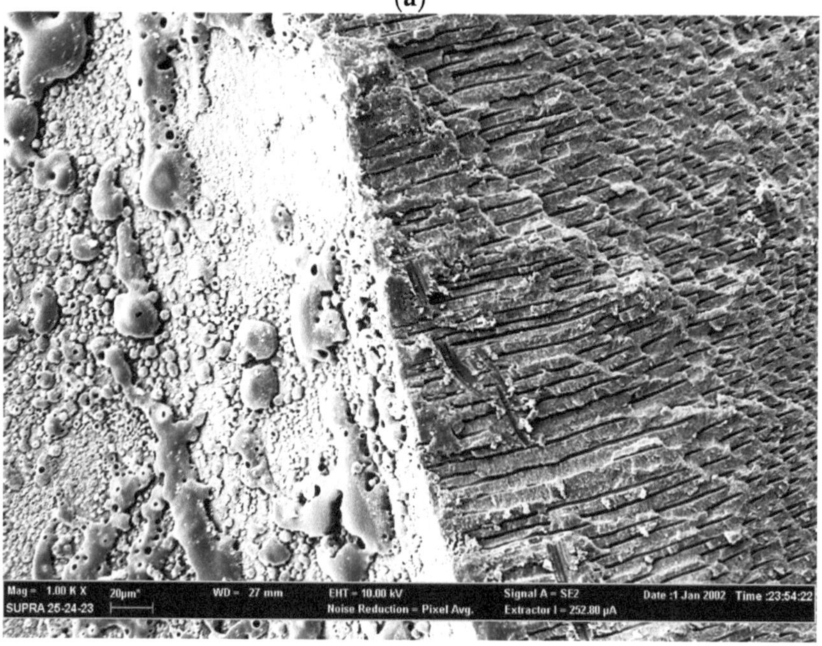

(**b**)

Figure 15. *Cont.*

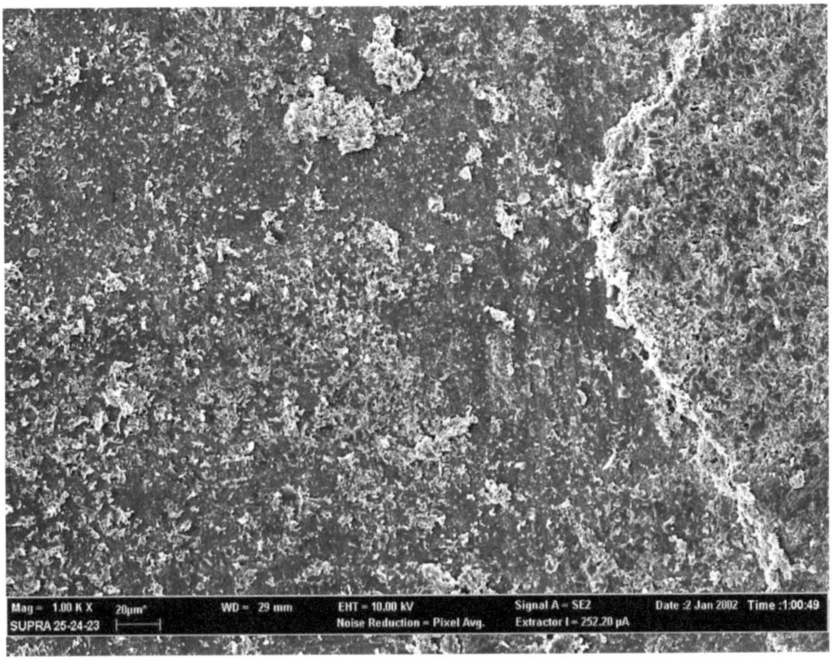

(c)

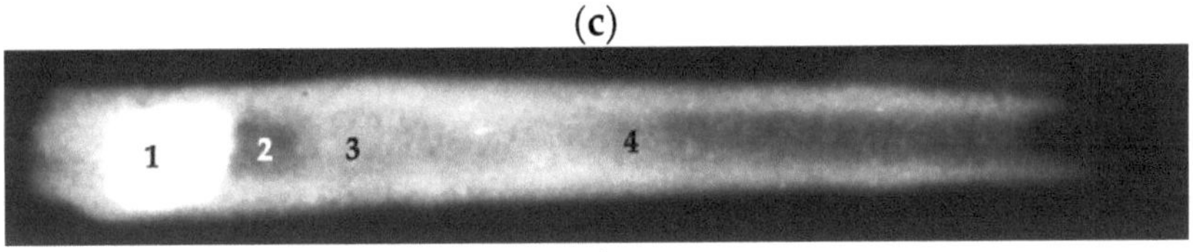

(d)

Figure 15. SEM and Radiographic Evaluation of Propolis in endodontics. (**a**) SEM analysis of canal dentin following ex vivo treatment with 10% alcoholic propolis as an irrigant. The image reveals the effective removal of the smear layer and the sealing of dentinal tubule entrances by the propolis solution, highlighting its potential to enhance the integrity and cleanliness of the treated dentin surface. (**b**) SEM image at 1000× magnification of the apical dentin section, illustrating localized penetration of 10% alcoholic propolis a few microns deep into the dentinal tubules. The treated areas show visible infiltration of the propolis within the tubular openings. (**c**) SEM image at 1000× magnification of the mid-root dentin section, showing widespread surface deposits and limited visibility of dentinal tubules. The image reveals evidence of surface impregnation by 10% alcoholic propolis on the dentin substrate. (**d**) X-ray image of an extracted piglet tooth after in vivo treatment with propolis. The image highlights the following attributes: 1. Definitive filling: The final restorative material used to seal the tooth. 2. Propolis paste: The applied propolis mixture, visible as a radiopaque area. 3. Dentin bridge: Newly formed dentin bridging the treated area. 4. Lumen canal: The main canal of the tooth. This X-ray demonstrates the effectiveness of propolis in dental treatment, showcasing its role in promoting dentin formation and effectively sealing the treated area. Credit: © Agron Meto, used with permission.

Its ability to reduce inflammation in periapical tissues and promote tissue regeneration supports faster healing and improves treatment outcomes. Propolis is also used in pulp capping procedures, where it aids in maintaining pulp vitality and stimulating reparative dentin formation [44,45].

In 2016, Meto et al. [45] conducted a study to explore the anti-inflammatory and regenerative effects of Albanian propolis in the setting of experimental vital amputations. The research aimed to assess the therapeutic potential of propolis in promoting healing and tissue regeneration following dental pulp injuries. Using an animal model to replicate conditions of vital amputation, a procedure that mimics the exposure and injury of dental pulp, the authors applied Albanian propolis directly to the injured pulp tissue. The study found that propolis exhibited significant anti-inflammatory properties, effectively reducing the inflammatory response commonly associated with pulp injuries (Figure 15d). Furthermore, the treatment with propolis enhanced tissue regeneration, indicating its potential as a valuable adjunct in endodontic procedures, especially in cases where pulp healing and protection are critical.

Wound healing in dentistry: Propolis's wound-healing properties are particularly beneficial in postoperative dental care. Its antimicrobial, anti-inflammatory, antioxidant, and regenerative effects facilitate the faster healing of oral wounds, such as those resulting from tooth extractions or surgical procedures. Propolis-based wound dressings and topical applications help in reducing microbial contamination, controlling inflammation, and promoting tissue regeneration, thereby improving healing outcomes [46,47].

Oral hygiene: Propolis has become a popular ingredient in oral hygiene products due to its ability to maintain oral health and prevent various oral diseases. It is incorporated into toothpaste, mouthwashes, and oral sprays to provide continuous antimicrobial protection, reduce inflammation, and enhance the overall health of the oral cavity. Regular use of these products helps in preventing dental plaque formation, reducing the risk of dental caries, gingivitis, and periodontitis, and maintaining fresh breath [48,49].

Propolis in the treatment of denture stomatitis: Denture stomatitis, an inflammatory condition affecting the oral mucosa under dentures, is often associated with Candida infection. Propolis has shown promise in treating this condition due to its strong antifungal activity against *Candida* spp., its ability to reduce inflammation, and its promotion of mucosal healing. Propolis-based gels, pastes, and sprays are applied to the fitting surfaces of dentures and the affected oral mucosa, providing direct antimicrobial action and enhancing tissue repair. This treatment is particularly beneficial for denture wearers, as it reduces symptoms and improves oral comfort [50,51].

Dental hypersensitivity: Propolis is effective in managing dental hypersensitivity by occluding exposed dentinal tubules, which are responsible for transmitting pain in response to stimuli. The compounds in propolis form a protective layer over the dentin surface, reducing fluid movement within the tubules and preventing external stimuli from reaching the nerves. This results in a significant reduction in sensitivity and discomfort. Propolis-based varnishes, toothpastes, and gels are used to provide relief from hypersensitivity, making it easier for individuals to maintain their oral hygiene without pain [52,53].

Immunomodulatory Properties of Propolis in the Oral Cavity

The oral cavity is a complex immunological environment in which constant exposure to microbial antigens demands a carefully balanced host response, strong enough to control pathogenic microorganisms but regulated to prevent excessive tissue destruction. Propolis, with its diverse array of flavonoids, phenolic acids, and terpenoids, exerts profound effects on both innate and adaptive immune mechanisms, thereby influencing periodontal and mucosal health.

A key aspect of this modulation is its impact on innate immunity. Compounds such as caffeic acid phenethyl ester (CAPE), artepillin C, and chrysin have been shown to influence macrophage polarization, shifting it toward an anti-inflammatory M2 phenotype that limits the overproduction of pro-inflammatory mediators like TNF-α and IL-1β [9,54]. Propolis also reduces harmful neutrophil-driven responses by inhibiting myeloperoxidase activity and excessive reactive oxygen species (ROS) production, which mitigates collateral tissue damage within gingival and periodontal sites [8]. Furthermore, certain flavonoid fractions have demonstrated the ability to downregulate complement C3 convertase activity, potentially dampening the inflammatory cascade that drives periodontal tissue destruction.

Propolis also shapes adaptive immune responses, which are pivotal in maintaining periodontal tissue homeostasis. CAPE suppresses nuclear factor kappa B (NF-κB) signaling, leading to the reduced production of pro-inflammatory Th1/Th17 cytokines such as IL-2, IFN-γ, and IL-17, while simultaneously enhancing the activity of regulatory T cells (Tregs) that help counteract destructive immune reactions in periodontal lesions [37]. In addition, in vitro studies suggest that propolis may stimulate salivary IgA secretion, thereby improving mucosal immune surveillance against cariogenic bacteria [36].

The influence of propolis extends to the regulation of cytokines and growth factors that govern inflammation and tissue repair. Treatment with propolis extracts has been shown to downregulate central pro-inflammatory mediators, including IL-1β, IL-6, and TNF-α, in gingival fibroblast cultures, thereby attenuating the inflammatory burden characteristic of periodontitis [55]. Conversely, it enhances the levels of anti-inflammatory cytokines, notably IL-10 and transforming growth factor-beta (TGF-β), which facilitate healing and connective tissue regeneration. Importantly, propolis phenolic compounds can also stimulate the expression of vascular endothelial growth factor (VEGF), supporting angiogenesis in post-extraction sockets and surgical wounds [56,57].

These immunomodulatory effects are supported by a growing body of clinical evidence. In periodontal therapy, studies show that propolis-containing mouthwashes and subgingival gels, when used adjunctively with scaling and root planing (SRP), significantly reduce gingival crevicular fluid (GCF) concentrations of IL-1β and TNF-α, alongside marked improvements in clinical attachment gain and pocket-depth reduction [37]. In endodontic applications, propolis used as an intracanal medicament has demonstrated a decrease in periapical inflammatory cytokines while promoting reparative dentinogenesis [36,58]. Moreover, in cases of mucositis and denture stomatitis, the application of propolis sprays has been associated with significant reductions in erythema and ulceration scores, likely due to a combined antifungal and anti-inflammatory immunomodulatory action [51,59].

4.4.3. Synergistic Effects with Other Natural Dental Agents

The interest in combining propolis with other natural dental agents arises from its polymodal properties, notably its antimicrobial, anti-inflammatory, antioxidant, and pro-healing activities. Pairing propolis with agents that act on complementary mechanisms has the potential to expand the antimicrobial spectrum, reduce oral dysbiosis, and enhance soft-tissue healing.

One promising pairing is propolis with aloe vera, especially for periodontal therapy and wound healing. Aloe vera contributes mucopolysaccharides that soothe tissues and attenuate local inflammatory mediators, while propolis adds polyphenol-driven antimicrobial effects and NF-κB modulation. Together, they appear to combine surface biofilm control with accelerated epithelialization. Clinical reviews show that propolis enhances plaque and gingival index scores when used as an adjunct, while aloe vera gels and rinses similarly demonstrate improvements in gingival indices during non-surgical periodontal therapy. Although robust RCTs directly testing the combination remain scarce, the biological rationale for additive benefits is strong, particularly for site-specific gels or irrigants. Both agents are generally well tolerated, but screening for contact reactions, especially in atopic patients, is advisable [36].

Another potential synergy is observed with propolis and tea tree oil (TTO; *Melaleuca alternifolia*), aimed at broadening anti-biofilm activity. TTO, rich in terpinen-4-ol, disrupts microbial cell membranes of Gram-positive and Gram-negative bacteria as well as Candida species. Propolis complements these actions by inhibiting glucosyltransferase (Gtf) activity in *Streptococcus mutans* and destabilizing biofilm matrices. Both agents have shown benefits individually: propolis mouthrinses reduce plaque and gingival bleeding, while TTO rinses demonstrate anti-plaque effects in smaller trials. Although evidence of direct synergistic efficacy is still limited, the complementary mechanisms suggest a combined low-TTO formulation may be useful for patient's intolerant to chlorhexidine, provided the risk of TTO sensitivity is addressed [8,36].

The combination of propolis and myrrh (*Commiphora* spp.) represents another traditional pairing, particularly for gingival conditioning and halitosis control. Myrrh resins, known for their antimicrobial and astringent properties, have long been used in gingival tonics. Propolis contributes sustained anti-inflammatory activity and further disrupts EPS biofilms, offering potential benefits for reducing gingival bleeding and improving breath quality. While narrative reviews support each agent's adjunctive role in non-surgical periodontal therapy, no high-quality RCTs have yet tested their combined effects, underscoring the need for more rigorous clinical studies [37].

Further possibilities include combining propolis with polyphenol-rich agents, such as green tea catechins (EGCG) or cranberry proanthocyanidins (PACs). These compounds interfere with bacterial adhesins and glucan synthesis, limiting *S. mutans* adherence and co-aggregation in plaque biofilms. Propolis complements these mechanisms with host–response modulation and biofilm matrix weakening, offering a plausible strategy for reducing periopathogen colonization and gingival inflammation. While in vitro studies and early clinical work on polyphenol-based rinses report reductions in key periopathogens and plaque indices, controlled trials evaluating their combination with propolis remain an unmet need [13,36].

Propolis also shows significant promise in endodontic and post-surgical applications. Its intracanal antimicrobial and anti-inflammatory activity has been well documented, and combining it postoperatively with gentle natural antimicrobials, such as low-percentage TTO or polyphenol-based rinses, may help suppress planktonic recolonization without increasing tissue irritation. While early evidence is encouraging, such applications should continue to follow standard endodontic protocols until more robust data emerge [36].

Current evidence supports the best use of propolis combinations as adjuncts to scaling and root planing (SRP) and home care, particularly in patients unable to tolerate chlorhexidine or requiring long-term maintenance for plaque control and gingival health. Those likely to benefit most include plaque-prone individuals with gingival inflammation, halitosis, or mild candidiasis risk, as well as patients in post-surgical soft-tissue recovery. Nonetheless, well-designed RCTs directly testing propolis combined with aloe vera, tea tree oil, and myrrh, compared with single agents and chlorhexidine controls, are still urgently needed. Future studies should evaluate clinical outcomes, such as plaque index, bleeding on probing (BOP), pocket depth reduction, microbiome shifts, and mucosal tolerance to confirm and refine these promising synergistic approaches [37,52,53].

4.4.4. Optimized Formulations for Propolis in Dental Care

The integration of propolis into contemporary dental formulations aims to harness its antimicrobial, anti-inflammatory, antioxidant, and wound-healing activities while ensuring sustained release, optimal bioavailability, and patient-friendly application. The choice of delivery system is tailored to the intended clinical objective, whether plaque control, mucosal healing, caries prevention, periodontal therapy, or endodontic treatment. Recent advances in formulation technologies have expanded the potential of propolis by improving solubility, stability, and contact time within the oral cavity.

Mouthwashes remain one of the most common delivery forms, typically employing hydroalcoholic or glycolic extracts at concentrations between 0.2% and 10%, with alcohol content kept below 10% to minimize mucosal irritation. Innovative nanoemulsion-based rinses are being developed to enhance dispersion and phenolic stability in aqueous environments. Recent studies show encouraging results, reporting that a propolis mouthwash produced gingival inflammation reductions comparable to chlorhexidine but with fewer side effects, such as taste alteration and staining [60,61]. While others found significant decreases in plaque indices and bleeding on probing in both gingivitis and periodontitis patients [36,55,61]. Although convenient and well accepted by patients, rinses provide only brief contact time, and their polyphenol-rich extracts are prone to oxidation in aqueous solutions, potentially diminishing long-term efficacy.

Toothpastes offer a complementary route for continuous low-dose exposure, especially valuable for caries-prone individuals. These formulations incorporate 0.5–2% w/w propolis powders or lyophilized extracts into standard silica-based abrasives and humectants; some combine propolis with fluoride or other herbal agents for added benefit. A Cochrane review by Pradeep et al. (2024) provided moderate-certainty evidence that propolis-enriched toothpaste lowers S. mutans counts and improves plaque control compared with fluoride-only pastes [11]. Likewise, fluoride–propolis combinations have demonstrated enhanced enamel remineralization, offering additional protective benefits against early carious lesions. While toothpaste formulations integrate seamlessly into routine oral hygiene practices, they are generally less effective for managing acute periodontal inflammation compared with site-specific gels or therapeutic rinses [62].

For periodontal pockets, carbomer- or hydroxyethylcellulose-based gels containing 2–10% propolis extract, often enriched with hyaluronic acid or aloe vera, allow prolonged local drug retention without significant systemic absorption [63]. These gels are generally applied subgingivally after scaling and root planing (SRP). Pezzella et al. (2025) showed that such gels maintained effective antimicrobial concentrations for up to seven days, significantly reducing P. gingivalis and T. forsythia levels [37]. Their principal limitation lies in the need for professional application and potential enzyme-mediated degradation within saliva.

For patients with root caries or dentin hypersensitivity, resin-based varnishes containing 5–10% propolis extract are applied to exposed dentin or root surfaces. These formulations enable the slow release of bioactive compounds for one to two weeks, forming a protective layer, demonstrating that propolis varnishes help reduce hypersensitivity and inhibit recolonization by cariogenic bacteria following SRP [52]. Despite their long-lasting effect, the need for chairside application and potential discoloration from the natural pigments remains a consideration.

In endodontics, propolis has gained attention as both an irrigant and intracanal medicament. Typical preparations include a 10% alcoholic solution or aqueous nanoemulsion for irrigation and paste mixtures often blended with calcium hydroxide for medicament use. These studies found these propolis-based medicaments to be comparable or superior to calcium hydroxide, achieving significant reductions in microbial load and postoperative pain in cases of necrotic pulp, while promoting reparative dentinogenesis [44,45].

For post-extraction sites and mucosal healing, propolis is applied as ointments, sprays, or bioadhesive patches at 5–10% concentrations. These delivery systems provide localized anti-inflammatory and antimicrobial action, supporting angiogenesis, collagen synthesis, and epithelial closure [46,49,54].

4.5. Ongoing Research

The therapeutic potential of propolis has garnered significant scientific interest, leading to a growing body of research aimed at understanding its full spectrum of biological activities. While substantial progress has been made in validating the traditional uses of propolis, ongoing research continues to explore new applications, optimize its use in clinical settings, and enhance its efficacy through novel formulations. This section delves into the latest trends in propolis research and the future directions that hold promise for its broader adoption in medicine and dentistry.

Molecular mechanisms of action: One of the primary areas of ongoing research is the elucidation of the molecular mechanisms underlying the biological effects of propolis. While the antimicrobial, anti-inflammatory, and antioxidant properties of propolis are well documented, scientists are increasingly focused on identifying the specific compounds responsible for these effects and understanding how they interact with cellular pathways. Advanced techniques in molecular biology, such as genomics, proteomics, and metabolomics, are being employed to map out these interactions at a detailed level. Recognizing these mechanisms could lead to the development of more targeted and effective therapeutic applications, particularly in the management of chronic diseases and infections [64].

Standardization and quality control: Another critical area of research is the standardization of propolis extracts. Given that the chemical composition of propolis can vary significantly depending on its geographic origin, botanical source, and method of extraction, there is a need for standardized products to ensure consistent therapeutic outcomes. Researchers are working on developing reliable methods for the standardization and quality control of propolis, which include identifying key bioactive compounds and setting benchmarks for their concentrations in commercial preparations. This standardization is essential for the integration of propolis into mainstream medicine and for ensuring the safety and efficacy of propolis-based products [65,66].

Novel delivery systems: To enhance the bioavailability and therapeutic efficacy of propolis, researchers are exploring innovative delivery systems. Traditional forms of propolis, such as tinctures and ointments, are being supplemented with advanced formulations, including nanoemulsions, liposomes, and hydrogels. These delivery systems are designed to improve solubility, stability, and absorption of propolis, allowing for more precise and effective targeting of tissues. For instance, nanoemulsions of propolis are being developed to increase its antimicrobial activity and facilitate deeper penetration into tissues, making it more effective in treating infections and promoting wound healing [66,67].

Synergistic effects with conventional therapies: Research is also focused on exploring the synergistic effects of propolis when used in combination with conventional therapies. Preliminary studies suggest that propolis can enhance the efficacy of antibiotics, reduce the side effects of chemotherapy, and improve the outcomes of surgical procedures. For example, propolis has been shown to potentiate the effects of certain antibiotics against resistant bacterial strains, making it a valuable adjunct in the fight against antibiotic resistance. Additionally, its anti-inflammatory and antioxidant properties can help mitigate the toxic effects of chemotherapy, potentially improving the quality of life for cancer patients [68,69].

Clinical trials and human studies: While much of the research on propolis has been conducted in vitro and in vivo models, there is a growing emphasis on conducting clinical trials to validate its efficacy in humans. These trials are essential for establishing the therapeutic benefits of propolis in various conditions, ranging from oral health issues like gingivitis and periodontitis to systemic diseases such as diabetes and cancer. Ongoing and future clinical trials aim to provide robust data on the safety, dosage, and efficacy of propolis in human populations, paving the way for its broader use in clinical practice.

Environmental and sustainability considerations: As the demand for propolis increases, researchers are also focusing on the environmental and sustainability aspects of its production. This includes studying the impact of propolis harvesting on bee populations and developing sustainable practices that ensure the long-term availability of this valuable resource. Additionally, research is being conducted on synthetic and semi-synthetic alternatives to propolis, which could reduce the pressure on natural bee populations while maintaining the therapeutic benefits of the natural product.

4.6. Conclusions

Propolis, a natural substance produced by bees, has long been valued for its extensive therapeutic properties. Modern research has expanded our understanding of its chemical composition, revealing a complex array of bioactive compounds including flavonoids, phenolic acids, and essential oils, each contributing to its antimicrobial, anti-inflammatory, antioxidant, and immunomodulatory effects. These properties have facilitated the integration of propolis into various medical and dental applications, where it is used to prevent and treat conditions ranging from dental caries and periodontal diseases to systemic infections and chronic inflammatory conditions. The growing body of scientific validation underscores its potential as a powerful natural adjunct in both traditional and modern therapeutic practices.

The ongoing research into the molecular mechanisms of propolis, coupled with efforts to standardize its composition and improve delivery methods, promises to enhance its therapeutic efficacy and broaden its applications. Additionally, the exploration of synergistic effects with conventional therapies and the focus on sustainable harvesting practices will be crucial in ensuring the long-term viability of propolis as a therapeutic agent. As we look to the future, the integration of propolis into mainstream healthcare offers a promising avenue for natural and effective treatment options that align with the growing trend toward holistic and sustainable medicine. Continued exploration and innovation in the use of propolis will undoubtedly contribute to its enduring legacy as a vital natural remedy in modern medicine and dentistry.

References

1. Nunn, J. Egyptian Medicine. In *The Cambridge History of Science*; Jones, A., Taub, L., Eds.; Cambridge University Press: Cambridge, UK, 2018; pp. 120–130. [CrossRef]
2. Kleisiaris, C.F.; Sfakianakis, C.; Papathanasiou, I.V. Health care practices in ancient Greece: The Hippocratic ideal. *J. Med. Ethics Hist. Med.* **2014**, *7*, 6. [PubMed]
3. Santacroce, L.; Bottalico, L.; Charitos, I.A. Greek Medicine Practice at Ancient Rome: The Physician Molecularist Asclepiades. *Medicines* **2017**, *4*, 92. [CrossRef]
4. Rojczyk, E.; Klama-Baryła, A.; Łabuś, W.; Wilemska-Kucharzewska, K.; Kucharzewski, M. Historical and modern research on propolis and its application in wound healing and other fields of medicine and contributions by Polish studies. *J. Ethnopharmacol.* **2020**, *262*, 113159. [CrossRef]
5. Toreti, V.C.; Sato, H.H.; Pastore, G.M.; Park, Y.K. Recent progress of propolis for its biological and chemical compositions and its botanical origin. *Evid.-Based Complement. Altern. Med.* **2013**, *2013*, 697390. [CrossRef] [PubMed]
6. Kuropatnicki, A.K.; Szliszka, E.; Krol, W. Historical aspects of propolis research in modern times. *Evid.-Based Complement. Alternat Med.* **2013**, *2013*, 964149. [CrossRef]
7. Hossain, R.; Quispe, C.; Khan, R.A.; Saikat, A.S.M.; Ray, P.; Ongalbek, D.; Yeskaliyeva, B.; Jain, D.; Smeriglio, A.; Trombetta, D.; et al. Propolis: An update on its chemistry and pharmacological applications. *Chin. Med.* **2022**, *17*, 100. [CrossRef] [PubMed]
8. Wezgowiec, J.; Wieczynska, A.; Wieckiewicz, W.; Kulbacka, J.; Saczko, J.; Pachura, N.; Wieckiewicz, M.; Gancarz, R.; Wilk, K.A. Polish Propolis—Chemical Composition and Biological Effects in Tongue Cancer Cells and Macrophages. *Molecules* **2020**, *25*, 2426. [CrossRef]
9. Šturm, L.; Ulrih, N.P. Advances in the Propolis Chemical Composition between 2013 and 2018: A Review. *eFood* **2020**, *1*, 24–37. [CrossRef]

10. López-Valverde, N.; Pardal-Peláez, B.; López-Valverde, A.; Flores-Fraile, J.; Herrero-Hernández, S.; Macedo-de-Sousa, B.; Herrero-Payo, J.; Ramírez, J.M. Effectiveness of Propolis in the Treatment of Periodontal Disease: Updated Systematic Review with Meta-Analysis. *Antioxidants* **2021**, *10*, 269. [CrossRef]
11. Pradeep, P.; Thomas, A.R.; Kaur, K.; Sarah Samson, R.; Mayya, A.; Adiga, S.; Kumbargere Nagraj, S. Herbal medicines to prevent dental caries. *Cochrane Database Syst. Rev.* **2024**, *5*, CD015832. [CrossRef]
12. Popravko, S.A.; Gurevich, A.I.; Kolosov, M.N. Flavonoid components of propolis. *Chem. Nat. Compd.* **1969**, *5*, 397–401. [CrossRef]
13. Altuntaş, Ü.; Güzel, İ.; Özçelik, B. Phenolic Constituents, Antioxidant and Antimicrobial Activity and Clustering Analysis of Propolis Samples Based on PCA from Different Regions of Anatolia. *Molecules* **2023**, *28*, 1121. [CrossRef]
14. Woźniak, M.; Sip, A.; Mrówczyńska, L.; Broniarczyk, J.; Waśkiewicz, A.; Ratajczak, I. Biological Activity and Chemical Composition of Propolis from Various Regions of Poland. *Molecules* **2022**, *28*, 141. [CrossRef]
15. Liu, G.; Zhang, C.P.; Lu, Y.Y.; Niu, D.F.; Hu, F.L. Biotransformation and metabolite activity analysis of flavonoids from propolis in vivo. *J. Asian Nat. Prod. Res.* **2024**, *26*, 1–15. [CrossRef] [PubMed]
16. Rivera-Yañez, C.R.; Ruiz-Hurtado, P.A.; Mendoza-Ramos, M.I.; Reyes-Reali, J.; García-Romo, G.S.; Pozo-Molina, G.; Reséndiz-Albor, A.A.; Nieto-Yañez, O.; Méndez-Cruz, A.R.; Méndez-Catalá, C.F.; et al. Flavonoids Present in Propolis in the Battle against Photoaging and Psoriasis. *Antioxidants* **2021**, *10*, 2014. [CrossRef]
17. Cui, J.; Duan, X.; Ke, L.; Pan, X.; Liu, J.; Song, X.; Ma, W.; Zhang, W.; Liu, Y.; Fan, Y. Extraction, purification, structural character and biological properties of propolis flavonoids: A review. *Fitoterapia* **2022**, *157*, 105106. [CrossRef]
18. Grinn-Gofroń, A.; Kołodziejczak, M.; Hrynkiewicz, R.; Lewandowski, F.; Bębnowska, D.; Adamski, C.; Niedźwiedzka-Rystwej, P. Antimicrobial Potential of Bee-Derived Products: Insights into Honey, Propolis and Bee Venom. *Pathogens* **2025**, *14*, 780. [CrossRef]
19. Ramanauskiene, K.; Savickas, A.; Ivanauskas, L.; Kalveniene, Z.; Kasparaviciene, G.; Banionyte, I.; Amsiejus, A.; Martirosyan, M. Danik, Analysis of Phenolic Acids in Propolis Using the High-Performance Liquid Chromatography Technique. *Curr. Nutr. Food Sci.* **2008**, *4*, 209–212. [CrossRef]
20. Tolba, M.F.; Azab, S.S.; Khalifa, A.E.; Abdel-Rahman, S.Z.; Abdel-Naim, A.B. Caffeic acid phenethyl ester, a promising component of propolis with a plethora of biological activities: A review on its anti-inflammatory, neuroprotective, hepatoprotective, and cardioprotective effects. *IUBMB Life* **2013**, *65*, 699–709. [CrossRef] [PubMed]
21. Kurek-Górecka, A.; Rzepecka-Stojko, A.; Górecki, M.; Stojko, J.; Sosada, M.; Swierczek-Zieba, G. Structure and antioxidant activity of polyphenols derived from propolis. *Molecules* **2014**, *19*, 78–101. [CrossRef] [PubMed]
22. Saleh, S.; Salama, A.; Ali, A.M.; Saleh, A.K.; Elhady, B.A.; Tolba, E. Egyptian propolis extract for functionalization of cellulose nanofiber/poly(vinyl alcohol) porous hydrogel along with characterization and biological applications. *Sci. Rep.* **2023**, *13*, 7739. [CrossRef] [PubMed]

23. Kasote, D.; Bankova, V.; Viljoen, A.M. Propolis: Chemical diversity and challenges in quality control. *Phytochem. Rev.* **2022**, *21*, 1887–1911. [CrossRef]
24. Santos, M.S.; Estevinho, L.M.; Carvalho, C.A.L.; Morais, J.S.; Conceição, A.L.S.; Paula, V.B.; Magalhães-Guedes, K.; Almeida, R.C.C. Probiotic Yogurt with Brazilian Red Propolis: Physicochemical and Bioactive Properties, Stability, and Shelf Life. *J. Food Sci.* **2019**, *84*, 3429–3436. [CrossRef]
25. Naik, R.R.; Shakya, A.K.; Oriquat, G.A.; Katekhaye, S.; Paradkar, A.; Fearnley, H.; Fearnley, J. Fatty Acid Analysis, Chemical Constituents, Biological Activity and Pesticide Residues Screening in Jordanian Propolis. *Molecules* **2021**, *26*, 5076. [CrossRef]
26. Wieczorek, P.P.; Hudz, N.; Yezerska, O.; Horčinová-Sedláčková, V.; Shanaida, M.; Korytniuk, O.; Jasicka-Misiak, I. Chemical Variability and Pharmacological Potential of Propolis as a Source for the Development of New Pharmaceutical Products. *Molecules* **2022**, *27*, 1600. [CrossRef] [PubMed]
27. Inci, H.; Sogut, B.; Sengul, T.; Yucel, B.; Kokten, K.; Tunca, R.I.; Ayasan, T.; Bengu, A.S.; Ul, A.G.; Celik, S.; et al. Comparison of fatty acid properties of Bingol Propolis. *S. Afr. J. Anim. Sci.* **2022**, *52*, 392–399. [CrossRef]
28. Vyssotski, M.; Lagutin, K.; Catchpole, O. Simple lipids and hydrocarbons of New Zealand propolis wax. *J. Apic. Res.* **2017**, *57*, 271–277. [CrossRef]
29. Zullkiflee, N.; Taha, H.; Usman, A. Propolis: Its Role and Efficacy in Human Health and Diseases. *Molecules* **2022**, *27*, 6120. [CrossRef]
30. Luo, X.; Li, J.; Cen, Z.; Feng, G.; Hong, M.; Huang, L.; Long, Q. Exploring the therapeutic potential of lupeol: A review of its mechanisms, clinical applications, and advances in bioavailability enhancement. *Food Chem Toxicol.* **2025**, *196*, 115193. [CrossRef]
31. Bobiş, O. Plants: Sources of Diversity in Propolis Properties. *Plants* **2022**, *11*, 2298. [CrossRef] [PubMed]
32. Berretta, A.A.; Arruda, C.; Miguel, F.G.; Baptista, N.; Nascimento, A.P.; Marquele-Oliveira, F.; Hori, J.I.; da Silva Barud, H.; Damaso, B.; Ramos, C.; et al. Functional Properties of Brazilian Propolis: From Chemical Composition Until the Market [Internet]. In *Superfood and Functional Food—An Overview of Their Processing and Utilization*; InTech: London, UK, 2017. [CrossRef]
33. Mountford-McAuley, R.; Robertson, A.; Taylor, M.; Clavijo McCormick, A. Characterisation of New Zealand Propolis from Different Regions Based on Its Volatile Organic Compounds. *Molecules* **2024**, *29*, 3143. [CrossRef] [PubMed]
34. Meto, A.; Colombari, B.; Meto, A.; Boaretto, G.; Pinetti, D.; Marchetti, L.; Benvenuti, S.; Pellati, F.; Blasi, E. Propolis Affects *Pseudomonas aeruginosa* Growth, Biofilm Formation, eDNA Release and Phenazine Production: Potential Involvement of Polyphenols. *Microorganisms* **2020**, *8*, 243. [CrossRef]
35. Wilson, M.B.; Brinkman, D.; Spivak, M.; Gardner, G.; Cohen, J.D. Regional variation in composition and antimicrobial activity of US propolis against Paenibacillus larvae and Ascosphaera apis. *J. Invertebr. Pathol.* **2015**, *124*, 44–50. [CrossRef]
36. Alghutaimel, H.; Matoug-Elwerfelli, M.; Alhaji, M.; Albawardi, F.; Nagendrababu, V.; Dummer, P.M.H. Propolis Use in Dentistry: A Narrative Review of Its Preventive and Therapeutic Applications. *Int. Dent. J.* **2024**, *74*, 365–386. [CrossRef]

37. Pezzella, V.; Cuozzo, A.; Mauriello, L.; Polizzi, A.; Iorio Siciliano, V.; Ramaglia, L.; Blasi, A. Propolis as an Adjunct in Non-Surgical Periodontal Therapy: Current Clinical Perspectives from a Narrative Review. *J. Funct. Biomater.* **2025**, *16*, 265. [CrossRef]
38. Przybyłek, I.; Karpiński, T.M. Antibacterial Properties of Propolis. *Molecules* **2019**, *24*, 2047. [CrossRef]
39. Zulhendri, F.; Lesmana, R.; Tandean, S.; Christoper, A.; Chandrasekaran, K.; Irsyam, I.; Suwantika, A.A.; Abdulah, R.; Wathoni, N. Recent Update on the Anti-Inflammatory Activities of Propolis. *Molecules* **2022**, *27*, 8473. [CrossRef]
40. Bhargava, P.; Mahanta, D.; Kaul, A.; Ishida, Y.; Terao, K.; Wadhwa, R.; Kaul, S.C. Experimental Evidence for Therapeutic Potentials of Propolis. *Nutrients* **2021**, *13*, 2528. [CrossRef] [PubMed]
41. Magnavacca, A.; Sangiovanni, E.; Racagni, G.; Dell'Agli, M. The antiviral and immunomodulatory activities of propolis: An update and future perspectives for respiratory diseases. *Med. Res. Rev.* **2022**, *42*, 897–945. [CrossRef] [PubMed]
42. Forma, E.; Bryś, M. Anticancer Activity of Propolis and Its Compounds. *Nutrients* **2021**, *13*, 2594. [CrossRef]
43. Altabbal, S.; Athamnah, K.; Rahma, A.; Wali, A.F.; Eid, A.H.; Iratni, R.; Al Dhaheri, Y. Propolis: A Detailed Insight of Its Anticancer Molecular Mechanisms. *Pharmaceuticals* **2023**, *16*, 450. [CrossRef]
44. Naeem, M.M.; Sarwar, H.; Nisar, A.; Ahmed, S.; Shabbir, J.; Khurshid, Z.; Palma, P.J. Effect of Propolis on Root Dentine Microhardness When Used as an Intracanal Medicament: An In Vitro Study. *J. Funct. Biomater.* **2023**, *14*, 144. [CrossRef]
45. Meto, A.; Meto, A.; Bimbari, B.; Shytaj, K.; Özcan, M. Anti-Inflammatory and Regenerative Effects of Albanian Propolis in Experimental Vital Amputations. *Eur. J. Prosthodont. Restor. Dent.* **2016**, *24*, 145–151. [CrossRef]
46. El-Sakhawy, M.; Salama, A.; Tohamy, H.S. Applications of propolis-based materials in wound healing. *Arch. Dermatol. Res.* **2023**, *316*, 61. [CrossRef]
47. Lisbona-González, M.J.; Muñoz-Soto, E.; Lisbona-González, C.; Vallecillo-Rivas, M.; Diaz-Castro, J.; Moreno-Fernandez, J. Effect of Propolis Paste and Mouthwash Formulation on Healing after Teeth Extraction in Periodontal Disease. *Plants* **2021**, *10*, 1603. [CrossRef]
48. Duane, B.; Yap, T.; Neelakantan, P.; Anthonappa, R.; Bescos, R.; McGrath, C.; McCullough, M.; Brookes, Z. Mouthwashes: Alternatives and Future Directions. *Int. Dent. J.* **2023**, *73*, S89–S97. [CrossRef] [PubMed]
49. Saeed, M.A.; Khabeer, A.; Faridi, M.A.; Makhdoom, G. Effectiveness of propolis in maintaining oral health: A scoping review. *Can. J. Dent. Hyg.* **2021**, *55*, 167–176. [PubMed]
50. Sokolonski, A.R.; Fonseca, M.S.; Machado, B.A.S.; Deegan, K.R.; Araújo, R.P.C.; Umsza-Guez, M.A.; Meyer, R.; Portela, R.W. Activity of antifungal drugs and Brazilian red and green propolis extracted with different methodologies against oral isolates of *Candida* spp. *BMC Complement. Med. Ther.* **2021**, *21*, 286. [CrossRef] [PubMed]

51. Pina, G.M.; Lia, E.N.; Berretta, A.A.; Nascimento, A.P.; Torres, E.C.; Buszinski, A.F.; de Campos, T.A.; Coelho, E.B.; Martins, V.P. Efficacy of Propolis on the Denture Stomatitis Treatment in Older Adults: A Multicentric Randomized Trial. *Evid.-Based Complement. Altern. Med.* **2017**, *2017*, 8971746. [CrossRef]
52. AlQahtani, S.M.; Nagate, R.R.; Al-Ahmari, M.M.M.; Magbol, M.A.; Gokhale, S.T.; Tikare, S.; Chaturvedi, S. Evaluation of Propolis Hydrogel for the Treatment of Dentinal Sensitivity: A Clinical Study. *Gels* **2023**, *9*, 483. [CrossRef] [PubMed]
53. Naghsh, N.; Mazrooei, F.; Hosseini, A.; Kiani, S.; Sahebkar, A. Effects of Propolis-Based Herbal Toothpaste on Dentine Hypersensitivity. *Int. Dent. J.* **2024**, *74*, 559–565. [CrossRef]
54. Armutcu, F.; Akyol, S.; Ustunsoy, S.; Turan, F.F. Therapeutic potential of caffeic acid phenethyl ester and its anti-inflammatory and immunomodulatory effects (Review). *Exp. Ther. Med.* **2015**, *9*, 1582–1588. [CrossRef]
55. Luque-Bracho, A.; Rosales, Y.; Vergara-Buenaventura, A. The benefits of propolis in periodontal therapy. A scoping review of preclinical and clinical studies. *J. Ethnopharmacol.* **2023**, *303*, 115926. [CrossRef]
56. Bertolucci, V.; Ninomiya, A.F.; Longato, G.B.; Kaneko, L.O.; Nonose, N.; Scariot, P.P.M.; Messias, L.H.D. Bioactive Compounds from Propolis on Bone Homeostasis: A Narrative Review. *Antioxidants* **2025**, *14*, 81. [CrossRef]
57. Zarei, M.; Jafarian, A.H.; Harandi, A.; Javidi, M.; Gharechahi, M. Evaluation of the expression of VIII factor and VEGF in the regeneration of non-vital teeth in dogs using propolis. *Iran. J. Basic Med. Sci.* **2017**, *20*, 172–177. [CrossRef]
58. Aldosari, A.Y.; Aljared, A.M.; Alqurshy, H.S.; Alfarran, A.M.; Alnahdi, M.G.; Alharbi, S.S.; Alharbi, W.S.; Alghamdi, F.T. The Clinical Effectiveness of Propolis on the Endodontic Treatment of Permanent Teeth: A Systematic Review of Randomized Clinical Trials and Updates. *Cureus* **2025**, *17*, e77430. [CrossRef] [PubMed]
59. Maria Parro, Y.; de Mendonça Guimarães, D.; Sampaio Muller, H.; Barbosa Coelho, E.; Aparecida Berretta, A.; Aparecida de Lima, J.; De Jong, D.; de Paulo Martins, V.T.; Negrini Lia, E. Efficacy of a 0.5% Propolis -0.9% Pomegranate Buccal Spray Treatment Compared with 2% Miconazole Gel for Denture Stomatitis Treatment in Elderly Patients: A Randomized Clinical Trial. *J. Dent.* **2022**, *23*, 472–479. [CrossRef]
60. Gunjal, S.; Pateel, D.G.S. Comparative effectiveness of Propolis with chlorhexidine mouthwash on gingivitis—A randomized controlled clinical study. *BMC Complement. Med. Ther.* **2024**, *24*, 154. [CrossRef]
61. Sycińska-Dziarnowska, M.; Szyszka-Sommerfeld, L.; Bugajska, M.; Ziąbka, M.; Szućko-Kociuba, I.; Spagnuolo, G.; Woźniak, K.; Park, H.-S. Propolis as a Natural Remedy in Reducing Dental Plaque and Gingival Inflammation: A Systematic Review and Meta-Analysis. *J. Funct. Biomater.* **2025**, *16*, 336. [CrossRef] [PubMed]
62. Ali, S.; Farooq, I.; Bugshan, A.; Siddiqui, I.A.; Al-Khalifa, K.S.; Al-Hariri, M. Efficacy of propolis in remineralising artificially induced demineralisation of human enamel—An in-vitro study. *J. Taibah Univ. Med. Sci.* **2020**, *16*, 283–287. [CrossRef]
63. Fraire-Reyes Irma, A.; Gaitán-Fonseca, C.; Cepeda-Argüelles, Ó.; Esparza-Villalpando, V.; Aguilera-Galavíz, L.; Bermúdez-Jiménez, C. Use and effectiveness of propolis on chronic periodontitis: A systematic review. *Odovtos Int. J. Dent. Sci.* **2022**, *24*, 32–43. [CrossRef]

64. Ayad, A.S.; Benchaabane, S.; Daas, T.; Smagghe, G.; Loucif-Ayad, W. Propolis Stands out as a Multifaceted Natural Product: Meta-Analysis on Its Sources, Bioactivities, Applications, and Future Perspectives. *Life* **2025**, *15*, 764. [CrossRef]
65. Contieri, L.S.; de Souza Mesquita, L.M.; Sanches, V.L.; Viganó, J.; Martinez, J.; da Cunha, D.T.; Rostagno, M.A. Standardization proposal to quality control of propolis extracts commercialized in Brazil: A fingerprinting methodology using a UHPLC-PDA-MS/MS approach. *Food Res. Int.* **2022**, *161*, 111846. [CrossRef]
66. Suhandi, C.; Wilar, G.; Lesmana, R.; Zulhendri, F.; Suharyani, I.; Hasan, N.; Wathoni, N. Propolis-Based Nanostructured Lipid Carriers for α-Mangostin Delivery: Formulation, Characterization, and In Vitro Antioxidant Activity Evaluation. *Molecules* **2023**, *28*, 6057. [CrossRef]
67. Kustiawan, P.M.; Syaifie, P.H.; Al Khairy Siregar, K.A.; Ibadillah, D.; Mardliyati, E. New insights of propolis nanoformulation and its therapeutic potential in human diseases. *ADMET DMPK* **2024**, *12*, 1–26. [CrossRef] [PubMed]
68. Hossain, S.; Yousaf, M.; Liu, Y.; Chang, D.; Zhou, X. An Overview of the Evidence and Mechanism of Drug-Herb Interactions Between Propolis and Pharmaceutical Drugs. *Front. Pharmacol.* **2022**, *13*, 876183. [CrossRef] [PubMed]
69. Salatino, A. Perspectives for Uses of Propolis in Therapy against Infectious Diseases. *Molecules* **2022**, *27*, 4594. [CrossRef] [PubMed]

5. Advancements in Copper–Calcium Hydroxide (Cupral) Research and Its Applications in Dentistry

5.1. Problems of Endodontic Treatment of Teeth

Building on the in-depth exploration of oral biofilms and their impact on health and disease in the previous chapters, Chapter 4 focused on the use of natural products like propolis in dentistry, particularly within endodontics. While propolis has demonstrated significant benefits, copper–calcium hydroxide (Cupral) has proven to be even more effective in various dental treatments, offering a superior alternative for those seeking additional solutions. The upcoming sections will examine this in detail, following a brief overview of the challenges encountered in dental scenarios.

Figure 16a illustrates the progression from dental caries to pulpitis and periodontitis and can visually highlight the critical steps in endodontic treatment, emphasizing the importance of thorough canal cleaning, shaping, and obturation in preventing further complications.

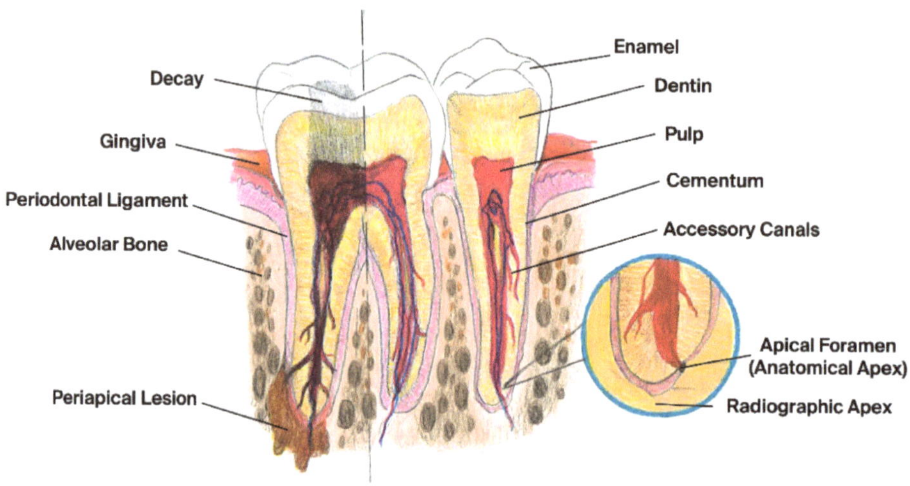

(a)

Figure 16. *Cont.*

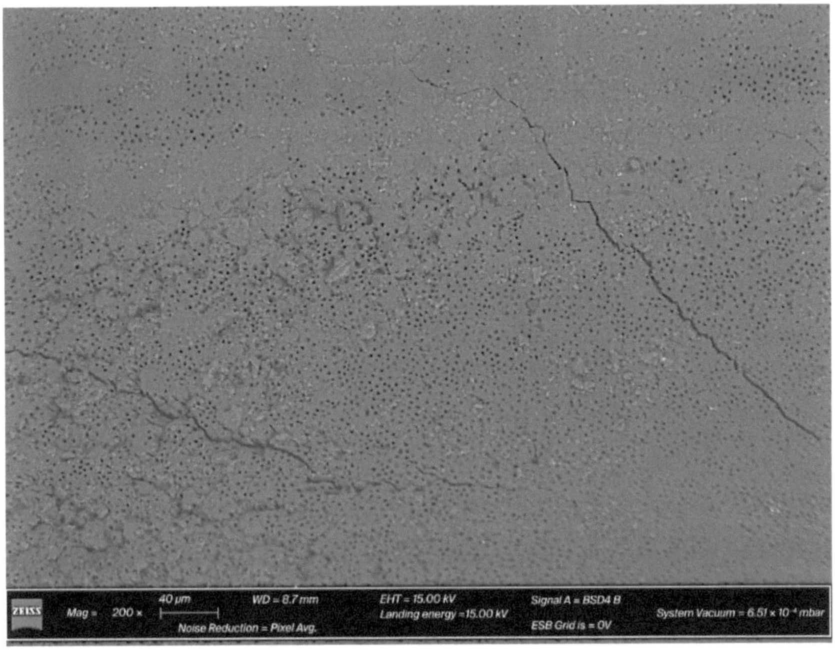

(b)

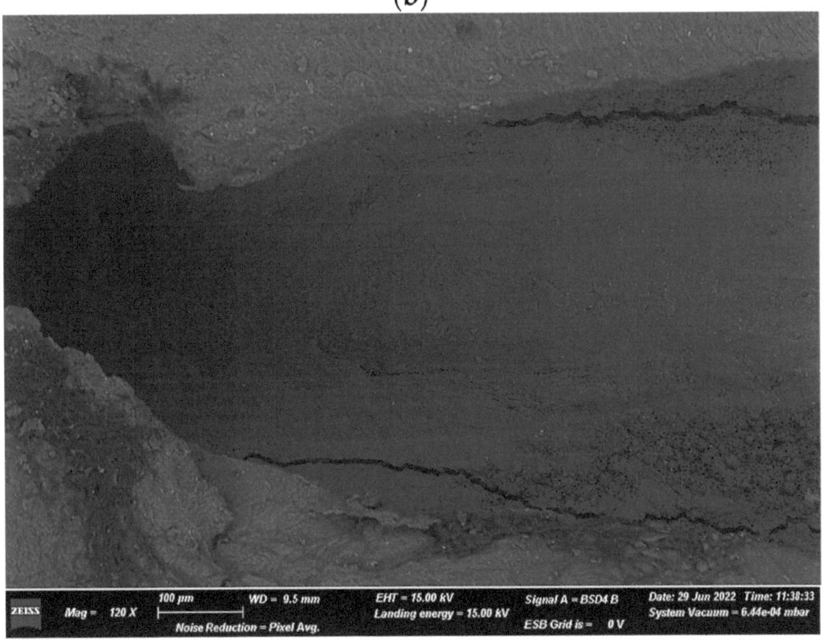

(c)

Figure 16. (**a**) Schematic representation of the progression from untreated dental caries to pulpitis and periodontitis, emphasizing the need for timely endodontic intervention. This figure provides a detailed depiction of tooth anatomy, illustrating key structures such as enamel, dentin, pulp, cementum, gingiva, PDL, and alveolar bone. The left side of the diagram depicts the development of decay leading to a periapical lesion, characterized by inflammation and infection at the root apex. A magnified inset on the right highlights the complex root anatomy, distinguishing between the anatomical apex (apical foramen) and the radiographic apex, underscoring the importance of precise diagnosis and treatment to prevent the spread of infection and the healing of periapical tissues. Credit: © Nensi Kallfani, used with permission. (**b**) SEM of canal dentin from an extracted, untreated tooth at 200× magnification. This image vividly displays the intricate microstructure of the dentin, revealing the dense network of dentinal tubules and the inherent porosity of the tooth's canal system. This micrograph underscores the importance of understanding dentin's structural complexity for optimizing endodontic therapies and improving clinical outcomes. Source: Picture by author. (**c**) SEM image of the root surface of an extracted maxillary canine at 120× magnification. The image shows the cementum surface with irregular topography and exposed dentinal structures, illustrating typical micro-morphological features of the root surface. Source: Picture by author.

Complications from dental caries, such as pulpitis and periodontitis, account for a significant portion of dental practice, representing nearly one-third of all cases and serving as primary causes of tooth extraction, thereby highlighting the need for effective endodontic strategies. If untreated, these conditions can intensify, leading to severe complications like abscess formation or systemic involvement, underscoring the importance of thorough endodontic treatment [1]. The treatment of the root canal system is a primary goal in endodontics, aiming to eliminate the infection within the canal and prevent its recurrence. Mechanical instrumentation, utilizing endodontic files, is crucial for removing infected tissue and shaping the canal for effective sealing, while antimicrobial agents target residual microflora and neutralize microbial byproducts, both of which are essential for preventing treatment failure [2]. Once the canal has been adequately cleaned and shaped, it must be obturated, or filled, with materials that prevent reinfection. A well-obturated canal creates a hermetic seal, effectively blocking microorganisms and their byproducts from entering or leaving the root canal system [3]. Poor obturation, characterized by voids, gaps, or inadequate sealing, is often associated with higher rates of treatment failure and persistent infection. These issues compromise the treatment's effectiveness and can lead to recurrent symptoms and the need for retreatment [4,5]. One of the critical challenges in endodontics is achieving a hermetic seal throughout the entire canal system, including the lateral canals and dentinal tubules, which are often difficult to access and fill completely (Figure 16b,c).

Achieving a comprehensive seal, especially in lateral canals and dentinal tubules, is a critical challenge in endodontics, particularly in cases of apical periodontitis where infection and inflammation complicate the sealing process. Insufficient obturation has been frequently identified as a cause of endodontic complications, leading to persistent or recurrent periapical lesions [6]. Long-term studies, such as the 18-year follow-up by Pontoriero et al. (2021), have shown high success rates for well-obturated teeth, regardless of whether posts were used, reinforcing the need for personalized treatment strategies [7]. Moreover, inadequate obturation remains a significant contributor to treatment failure, as evidenced by the work of Tabassum and Khan (2016), who provide practical guidance for improving obturation techniques [8].

To address these challenges, the adoption of advanced techniques and materials is crucial. Geurtsen and Leyhausen's (1997) extensive research on the biological properties of various root canal filling materials underscored the critical need for materials that not only effectively seal the root canal system but also ensure biocompatibility, minimizing adverse reactions in surrounding tissues and thereby enhancing the long-term success of endodontic treatments [9].

Modern endodontics increasingly focuses on materials that not only seal the canal system but also support regeneration, especially in managing chronic periodontitis, where eliminating infection and stimulating bone regeneration are critical goals [10]. To enhance the efficiency of endodontic treatments and reduce overall treatment time, the incorporation of materials that contain antibiotics, sulfanilamides, and other bioactive agents has been proposed. These materials are specifically designed to extend beyond the apex of the root canal, where they can exert potent antimicrobial effects and stimulate phagocytosis [11]. This process is crucial for the transformation of granulation tissue into fibrous tissue, a key step in the healing process.

In cases where root canals are particularly challenging due to their impassable nature or complex anatomy, techniques such as iontophoresis and electrophoresis have become integral to both international and national dental practices [12]. Electrophoresis, in particular, has been effectively utilized to introduce therapeutic agents like iodine, decamethoxine, and dimexide directly into the tooth canal and periodontium, enhancing the penetration and efficacy of the treatment [13,14]. This technique has also proven beneficial in treating cold abscesses, particularly in chronic cases where symptoms are not overt, by increasing the overall effectiveness of the endodontic treatment. Furthermore, Mironova's (1977) work with transcanal ultraphonophoresis demonstrated significant improvements in the penetration of medicinal substances into the periodontium [15]. This method, although complex and requiring the tooth to be encased in a titanium shell to improve bone contact, offers a promising approach to enhancing treatment outcomes, especially in challenging cases like apical periodontitis [15].

For dental clinicians, a deep understanding of the factors influencing canal filling quality is paramount, and continuous education on evidence-based obturation practices is crucial for improving long-term treatment outcomes and patient satisfaction.

Introduction to Copper–Calcium Hydroxide (Cupral)

Copper–calcium hydroxide (commonly known as Cupral) is an advanced endodontic medicament that combines copper (Cu) and calcium hydroxide [$Ca(OH)_2$] in a synergistic formulation. Chemically, it typically exists as a paste or suspension in which finely dispersed copper compounds are integrated with calcium hydroxide, producing a dual-action therapeutic effect. The copper component provides broad-spectrum antimicrobial properties through the sustained release of Cu^{2+} ions, which disrupt bacterial cell membranes, denature proteins, and interfere with microbial enzyme systems, effectively targeting even resistant biofilm-forming species such as *E. faecalis* and *C. albicans* [16–18].

In parallel, the high alkalinity of $Ca(OH)_2$ (pH $\approx$ 12.4) creates an inhospitable environment for most oral pathogens, denatures bacterial endotoxins, and stimulates hard tissue formation. This combination not only eliminates existing infections but also inhibits recolonization within the root canal system [19,20].

A distinguishing feature of Cupral over traditional calcium hydroxide lies in its enhanced and prolonged antimicrobial effect. While $Ca(OH)_2$'s antibacterial efficacy diminishes over time due to buffering by dentinal fluid and organic matter, the copper ions in Cupral maintain sustained antimicrobial activity, even in challenging anaerobic and necrotic environments [17,21]. Studies have shown that Cupral achieves deeper penetration into dentinal tubules, especially when applied with electrophoretic or depotphoresis techniques, resulting in superior biofilm disruption compared to $Ca(OH)_2$ alone [18,22,23].

From a regenerative standpoint, Cupral's alkaline environment stimulates osteoblastic and odontoblastic activity, aiding in the repair of periapical bone and cementum. In clinical contexts, its use has been associated with faster resolution of periapical lesions, reduced postoperative pain, and improved long-term treatment stability [22,24]. Furthermore, its bioactivity extends to encouraging mineralized tissue deposition, an essential factor in apexification and apical barrier formation in immature teeth [18,20].

Given its broad-spectrum antimicrobial potency, biofilm penetration capacity, tissue regenerative potential, and compatibility with advanced delivery systems, Cupral is increasingly regarded as a superior alternative to traditional calcium hydroxide in endodontics, especially in cases of persistent or complex infections where conventional methods may fail.

5.2. Composition of Cupral

Achieving successful dental treatment is often hindered by various challenges, such as complex anatomy, obliterated canals, fractured instruments within root canals, and impassable pathways [25]. Additionally, patient allergies to certain endodontic materials can further complicate treatment outcomes. To address these issues, Cupral, a compound consisting of Cu and $Ca(OH)_2$, offers a versatile solution for a range of clinical scenarios. The unique properties and applications of Cupral are explored in detail in the following sections.

5.2.1. Cu in Dentistry

Cu is a versatile metal with significant applications across healthcare, technology, and industry, driven by its unique properties and benefits. Recent research and developments have highlighted its diverse applications, particularly emphasizing its antimicrobial properties and its role in enhancing the performance of various materials.

One of the primary areas of research focuses on Cu's potent antimicrobial properties, which are effective against a broad spectrum of pathogens, including bacteria, viruses, and fungi. Studies have demonstrated that copper surfaces can kill microorganisms upon contact, significantly reducing the spread of infections, especially in healthcare settings. This makes Cu a valuable asset in infection control, particularly in hospitals where preventing the transmission of pathogens is critical. The integration of copper surfaces in medical facilities has been shown to substantially lower microbial loads, leading to reduced infection rates among patients, thereby enhancing overall patient safety and care quality [16].

In dentistry, Cu's integration has garnered considerable attention due to its antimicrobial properties and its ability to improve the physical and chemical characteristics of dental materials. Cu-containing nanoparticles, for instance, have been shown to inhibit microbial growth when added to dental materials, primarily through the release of copper ions. These ions disrupt microbial cell walls and metabolic processes, thereby significantly reducing the risk of infections associated with dental procedures and improving patient outcomes [21].

Furthermore, the incorporation of copper nanoparticles into dental amalgams, cements, and polymers has demonstrated improvements in mechanical strength, wear resistance, and antimicrobial efficacy. These enhancements make dental restorations more durable and resistant to microbial colonization, ultimately leading to longer-lasting dental work and improved oral health [26].

Cu also plays a crucial role in preventing gum disease and tooth decay by combating harmful microorganisms. The antimicrobial properties of Cu contribute to healthier gums by reducing the risk of periodontal diseases and gingivitis, which are often exacerbated by bacterial plaque. In endodontics, Cu bands are used to create resin cores in teeth with subgingival margins. These copper bands can be precisely shaped to fit the dental structure, providing a secure fit and effective isolation for resin core buildup, which is crucial for the success of endodontic treatments. This method improves the precision and reliability of endodontic restorations, contributing to better long-term outcomes for patients [27].

Ongoing research continues to support Cu's potential in improving dental treatments, reducing infections, and promoting overall oral health, making it a vital component in modern dental practice.

5.2.2. $Ca(OH)_2$ in Dentistry

$Ca(OH)_2$ has been a cornerstone in dentistry for over a century, valued for its high pH and therapeutic properties, particularly in endodontics and pulp therapy. Its versatile applications have made it an essential component in various dental treatments.

One of the primary uses of $Ca(OH)_2$ is as an intracanal medicament during endodontic therapy. Its high pH creates an alkaline environment within the root canal system, effectively inhibiting bacterial growth and aiding in the dissolution of necrotic tissue. This makes it an invaluable tool for disinfecting root canals, contributing to the success of endodontic treatments [19,28].

Additionally, $Ca(OH)_2$ is widely used as a component in root canal sealers, enhancing their antimicrobial properties. By providing additional protection against residual bacteria, it helps to ensure a hermetic seal after root canal therapy, reducing the risk of reinfection and improving treatment outcomes [29,30].

In pulp therapy, $Ca(OH)_2$ plays a crucial role in pulp capping procedures, where it is applied directly over exposed pulp tissue to promote healing and maintain vitality. The compound induces the formation of a reparative dentin bridge, which protects the pulp and facilitates its recovery [20]. Furthermore, in young permanent teeth with incomplete root formation, $Ca(OH)_2$ is used in apexification procedures to stimulate the formation of a calcified barrier at the root apex. This process enables subsequent root canal therapy, ensuring the long-term preservation of the tooth.

$Ca(OH)_2$ is also employed in the management of root perforations, where its ability to promote calcification helps seal the perforation and restore the integrity of the tooth structure. This application is particularly beneficial in preserving teeth that might otherwise be lost due to structural damage [31].

5.2.3. Cupral's Role in Dentistry

Cupral has emerged as a crucial agent in dentistry, particularly within the field of endodontics, due to its potent antimicrobial properties and excellent biocompatibility. These characteristics make it especially effective in managing root canal infections and promoting the healing of periapical tissues. Cupral has been developed in various formulations, such as pastes and solutions, designed to disinfect root canals thoroughly and support the healing process. Research has shown that in vitro, Cupral exhibits high effectiveness against a wide range of pathogens commonly associated with endodontic infections, including *S. aureus*, *P. aeruginosa*, and *C. albicans* [17]. The study found that Cupral paste exhibited significant antimicrobial activity against all tested microorganisms. The paste was able to significantly inhibit microbial growth, both in planktonic form and in biofilms. In particular, Cupral paste demonstrated antibiofilm activity, disrupting the biofilm structure and reducing the viability of microorganisms within the biofilm. This dual action of antimicrobial and antibiofilm efficacy highlights the potential of Cupral-based materials in the management of endodontic infections. The study suggests that Cupral may serve as an effective adjunct in root canal disinfection, particularly in cases where conventional treatments have failed or when dealing with persistent infections [17].

Beyond its disinfection capabilities, Cupral has also demonstrated promise in enhancing periapical healing, particularly when used in conjunction with advanced techniques like permanent electrophoretic current. This innovative approach has been shown to be effective in treating apical periodontitis, a challenging condition often exacerbated by the complex anatomy of the root canal system and the persistence of microbial biofilms. By using electrophoretic current, Cupral's antimicrobial agents are more thoroughly delivered into the infected tissues, resulting in more comprehensive disinfection and improved clinical outcomes [22].

Ex vivo studies further validate the efficacy of Cupral, particularly when employed in combination with depotphoresis—a method that enhances the diffusion of disinfectants into the root canal system through electrochemical techniques. This method has proven effective in eradicating pathogens from hard-to-reach areas, thereby supporting more thorough root canal disinfection [32]. Moreover, studies comparing the efficacy of Cupral with other disinfection methods, such as electrophoresis, have shown Cupral to be highly effective in reducing microbial loads, including in complex scenarios like canals blocked by separated instruments [33].

The antimicrobial action of Cupral is primarily driven by the release of Cu ions, which, when combined with the high pH environment provided by $Ca(OH)_2$, create conditions that are lethal to bacteria, ensuring effective root canal disinfection. Additionally, Cupral has been shown to promote the formation of mineralized tissue, which aids in the repair of periapical lesions and further supports the healing process.

Cupral's utility is not limited to endodontics; it also holds promise in other areas of dentistry. For example, a case report by Meto et al. (2019) demonstrated the effectiveness of Cupral solution in reducing microbial plaque on orthodontic clear aligners [34]. The study revealed that the application of Cupral significantly reduced plaque accumulation, thereby mitigating the risk of caries and gingivitis associated with the use of clear aligners. This finding suggests that Cupral could be an important adjunct in orthodontic care, helping to maintain oral hygiene and prevent complications during treatment. Figure 17 illustrates the diverse microbial species commonly found on orthodontic clear aligners, as reported by Meto et al. (2019), and demonstrates how the application of Cupral solution effectively reduces microbial plaque on these aligners [34]. The study demonstrated significant antimicrobial activity against several oral pathogens, including *Streptococcus sanguinis*, *Streptococcus mitis/oralis*, *Rothia aeria*, *Staphylococcus aureus*, *Neisseria mucosa/sicca*, and *Haemophilus parainfluenzae*. The results underline the importance of using effective antimicrobial agents in maintaining the hygiene of orthodontic devices, potentially preventing oral health complications associated with biofilm formation on aligners.

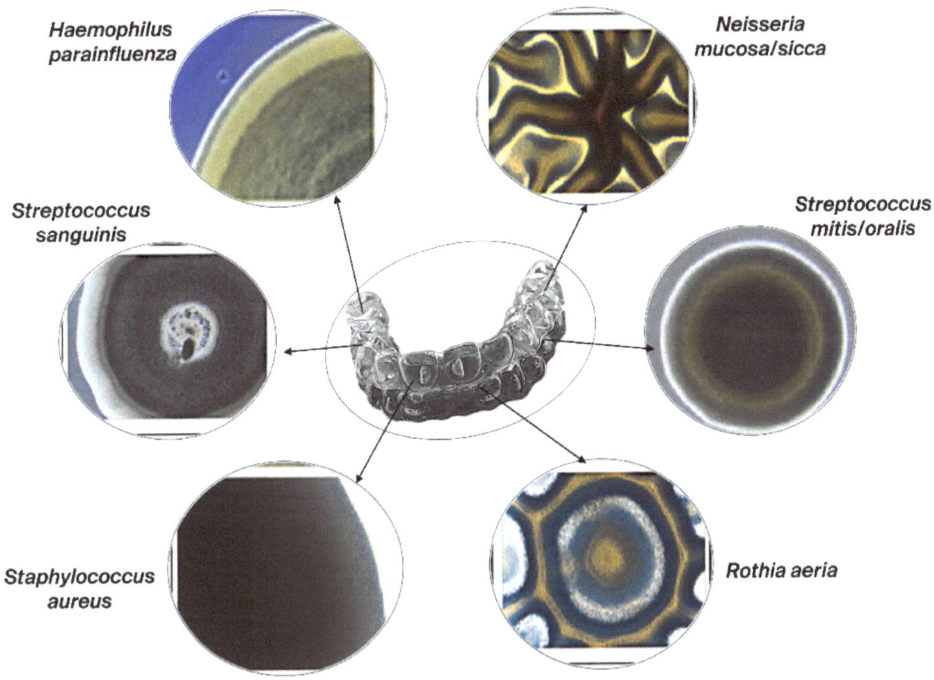

Figure 17. Microbial species isolated from orthodontic clear aligners. The figure illustrates the diverse range of oral pathogens commonly found on clear aligners, with the central image showcasing the aligner itself. Surrounding close-ups highlight the distinct colonies of each microorganism, underscoring the microbial diversity on these dental devices. The pathogens identified include *S. sanguinis*, *Streptococcus mitis/oralis*, *Rothia aeria*, *S. aureus*, *Neisseria mucosa/sicca*, and *Haemophilus parainfluenzae* [34]. Source: Figure by author.

Further supporting these findings, several studies have explored the use of Cupral in conjunction with depotphoresis for treating challenging endodontic cases. Research by Enginalev and Gura (1985) highlighted the effectiveness of depotphoresis materials as galvanic post elements, particularly in hard-to-reach or blocked canals [35]. Knappwost (1998) emphasized the importance of physicochemical techniques like depotphoresis in advancing endodontic outcomes, highlighting its role in the evolution of modern endodontic practices [36].

In addition, Zhdanov et al. (2002) demonstrated the effectiveness of Cupral depotphoresis in delivering medicaments to impassable and hard-to-reach root canals, significantly improving treatment success rates [37]. Similarly, a study by Moradi et al. (2023) demonstrated that depotphoresis, when combined with Cupral, was significantly more effective than traditional irrigation methods in reducing bacterial counts, particularly against *E. faecalis*, a common and resilient pathogen in root canal infections [32]. However, Rumiantsev et al. (2013) employed electron microscopy to evaluate the effectiveness of endodontic electrophoresis, demonstrating that this technique is highly proficient in eliminating bacteria and debris from the root canal system [38].

Recent research has significantly expanded our understanding of Cupral's efficacy and its comparison to other antimicrobial agents like calcium hydroxide in various clinical scenarios. For instance, a systematic review conducted by Lina et al. (2023) meticulously analyzed the use of Cu-$Ca(OH)_2$ nanoparticles, particularly in the treatment of apical periodontitis [18]. The review highlighted the unique advantages of these nanoparticles, noting their potent antimicrobial activity, which is crucial in reducing the microbial load in infected root canals. Apical periodontitis is notoriously difficult to treat due to the complexity of the root canal system and the presence of resistant bacterial strains. The review by Lina et al. emphasized how the incorporation of Cu into $Ca(OH)_2$ not only enhances the antimicrobial properties but also supports tissue healing and regeneration. This dual action makes Cu-$Ca(OH)_2$ nanoparticles an attractive option for endodontic therapy, especially in cases where traditional materials may fall short in effectively managing infection and promoting recovery [18].

In another study, Aminsobhani et al. (2021) explored the safety and efficacy of Cu ion extrusion following electrophoresis in a clinical setting [39]. The study specifically measured the amount of copper ions extruded from the apex of human teeth with single canals after the application of electrophoresis. The findings demonstrated that the controlled extrusion of copper ions during the procedure was both safe and effective, contributing to the disinfection process without causing adverse effects on the surrounding tissues. This research is particularly significant as it addresses concerns related to the potential cytotoxicity of Cu ions, confirming that when properly managed, Cu-based treatments can be both potent and safe. The study underscores the importance of precise control in the application of electrophoresis to maximize therapeutic benefits while minimizing risks, reinforcing the role of Cu ions as a valuable component in endodontic therapy [39].

These studies collectively highlight the evolving landscape of endodontic materials and techniques, where the integration of advanced Cu-based compounds like Cupral offers promising alternatives to traditional approaches, particularly in the management of complex infections and in promoting optimal healing outcomes.

Overall, Cupral represents a powerful tool in modern dentistry, combining antimicrobial action with tissue-regenerative properties. Its applications span from endodontic therapy to orthodontic care, making it a versatile and valuable addition to the dental practitioner's armamentarium. Ongoing research continues to support its efficacy and potential in improving oral health outcomes.

5.3. Depotphoresis Methodology

Depotphoresis with Cupral, developed by Prof. Adolf Knappwost, represents a significant advancement in endodontic treatment, offering a more targeted and effective approach compared to traditional hydroxyl iontophoresis. This method involves the electrophoretic application of Cupral within the root canal system, where it forms a long-term reservoir that ensures complete sterility and promotes bone tissue regeneration. By shifting the pH within the canal to an alkaline environment, depotphoresis creates conditions conducive to healing and mineralization, making it a valuable tool in complex endodontic cases [23].

5.3.1. Methodology of Depotphoresis with Cupral

The depotphoresis treatment begins with the preparation of the root canal. In the first session, the canal is mechanically opened using ISO instruments from size 40 to approximately two-thirds of its length. Following this preparation, Cupral paste is introduced into the canal (Figure 18a) [23,36].

Cupral's formulation is highly potent due to the synergistic bactericidal properties of Cu and Ca ions, which disrupt microbial proteins and create an alkaline environment hostile to bacterial survival [23,36].

The key aspect of depotphoresis is the use of electrophoresis, an electrochemical process that drives Cupral deep into the root canal system. During the initial session, a controlled electrical current is applied through specialized electrophoresis equipment. This current facilitates the penetration of Cupral into the intricate structures of the root canal, including lateral canals and dentinal tubules, ensuring a thorough disinfection that exceeds the capabilities of conventional methods [23].

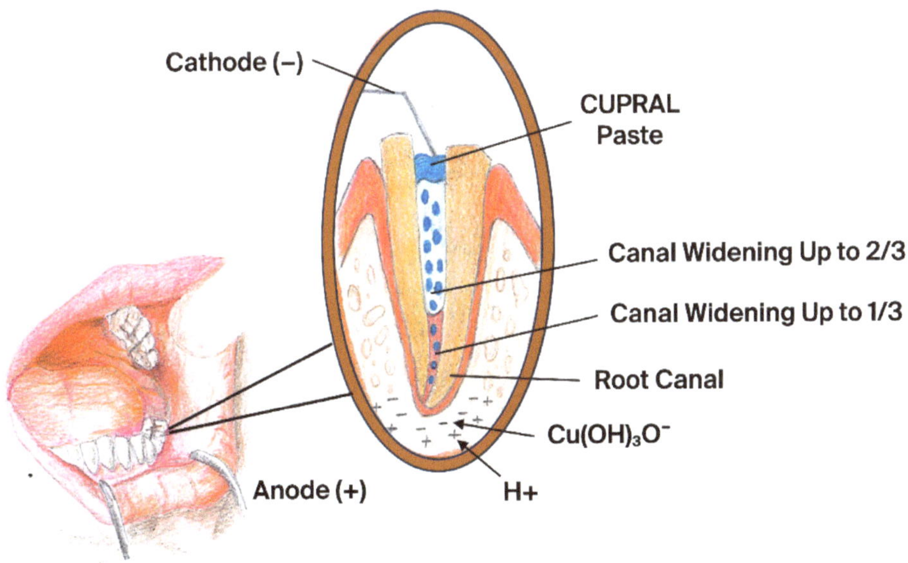

(a)

Figure 18. *Cont.*

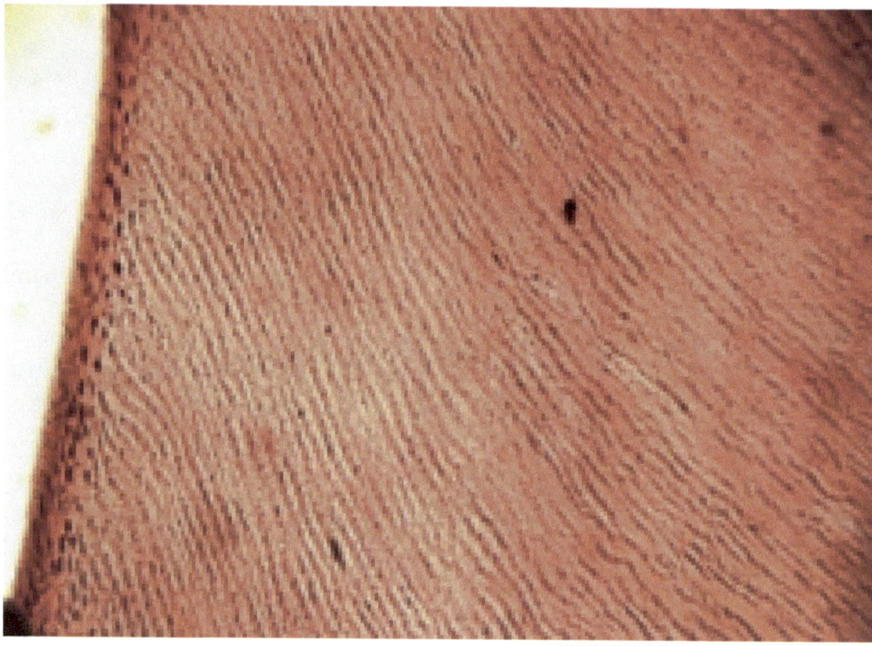

(b)

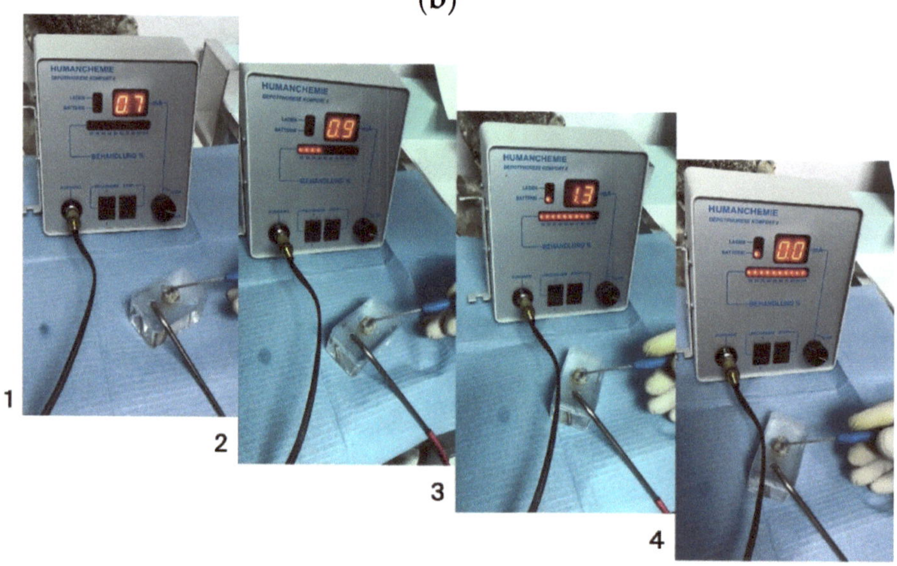

(c)

Figure 18. (**a**) Schematic representation of a depotphoresis session using cupral. This figure illustrates the detailed process of depotphoresis during endodontic treatment, where Cupral paste is applied within the root canal. The diagram shows the application of the cathode (−) and anode (+) electrodes, creating an electrophoretic environment that facilitates the movement of $Cu(OH)_3O^-$ ions into the dentinal tubules and the root canal system. The root canal is widened progressively up to two-thirds and one-third of its length, allowing for the effective penetration of the Cupral paste. The ions generated during the process play a critical role in disinfecting the canal and promoting healing. This visual also includes a cross-section of the tooth within the oral cavity, highlighting the placement of electrodes and their respective polarities. The illustration effectively captures the essential elements of the depotphoresis. Credit: © Nensi Kallfani, used with permission. (**b**) The longitudinal slide exhibits the blockage of dentinal radicular, which extend from the internal canal to the dentin-cementum junction. The image reveals light brown micro-crystals of Cu that characterize these obstructions, with the canal lumen matrix visibly impregnated with copper sulfide. This distribution of micro-crystals and the copper sulfide matrix indicates the extent of the copper-based treatment's penetration and its interaction with the dentinal structure. Credit: © Agron Meto, used with permission. (**c**) Sequential stages of depotphoresis methodology demonstrated ex vivo using an extracted tooth. The sequence illustrates the step-by-step process of the depotphoresis technique, simulating a clinical environment. The stages are as follows: (1) Device Activation—the depotphoresis device is activated, initiating the procedure with Cupral paste applied to the open root canal. (2) & (3) Voltage Monitoring—the procedure progresses with voltage readings displayed, ensuring effective iontophoresis within the canal during treatment. (4) Procedure Completion—the treatment concludes, marking the final phase of the depotphoresis as it would be performed in a clinical setting. Source: Picture by author.

In the subsequent sessions, typically the second and third, the procedure is repeated with an increased current strength, reaching up to 5 mA. This step ensures that any remaining microorganisms are eradicated and that the Cupral paste continues to act as a reservoir, releasing ions that contribute to ongoing disinfection and healing. By the end of the third session, the root canal system is expected to be fully sterilized and ready for final obturation [36].

Knappwost's methodology emphasizes creating a stable deposit of Cupral, which gradually releases ions into the canal system, sterilizing the tissues and promoting bone regeneration.

From a histopathological view, Figure 18b demonstrates the intricate patterning of blocked dentinal radicular microcanals, highlighting extensive Cu crystal deposition within the dentin. The light brown coloration indicates the presence of Cu micro-crystals, which are systematically arranged throughout the microcanals and further impregnated with a copper sulfide matrix. This microscopic view provides valuable insight into the penetration of copper-based treatment within the dentinal structure, effectively sealing the microcanals from the internal canal to the dentin-cementum junction. Visualization underscores the potential of Cu compounds to enhance the durability and antimicrobial efficacy of endodontic treatments.

The use of an electrophoresis apparatus enables precise control of current strength and treatment duration. Figure 18c presents a sequential ex vivo demonstration of the depotphoresis methodology using an extracted tooth, highlighting the key stages of device activation, voltage monitoring, and the final procedure completion, effectively simulating the application of this technique in a clinical environment.

5.3.2. Final Canal Sealing with Atacamit

After completing the depotphoresis treatment sessions, the next step is the permanent obturation of the root canal. This is achieved using Atacamit, a specialized cement known for its strong sealing properties and X-ray opacity. Atacamit plays a crucial role in preventing bacterial reinvasion after sterilization. The cement's powder component includes calcium oxide, calcium silicate, calcium aluminate, titanium oxide, copper oxide chloride, magnesium hexafluorosilicate, and polyvinyl pyrrolidone. The liquid component consists of high-dispersion $Ca(OH)_2$ powder mixed with distilled water.

To prepare Atacamit for use, the powder and liquid are mixed on a glass plate with a metal spatula until the paste achieves a consistency suitable for insertion into the canal using a lentulo spiral or filler instrument. It is essential to avoid the paste overflowing into the periapical region, as its high pH (11.5–12) can cause discomfort. However, once the paste hardens, it provides long-term protection against bacterial infiltration by maintaining an alkaline environment that continues to disinfect the canal [40].

Atacamit's robust sealing capability ensures that the sterilization achieved through depotphoresis is maintained, providing a complete and lasting seal. It is important to note that while Atacamit is effective for sealing, it lacks sufficient mechanical strength for securing intracanal posts on its own. Therefore, additional cement may be required if post-fixation is necessary.

5.3.3. Clinical Success and Applications

Depotphoresis with Cupral has shown significant clinical success in endodontic treatments, particularly in cases where traditional methods have failed or where the root canal system's anatomy presents challenges. Studies have reported increased mineralization in periapical tissues and a reduction in destructive foci, both critical indicators of successful treatment outcomes. For instance, a study by Meto et al. (2021) demonstrated the effectiveness of Cupral used in conjunction with permanent electrophoretic current for treating apical periodontitis [22]. This combined approach was found to be more effective in achieving the clinical and radiographic resolution of apical periodontitis compared to conventional methods. The use of electrophoresis with Cupral not only facilitated the eradication of pathogens but also promoted healing, making it a valuable option for resistant cases [22].

Moreover, depotphoresis reduces the need for extensive mechanical instrumentation, which is often associated with increased risks of complications. By focusing on thorough sterilization and effective canal filling, depotphoresis aligns with the principles of minimally invasive dentistry, offering a comprehensive yet conservative approach to endodontic therapy. This method is particularly indicated for use in canals with partial passability, teeth requiring retreatment, cases involving broken or stuck instruments, and scenarios where there is limited access due to a restricted oral opening. However, it is contraindicated in cases such as pregnancy, malignant neoplasms, severe autoimmune diseases, allergic reactions to copper, relapses of acute chronic periodontitis, purulent cysts, and the presence of silver pins [23].

In a randomized clinical trial conducted by Dalaei Moghadam et al. (2021), the comparative efficacy of depotphoresis and diode laser treatments was evaluated for their effectiveness in reducing microbial load, alleviating postoperative pain, and promoting the healing of periapical lesions [24]. The study demonstrated that both methods were effective in reducing microbial counts within the root canal system, but depotphoresis showed superior results in terms of sustained microbial suppression and faster healing of periapical tissues. Additionally, patients treated with depotphoresis reported lower levels of postoperative pain compared to those treated with diode laser, suggesting that depotphoresis may offer a more comprehensive and patient-friendly approach to managing endodontic infections and enhancing recovery [24].

The method offers an important advantage for endodontists, reducing the demand for extensive instrumentation and minimizing operative complications. It aligns with the principles of minimally invasive "biological" treatment, emphasizing the importance of comprehensive sterilization and effective canal filling.

5.4. Comparative Efficacy and Controlled Studies of Cupral

Research on the clinical performance of Cupral remains relatively limited, but several controlled studies provide important insights into its potential as an antimicrobial adjunct in endodontics. The best current evidence centers on its use in depotphoresis, a technique that employs electrophoretic delivery to enhance the penetration of Cupral into dentinal tubules and accessory canals.

A pivotal randomized clinical trial by Dalaei Moghadam et al. (2021) compared depotphoresis with Cupral to a diode laser protocol and conventional irrigation in 90 necrotic teeth with chronic apical periodontitis (98 roots) [24]. The study demonstrated that Cupral depotphoresis achieved greater microbial reduction, faster radiographic healing of periapical lesions, and lower postoperative pain scores compared with both diode laser and standard irrigation methods, highlighting its superiority in microbial suppression and early healing outcomes.

The safety profile of Cupral has also been evaluated. Aminsobhani et al. (2021) conducted an in vivo study to quantify copper ion extrusion from the apical foramen during depotphoresis in single-canal teeth [39]. The results indicated that, under controlled procedural parameters, the levels of copper ions remained within clinically safe limits, supporting the biocompatibility and procedural safety of Cupral when used with appropriate dosing and current regulations.

An important contribution to the evidence base comes from a 2023 systematic review by Lina et al., which examined copper–calcium hydroxide formulations, including nano-forms and electrophoretic delivery systems, for the management of apical periodontitis [18]. The review concluded that Cupral-based therapies exhibit enhanced antimicrobial efficacy and favorable tissue-healing effects when compared to conventional treatments, but it also underscored the scarcity of high-quality randomized controlled trials (RCTs) and emphasized the need for standardized treatment protocols to ensure reproducible outcomes.

While Cupral shows promising results in infected canal disinfection, its application in vital pulp therapy (VPT), such as direct pulp capping or partial pulpotomy, remains poorly studied. Currently, no robust head-to-head RCTs directly compare Cupral to other pulp-capping agents. In contrast, a substantial body of evidence supports the use of mineral trioxide aggregate (MTA) and calcium silicate-based bioceramics in VPT. A meta-analysis by Li et al. (2015) found that MTA demonstrated significantly higher long-term success rates for direct pulp capping compared with traditional calcium hydroxide, with an odds ratio of approximately 3.1, and these superior outcomes persisted at multi-year follow-up [41]. Similarly, a recent meta-analysis by Silva et al. (2025) confirmed that calcium silicate-based cements, including MTA and Biodentine, outperform calcium hydroxide in hard tissue bridge formation and long-term pulp vitality [42]. A triple-blinded randomized clinical trial by Mahapatra et al. (2024) further reported that Biodentine and MTA were superior to TheraCal LC in maintaining favorable clinical and radiographic outcomes in patients with pulpal exposure [43].

Collectively, these data position MTA and Biodentine as the current gold-standard agents for VPT, owing to their superior biocompatibility and dentinogenic potential, while Cupral's demonstrated strength remains focused on intra-canal disinfection rather than pulp-capping applications. There is currently a lack of well-designed comparative clinical trials directly evaluating Cupral-based protocols vs. conventional obturation systems, such as gutta-percha with resin or bioceramic sealers, in terms of long-term healing, retreatment rates, or tooth survival. Most of the available evidence for Cupral remains focused on short- to mid-term outcomes, namely microbial reduction and radiographic healing of periapical lesions, rather than definitive hard endpoints.

Notably, Cupral's electrophoretic delivery method offers certain clinical advantages in challenging cases. Studies indicate that depotphoresis improves penetration into dentinal tubules, lateral canals, and anatomically complex or partially blocked canals, leading to more effective microbial suppression and, in some cases, faster radiographic resolution compared to conventional irrigation or non-electrical adjuncts [24]. Furthermore, the ion-extrusion safety data confirm that, when current and duration are appropriately controlled, copper exposure remains within clinically acceptable thresholds, alleviating concerns about systemic toxicity [39].

In summary, the strongest evidence for Cupral lies in its role as an antimicrobial adjunct in infected canals, particularly when delivered by depotphoresis, where limited but compelling head-to-head data demonstrate advantages over diode laser disinfection in terms of microbial reduction, healing acceleration, and pain relief. However, the evidence remains insufficient to recommend Cupral for vital pulp therapy, where MTA and Biodentine continue to be the evidence-based first-line materials, or as a stand-alone root canal filling agent, given the absence of robust long-term comparative trials. Future research should prioritize multicenter, large-scale RCTs directly comparing Cupral-based depotphoresis protocols with state-of-the-art chemomechanical preparation and bioceramic sealers, focusing on clinically relevant outcomes such as healing at 12–24 months, retreatment rates, and tooth survival.

5.5. The Role of Nanotechnology in Enhancing Cupral Efficacy

Recent advances in nanotechnology have provided novel opportunities to improve the therapeutic performance of Cupral in endodontic treatment. By engineering the components of Cupral at the nanoscale, researchers aim to optimize antimicrobial potency, improve penetration into the intricate root canal system, and achieve sustained ion release, thereby enhancing its effectiveness against persistent infections and biofilms.

A key advantage of nano-Cupral formulations lies in their increased surface-to-volume ratio. When copper and calcium hydroxide are reduced to nanoscale particles, their reactive surface area expands dramatically, improving contact with bacterial biofilms and accelerating ion release kinetics. This facilitates more efficient disruption of microbial membranes and enhances the ability to eradicate pathogens that inhabit the depths of dentinal tubules and accessory canals. Copper nanoparticles have demonstrated broad-spectrum antimicrobial properties, showing activity even against resistant organisms such as *P. aeruginosa* and *C. albicans* [16,17].

Beyond enhancing antimicrobial potency, nanotechnology also enables targeted drug delivery systems. For example, polymeric or lipid-based nanoparticles can encapsulate copper–calcium hydroxide components, allowing for controlled and sustained release of copper and hydroxyl ions within the root canal environment. This sustained-release profile not only extends antimicrobial activity but also reduces the frequency of medicament re-application, potentially improving clinical efficiency and patient compliance [21,26].

When combined with electrophoretic delivery techniques such as depotphoresis, nano-Cupral formulations may penetrate more deeply into dentinal tubules and irregular canal anatomies compared with conventional bulk formulations. This combined approach could be particularly beneficial for the disinfection of anatomically complex canals, areas often inaccessible to traditional irrigation methods, thereby reducing the risk of persistent infection [18,22].

Biofilm disruption represents another critical mechanism through which nano-Cupral exerts its benefits. Studies have shown that nano-Cupral formulations disrupt mature biofilms more effectively than their conventional counterparts. The copper nanoparticles contribute by generating reactive oxygen species (ROS) and releasing copper ions that destabilize microbial membranes, while calcium hydroxide maintains a highly alkaline pH that is inhospitable to most endodontic pathogens. The dual action of copper's oxidative stress and calcium hydroxide's alkalinity may reduce biofilm resilience, lower the risk of reinfection, and promote favorable periapical healing outcomes [17,21,26].

Emerging research is also exploring innovative strategies to further enhance nano-Cupral formulations. The surface functionalization of nanoparticles with bioactive peptides is being investigated to enable specific targeting of bacterial adhesins or receptors, improving selectivity toward pathogenic species. Hybrid nanostructures that combine copper with silver or zinc oxide have demonstrated synergistic antimicrobial effects, potentially broadening the antimicrobial spectrum. Furthermore, the development of stimuli-responsive nanoparticles, engineered to release copper ions in response to pH shifts or enzymatic activity in infected tissues, may allow precise, on-demand antimicrobial release that enhances treatment specificity and safety [21,26].

Despite the promising laboratory and early preclinical findings, the clinical translation of nano-Cupral remains at an early stage. Before its widespread adoption in endodontic protocols, further work is needed to optimize ion-release profiles, establish long-term safety data, and conduct robust randomized clinical trials to validate both efficacy and biocompatibility in vivo. Long-term follow-up studies will be essential to assess the impact of these nano-formulations on healing outcomes, retreatment rates, and tooth survival.

Nanotechnology has the potential to transform Cupral from a conventional antimicrobial adjunct into a precision-targeted, sustained-release therapeutic platform in endodontics. By combining nanoscale engineering with established depotphoresis delivery methods, the next generation of nano-Cupral formulations may represent a significant advancement in root canal disinfection technology, improving outcomes for resistant infections and complex cases.

5.6. Biocompatibility and Safety of Cupral

Ensuring the biocompatibility of any intracanal medicament is critical to the safety and success of endodontic treatment. For Cupral, the safety profile encompasses local tissue compatibility, the risk of copper ion extrusion beyond the apical foramen, and patient-specific factors such as hypersensitivity reactions, pregnancy, systemic diseases, or malignancy that could increase susceptibility to adverse effects.

What does "biocompatibility" mean in endodontics? In endodontic practice, biocompatibility reflects a material's ability to eliminate infection without provoking harmful local or systemic effects. This includes demonstrating histocompatibility, minimal irritation to periradicular tissues, as well as low cytotoxicity and absence of mutagenic potential. These criteria, originally outlined by Geurtsen and Leyhausen (1997), remain the benchmark against which new intracanal agents and delivery technologies are evaluated [9].

Studies examining electrophoresis-based Cupral delivery show intimate interaction with dentin surfaces and effective penetration into the intricate canal anatomy, aiding in the removal of debris and biofilm from dentinal tubules. Rumiantsev et al. (2013), using scanning electron microscopy, reported that Cupral depotphoresis enhanced cleaning efficiency and established close apposition to dentin walls, which is therapeutically advantageous for disinfection [38]. However, such deep penetration also underscores the need to monitor periapical tissues during and after treatment to ensure that ion diffusion does not provoke local tissue damage [38].

A primary safety concern with Cupral depotphoresis is the potential extrusion of copper ions beyond the apical foramen. This has been directly investigated in a clinical in vivo study by Aminsobhani et al. (2021), who measured copper ion release from single-canal teeth following electrophoresis [39]. The study demonstrated that, when the electric current, exposure duration, and canal status were properly controlled, copper ion concentrations remained within clinically acceptable and non-toxic levels, supporting the procedural safety of Cupral-based protocols in standard endodontic practice [39].

Comparative evaluation of Cupral's safety profile benefits from historical data on calcium hydroxide and $Ca(OH)_2$-based sealers, which are well-characterized in terms of tissue responses, high pH, related irritation, and time-dependent effects on periapical tissues. Desai and Chandler (2009) and Mohammadi and Dummer (2011) emphasized that while calcium hydroxide is generally well tolerated, its high alkalinity can produce localized irritation if extruded into periapical tissues [30,31]. These studies provide a baseline reference for interpreting Cupral's performance in terms of local irritation and healing response [30,31].

Modern expert guidelines, such as those by Zou et al. (2024), highlight the importance of protocol standardization, controlled dosage, and careful delivery for intracanal medications [28]. These principles are directly applicable to Cupral, particularly when combined with electrophoretic delivery systems. Furthermore, recognized contraindications for Cupral depotphoresis, such as pregnancy, copper allergy, malignant neoplasms, or severe autoimmune disorders, should always be considered during patient assessment to minimize risks.

A practical safety framework for Cupral use involves several key measures:

- Dose and delivery control: Calibrating electrical current and application duration to minimize apical extrusion.
- Anatomy-aware application: Using microscopy-supported delivery to enhance cleaning while monitoring periapical tissues for adverse responses.
- Patient screening: Identifying individuals with allergy risks or systemic contraindications to reduce the likelihood of complications.
- Comparison of results: Interpreting healing and clinical signs in relation to established biocompatibility criteria for endodontic materials [44].

Current evidence, including direct ion-extrusion measurements, supports the idea that Cupral can be used safely in endodontics when protocols are standardized, dosage is well-controlled, and patient selection is appropriate. Nevertheless, the literature still lacks comprehensive histological studies that compare long-term tissue responses between Cupral, contemporary calcium silicate-based biomaterials, and $Ca(OH)_2$ sealers. Future research should focus on head-to-head histopathologic and clinical investigations to better define Cupral's long-term biocompatibility and guide evidence-based recommendations for its use in modern practice.

5.7. Addressing Barriers to Clinical Adoption of Cupral

Although Cupral has shown encouraging antimicrobial and clinical performance, particularly when delivered via depotphoresis (electrophoretic delivery), its widespread integration into routine endodontic practice remains limited. These barriers stem from a combination of evidence gaps, technical demands, perceived safety concerns, and workflow challenges. Addressing them requires a coordinated effort involving research standardization, clinician training, patient education, and institutional support.

One of the primary obstacles is the relative immaturity of the clinical evidence base. Much of the published literature on Cupral originates from in vitro and ex vivo investigations, supplemented by a handful of single-center randomized clinical trials. While these studies, comparing depotphoresis with diode laser protocols, indicate superior microbial reduction, faster periapical healing, and lower postoperative pain, systematic reviews emphasize the lack of multicenter trials and protocol harmonization [24]. This heterogeneity in dosing, current intensity, and session frequency contributes to inconsistent outcomes and has slowed guideline integration and clinician confidence [22,28,32].

The need for specialized depotphoresis equipment, combined with the requirement to control parameters such as electrical current, duration of application, and number of sessions, creates an additional barrier for many dental practices. This complexity entails longer chair time, additional procurement costs, and a learning curve for clinical staff. The perception that Cupral protocols are more cumbersome compared to conventional irrigants or medicaments contributes to hesitancy in adoption, especially in resource-limited or high-volume settings [40].

Despite evidence demonstrating that copper ion extrusion remains within safe limits when protocols are properly calibrated, as shown by Aminsobhani et al. (2021), many clinicians continue to harbor concerns about potential periapical irritation and systemic effects [39]. These perceptions often outweigh the data, highlighting the need for better risk communication strategies that transparently share real-world safety data, including baseline and follow-up radiographic monitoring to reassure patients and clinicians alike.

Unlike traditional single-phase sealers, Cupral typically serves as an antimicrobial medicament stage rather than a permanent obturation material. This necessitates a sequential workflow, where Cupral is followed by a separate sealer such as Atacamit for the final obturation. The additional steps and inventory requirements, coupled with the need for proper timing between medicament and sealer placement, can deter some practitioners, particularly those without prior training in combined protocols [22].

Another practical barrier is the requirement for rigorous patient screening. Cupral depotphoresis is contraindicated in individuals with copper allergy, pregnancy, malignant neoplasms, or severe systemic and autoimmune diseases. In some clinics, workflows for systematic pre-treatment screening and informed consent are either underdeveloped or absent, increasing medicolegal hesitation and contributing to underutilization.

Overcoming these obstacles requires a multi-pronged approach. The publication and dissemination of standardized clinical protocols, guided by frameworks such as the 2024 International Expert Consensus on Irrigation and Intracanal Medication (Zou et al., 2024), would provide practitioners with clear instructions on indications, current calibration, session counts, and follow-up imaging intervals [28]. Such guidelines, ideally developed and endorsed by national endodontic societies, could transform Cupral use from a niche technique into a mainstream adjunctive therapy.

Practical continuing education (CE) programs, including hands-on workshops, can address the technical learning curve by familiarizing clinicians with device setup, parameter control, case selection, and integration into conventional chemomechanical workflows. Mentorship models, where experienced Cupral users guide new adopters, could further facilitate skill acquisition and confidence.

The creation of consent templates and risk communication tools summarizing existing ion-extrusion safety data and monitoring protocols can mitigate both patient and practitioner concerns. Clinics might also benefit from implementation bundles, starter kits including the depotphoresis device, quick-reference protocol cards, and evidence-based case selection guides, to reduce logistical friction during initial adoption.

Finally, establishing multicenter registries to track short- and mid-term healing outcomes, retreatment rates, and patient-reported satisfaction would both accelerate evidence generation and support reimbursement discussions. Such registries would provide the large-scale data needed to complement RCTs and refine clinical decision-making for Cupral-based protocols.

The current barriers to Cupral's clinical adoption, chiefly protocol heterogeneity, equipment demands, safety perceptions, integration challenges, and patient-screening logistics, are surmountable through a coordinated strategy that emphasizes protocol standardization, professional training, transparent risk communication, and real-world evidence collection. As ongoing multicenter studies and outcomes registries address these gaps, the potential exists for Cupral to shift from a promising adjunct to a validated and widely accepted component of modern endodontic therapy.

5.8. Advanced Techniques for Delivering Cupral: Iontophoresis and Electrophoresis

The complex anatomy of the root canal system, characterized by ramifications, isthmuses, fins, and apical deltas, often limits the ability of conventional irrigation to completely eliminate microbial biofilms. To address these challenges, electrokinetic delivery methods such as iontophoresis and electrophoresis have emerged as powerful adjunctive approaches for enhancing the penetration and effectiveness of Cupral.

Both iontophoresis and electrophoresis rely on the application of a low-intensity electric current to mobilize ionized particles within a medicament, driving them beyond the main canal lumen into otherwise inaccessible microanatomical spaces. Iontophoresis specifically refers to the active transport of charged drug molecules across tissue barriers via electrorepulsion, a principle where like charges repel, allowing positively charged copper and calcium ions in Cupral to be propelled deep into dentinal tubules and lateral canals. Electrophoresis, a broader term that includes iontophoresis, describes the general migration of charged particles under an electric field. In endodontics, it is commonly associated with depotphoresis, where a suspension of Cupral is introduced into the canal and then subjected to a constant, low-intensity current. This technique creates a reservoir of antimicrobial ions within dentin, offering a prolonged effect that extends well beyond the period of application.

By harnessing these electrokinetic forces, both techniques overcome the limitations of passive diffusion, which typically restricts medicaments to the main canal lumen. As a result, electrokinetic delivery not only improves depth of penetration but also ensures a more uniform distribution of active ions throughout the intricate canal system.

The clinical value of these techniques lies in their ability to enhance disinfection in areas unreachable by conventional irrigation methods. By actively driving antimicrobial ions into dentinal tubules and accessory canals, iontophoresis and electrophoresis can achieve superior biofilm disruption and reduce microbial persistence, a key factor in recurrent infection. Furthermore, depotphoresis establishes a sustained antimicrobial reservoir within the dentin, maintaining ion activity between treatment sessions. These properties make electrokinetic Cupral delivery particularly useful in chronic apical periodontitis, retreatment cases with resistant infections, and teeth with complex or calcified anatomy where mechanical shaping alone is insufficient for adequate microbial control.

A growing body of research underpins the clinical promise of Cupral delivered through depotphoresis. In a randomized clinical trial involving necrotic teeth with chronic apical periodontitis, demonstrated that Cupral depotphoresis achieved significantly greater microbial reduction, the more rapid radiographic healing of periapical lesions, and reduced postoperative pain compared to both diode laser disinfection and conventional irrigation protocols [24]. The safety of the technique was corroborated by Aminsobhani et al. (2021), who quantified copper ion extrusion from single-canal teeth and found that the levels remained within clinically acceptable limits when current and exposure duration were carefully controlled [39].

Further clinical validation was provided by Meto et al. (2021), who reported marked radiographic resolution of chronic apical periodontitis lesions when copper–calcium hydroxide was used in combination with permanent electrophoretic current [22]. Complementing these findings, Moradi et al. (2023) conducted an ex vivo study that demonstrated deeper antimicrobial penetration of depotphoresis-delivered Cupral compared with traditional non-electrokinetic delivery methods [32]. Together, these studies reinforce that the electrokinetic approach is both efficacious and safe when standardized protocols are observed.

To realize the full benefits of iontophoresis and electrophoresis in Cupral delivery, protocol standardization is paramount. Current strength, the duration of application, and the number of sessions must be carefully controlled to ensure therapeutic efficacy while minimizing the risk of apical extrusion of ions. Case selection also plays a crucial role; the greatest clinical gains are observed in cases where mechanical instrumentation and standard irrigation cannot adequately reach all infected areas.

Clinicians are advised to adopt a combination strategy, in which mechanical shaping and conventional irrigation are performed first to reduce the bulk microbial load, followed by Cupral depotphoresis to disinfect inaccessible microanatomical regions, and completed with a suitable obturation material to achieve long-term canal sealing. Such a multi-step approach aligns with current principles of endodontic disinfection and provides more consistent long-term clinical outcomes.

Iontophoresis and electrophoresis represent a significant technological advancement in intracanal medicament delivery. By leveraging electrokinetic forces to drive Cupral ions deeply into dentinal tubules and lateral canals, these techniques offer enhanced antimicrobial reach, sustained ionic activity, and superior biofilm disruption compared to passive application alone. Clinical studies underscore not only their effectiveness in reducing microbial load and accelerating lesion healing but also their safety profile under controlled conditions. As standardized protocols become more widely adopted and training in electrokinetic delivery expands, these methods have the potential to transform Cupral from a localized medicament into a deep-penetrating, long-lasting therapeutic solution for the most challenging endodontic cases.

5.9. Current Guidelines and Standards for Cupral Use in Endodontics

Although Cupral is not yet incorporated into all international endodontic guidelines, there is a growing framework of expert consensus statements, national recommendations, and manufacturer-supported protocols that collectively inform its safe and effective clinical use. These guidelines are particularly relevant when Cupral is applied with depotphoresis, the electrophoretic delivery method that distinguishes its clinical performance from conventional intracanal medicaments.

5.9.1. Alignment with International Expert Consensus

The 2024 International Expert Consensus on Irrigation and Intracanal Medication in Root Canal Therapy emphasizes three core principles for modern disinfection strategies: the standardization of antimicrobial medicament delivery protocols, the importance of achieving deep penetration into dentinal tubules to eradicate resistant infections, and the systematic assessment of patient safety, including screening for contraindications. While Cupral is not mentioned by name in this document, its use via depotphoresis aligns closely with these priorities, particularly as it supports adjunctive antimicrobial strategies in persistent or anatomically complex cases where conventional methods may fail [28].

5.9.2. National and Manufacturer Protocols: The German Experience

In the absence of universal international recommendations, national and manufacturer-derived protocols have played a pivotal role in shaping clinical practice. Among the most influential are the German Depotphorese® guidelines provided by Humanchemie GmbH, which offer a step-by-step clinical workflow for Cupral application with depotphoresis. These protocols specify critical procedural parameters such as current intensity, exposure duration, and the recommended number of treatment sessions, while clearly delineating contraindications, including copper allergy, pregnancy, malignancies, and severe autoimmune diseases.

These validated protocols have been widely adopted in Germany, Eastern Europe, and parts of the Middle East, where they effectively serve as a de facto clinical standard for Cupral use. Their structured approach to treatment planning, dosage control, and contraindication screening provides an operational model that other regions may follow as Cupral gains wider acceptance [40].

5.9.3. Integration into Clinical Practice Frameworks

Drawing on the consensus recommendations and national protocols, clinicians have begun to integrate Cupral into specific clinical scenarios where conventional treatment alone is insufficient. The material has been particularly valuable in teeth with persistent apical periodontitis that have not responded to standard root canal therapy, in retreatment cases where conventional irrigation fails to clear microbial biofilms, and in anatomically complex teeth with isthmuses, apical deltas, or calcified canals.

Operational guidelines emphasize the need for pre-treatment screening to rule out hypersensitivity or systemic contraindications, as well as controlled delivery of depotphoresis parameters, including current, duration, and number of sessions, to ensure optimal safety and efficacy. Clinicians are also advised to conduct follow-up imaging at 6–12 months post-treatment to monitor radiographic evidence of periapical healing and long-term success [22,24,39].

5.9.4. Future Directions for International Guideline Development

The formal incorporation of Cupral into major international guidelines, such as those by the European Society of Endodontology (ESE) and the American Association of Endodontists (AAE), will depend on the availability of robust multicenter randomized controlled trials and long-term outcome studies. Current data already suggest that Cupral delivered via depotphoresis enhances microbial reduction and accelerates periapical healing compared with conventional irrigation and even diode laser adjuncts [24]. Until these findings are confirmed by large-scale clinical studies, clinicians can safely rely on the existing expert consensus for intracanal medicaments, supplemented by the structured depotphoresis protocols provided by manufacturers. This hybrid approach ensures that Cupral use remains both evidence-aligned and clinically responsible during this transitional period.

5.10. Future Directions and Research Gaps for Cupral

Although Cupral has shown robust antimicrobial efficacy and emerging regenerative potential, its widespread integration into contemporary endodontic practice remains incomplete. To transform Cupral from a promising adjunct into a standardized component of global endodontic protocols, several scientific, clinical, and technological gaps must be addressed. Future research will need to focus on three interconnected domains: formulation optimization, advances in delivery systems, and long-term clinical validation.

One of the most active areas of investigation involves improving Cupral's chemical and physical formulation. The development of nanoparticle-enhanced Cupral represents a key innovation. At the nanoscale, the copper–calcium hydroxide particles exhibit a dramatically increased surface-to-volume ratio, which enhances ion release kinetics, contact with microbial biofilms, and the ability to penetrate dentinal tubules. Such nano-engineering could amplify the antimicrobial effect while minimizing the amount of medicament required for clinical efficacy.

In addition to nanoscale modifications, research is exploring hybrid bioactive composites, which combine Cupral with other antimicrobial or regenerative agents, such as silver nanoparticles, zinc oxide, or bioceramic fillers. These composites may leverage synergistic effects, improving not only antimicrobial potency but also the regenerative capacity of dentin and periapical tissues. Another promising avenue involves pH modulation strategies. Since the antimicrobial efficacy of calcium hydroxide is linked to its alkalinity, fine-tuning the balance between high-pH antimicrobial activity and tissue biocompatibility could improve healing outcomes and reduce potential irritation to periapical tissues.

Future progress also depends on optimizing the delivery mechanisms that drive Cupral deeper into the complex architecture of the root canal. Although electrophoresis and iontophoresis have demonstrated impressive results by overcoming the limitations of passive diffusion, there is a pressing need to standardize key parameters such as current intensity, the duration of application, and session frequency. Standardization will not only enhance clinical efficacy but also improve procedural safety by minimizing copper ion extrusion beyond the apical foramen.

Emerging smart-carrier technologies are another frontier for exploration. These involve stimuli-responsive delivery platforms that release Cupral ions selectively in response to local pH changes, bacterial enzymatic activity, or inflammatory markers in infected tissues. By ensuring targeted and sustained antimicrobial release, these carriers have the potential to further reduce reinfection rates. Additionally, advances in single-visit protocols, where optimized delivery methods could achieve comprehensive disinfection and early healing without multiple appointments, may significantly improve patient compliance and chairside efficiency.

While Cupral's primary use has been in intracanal disinfection, future research must assess its comparative performance in other endodontic procedures. In VPT, for example, controlled trials are needed to evaluate Cupral's clinical success as a direct pulp capping or partial pulpotomy material, particularly in comparison to current gold standards like MTA and Biodentine.

There is also growing interest in Cupral's potential role in regenerative endodontics, where its antimicrobial and possible bioactive properties could support the re-establishment of a functional pulp–dentin complex. Furthermore, targeted studies should investigate the outcomes and safety of Cupral use in medically compromised patients, such as those with diabetes, autoimmune disorders, or reduced healing capacity, since these populations often present with more complex endodontic challenges and may particularly benefit from enhanced disinfection protocols.

Despite encouraging short-term clinical data, long-term evidence remains limited. High-quality multicenter RCTs are urgently required to validate Cupral's reported advantages in healing rates, tooth survival, retreatment needs, and patient-reported outcomes over periods extending beyond 12–24 months. Such trials should also compare Cupral directly with other contemporary intracanal medicaments and obturation systems to establish clear clinical guidelines for its use.

In parallel, histological studies comparing tissue responses to Cupral with established agents such as calcium hydroxide-based sealers and bioceramics are critical to confirm long-term biocompatibility and safety. Additionally, establishing large-scale clinical registries that capture real-world outcomes across diverse geographic and practice settings would provide invaluable insights into effectiveness, safety, and cost–benefit considerations in routine dental care.

Taken together, Cupral's unique combination of antimicrobial power, potential for sustained ionic release, and compatibility with electrokinetic delivery makes it an exciting candidate for further exploration. However, its future as a mainstream endodontic material depends on two essential pillars: the development of innovative formulations and smarter delivery systems, and the generation of robust, long-term clinical evidence to secure its place in evidence-based guidelines. By addressing these research gaps through collaborative multicenter studies, translational nanotechnology, and standardized protocols, Cupral could evolve from a niche adjunctive therapy into a central component of modern endodontic practice worldwide.

5.11. Conclusions

This chapter highlights the growing clinical significance of Cupral as an antimicrobial adjunct in modern endodontic therapy, particularly when combined with depotphoresis (electrophoretic delivery). A synthesis of available evidence demonstrates that Cupral possesses potent and broad-spectrum antimicrobial activity, capable of penetrating dentinal tubules and complex root canal anatomies where conventional irrigants often fail. Its distinctive dual mechanism of copper-mediated microbial membrane disruption and calcium hydroxide–driven alkalinity underpins its strong performance in suppressing resistant biofilms and facilitating periapical healing.

Comparative clinical data, though still limited, suggest that Cupral delivered via depotphoresis can achieve greater microbial reduction, lower postoperative pain, and faster radiographic resolution of apical lesions than several conventional adjuncts, including diode lasers and standard irrigation protocols. These therapeutic gains appear particularly meaningful in retreatment cases, teeth with persistent apical periodontitis, and anatomically challenging canals. Importantly, direct measurements of copper ion extrusion confirm that Cupral can be used safely when delivery parameters, current intensity, exposure duration, and session count are standardized and contraindications such as pregnancy or copper hypersensitivity are respected.

Beyond its disinfection role, emerging innovations in nanotechnology offer exciting prospects for Cupral's evolution. Nanoscale formulations have demonstrated enhanced surface reactivity, more sustained ion release, and superior biofilm disruption, opening the door to precision-targeted, prolonged-release therapies. Such advancements may transform Cupral from a traditional medicament into a multifunctional agent with regenerative and antimicrobial benefits, especially when integrated into stimuli-responsive carriers or hybrid composites with other bioactive materials.

Nonetheless, several barriers to widespread adoption remain, including the lack of large multicenter randomized controlled trials, limited inclusion in international guidelines, and perceived workflow complexity of depotphoresis. Addressing these gaps through protocol harmonization, targeted clinician training, transparent risk communication, and multicenter outcome registries will be critical for integrating Cupral into mainstream practice.

The evidence presented here underscores that Cupral is a promising, biologically active adjunct capable of enhancing the predictability of endodontic disinfection, particularly in resistant or recurrent infections. Its future, however, hinges on continued innovation in formulation and delivery technologies, rigorous safety and biocompatibility validation, and the generation of high-quality long-term clinical data. With these developments, Cupral could transition from a niche alternative into a standardized, evidence-based component of global endodontic protocols, improving both treatment outcomes and patient quality of care.

References

1. Persoon, I.F.; Özok, A.R. Definitions and Epidemiology of Endodontic Infections. *Curr. Oral Health Rep.* **2017**, *4*, 278–285. [CrossRef] [PubMed]
2. Fouad, A.F.; Diogenes, A.R.; Torabinejad, M.; Hargreaves, K.M. Microbiome Changes during Regenerative Endodontic Treatment Using Different Methods of Disinfection. *J. Endod.* **2022**, *48*, 1273–1284. [CrossRef]
3. Ng, Y.L.; Mann, V.; Rahbaran, S.; Lewsey, J.; Gulabivala, K. Outcome of primary root canal treatment: Systematic review of the literature—Part 2. Influence of clinical factors. *Int. Endod. J.* **2008**, *41*, 6–31. [CrossRef] [PubMed]
4. Bhandi, S.; Mashyakhy, M.; Abumelha, A.S.; Alkahtany, M.F.; Jamal, M.; Chohan, H.; Raj, A.T.; Testarelli, L.; Reda, R.; Patil, S. Complete Obturation—Cold Lateral Condensation vs. Thermoplastic Techniques: A Systematic Review of Micro-CT Studies. *Materials* **2021**, *14*, 4013. [CrossRef]
5. Ray, H.A.; Trope, M. Periapical status of endodontically treated teeth in relation to the technical quality of the root filling and the coronal restoration. *Int. Endod. J.* **1995**, *28*, 12–18. [CrossRef]
6. Hoen, M.M.; Pink, F.E. Contemporary endodontic retreatments: An analysis based on clinical treatment findings. *J. Endod.* **2002**, *28*, 834–836. [CrossRef]
7. Pontoriero, D.I.K.; Grandini, S.; Spagnuolo, G.; Discepoli, N.; Benedicenti, S.; Maccagnola, V.; Mosca, A.; Ferrari Cagidiaco, E.; Ferrari, M. Clinical Outcomes of Endodontic Treatments and Restorations with and without Posts Up to 18 Years. *J. Clin. Med.* **2021**, *10*, 908. [CrossRef] [PubMed]

8. Tabassum, S.; Khan, F.R. Failure of endodontic treatment: The usual suspects. *Eur. J. Dent.* **2016**, *10*, 144–147. [CrossRef]
9. Geurtsen, W.; Leyhausen, G. Biological aspects of root canal filling materials--histocompatibility, cytotoxicity, and mutagenicity. *Clin. Oral. Investig.* **1997**, *1*, 5–11. [CrossRef]
10. Staffoli, S.; Plotino, G.; Nunez Torrijos, B.G.; Grande, N.M.; Bossù, M.; Gambarini, G.; Polimeni, A. Regenerative Endodontic Procedures Using Contemporary Endodontic Materials. *Materials* **2019**, *12*, 908. [CrossRef]
11. Bystrom, A.; Claesson, R.; Sundqvist, G. The antibacterial effect of camphorated paramonochlorophenol, camphorated phenol and calcium hydroxide in the treatment of infected root canals. *Endod. Dent. Traumatol.* **1985**, *1*, 170–175. [CrossRef] [PubMed]
12. Pohl, G. Zu praktischen Versuchen mit der Ionophorese nach Bernard [Practical experiments with Bernard's iontophoresis]. *Zahnarztl. Welt Zahnarztl. Reform. Zwr.* **1951**, *6*, 430–432. [PubMed]
13. Basharina, O.M. Elektroforez kornevykh kanalov pri lechenii peritsementitov [Electrophoresis of root canals in the treatment of pericementitis]. *Stomatologiia* **1967**, *46*, 96–97. [PubMed]
14. Shakun, S.L. Lechenie periodontitov metodom transkanal'nogo élektroforeza [Treatment of periodontitis by transcanal electrophoresis]. *Feldsher Akush.* **1988**, *53*, 60–62. [PubMed]
15. Mironova, V.V. Lechenie verkhushechnogo periodontita ul'tranfonoforezom [Treatment of apical periodontitis by ultraphonophoresis]. *Stomatologiia* **1977**, *56*, 63–65. [PubMed]
16. Grass, G.; Rensing, C.; Solioz, M. Metallic copper as an antimicrobial surface. *Appl. Environ. Microbiol.* **2011**, *77*, 1541–1547. [CrossRef]
17. Meto, A.; Colombari, B.; Sala, A.; Pericolini, E.; Meto, A.; Peppoloni, S.; Blasi, E. Antimicrobial and antibiofilm efficacy of a copper/calcium hydroxide-based endodontic paste against Staphylococcus aureus, Pseudomonas aeruginosa and Candida albicans. *Dent. Mater. J.* **2019**, *38*, 591–603. [CrossRef]
18. Lina, R.M.; Sindhu, R.; Bharathwaj, V.V.; Dhamodhar, D.; Sathiyapriya, S.; Prabu, D.; Rajmohan, M. Systematic Review on Copper Calcium Hydroxide Nanoparticles in the Treatment of Apical Periodontitis. *J. Pharm. Bioallied Sci.* **2023**, *15*, S105–S109. [CrossRef] [PubMed]
19. Ba-Hattab, R.; Al-Jamie, M.; Aldreib, H.; Alessa, L.; Alonazi, M. Calcium Hydroxide in Endodontics: An Overview. *Open J. Stomatol.* **2016**, *6*, 274–289. [CrossRef]
20. Reddy, S.; Prakash, V.; Subbiya, A.; Mitthra, S. 100 Years of Calcium Hydroxide in Dentistry: A Review of Literature. *Indian J. Forensic Med. Toxicol.* **2020**, *14*, 1203–1219. [CrossRef]
21. Ma, X.; Zhou, S.; Xu, X.; Du, Q. Copper-containing nanoparticles: Mechanism of antimicrobial effect and application in dentistry—A narrative review. *Front. Surg.* **2022**, *9*, 905892. [CrossRef]
22. Meto, A.; Droboniku, E.; Blasi, E.; Colombari, B.; Tragaj, E.; Cervino, G.; Fiorillo, L.; Meto, A. Copper-Calcium Hydroxide and Permanent Electrophoretic Current for Treatment of Apical Periodontitis. *Materials* **2021**, *14*, 678. [CrossRef]

23. Knappwost, A. The depotophoresis procedure with copper-calcium hydroxide used for systematic healing. A leading alternative in endodontics. *Ger. Dent. J.* **1993**, *102*, 618–628.
24. Dalaei Moghadam, M.; Saberi, E.A.; Farhad Molashahi, N.; Shahraki Ebrahimi, H. Comparative efficacy of Depotphoresis and diode laser for reduction of microbial load and postoperative pain, and healing of periapical lesions: A randomized clinical trial. *Giornale Italiano Di Endodonzia* **2021**, *35*. [CrossRef]
25. Mamat, R.; Nik Abdul Ghani, N.R. The Complexity of the Root Canal Anatomy and Its Influence on Root Canal Debridement in the Apical Region: A Review. *Cureus* **2023**, *15*, e49024. [CrossRef] [PubMed]
26. Xu, V.W.; Nizami, M.Z.I.; Yin, I.X.; Yu, O.Y.; Lung, C.Y.K.; Chu, C.H. Application of Copper Nanoparticles in Dentistry. *Nanomaterials* **2022**, *12*, 805. [CrossRef]
27. de la Peña, V.A.; Darriba, I.L.; Valea, M.C.; Santana-Mora, U. Use of a Copper Band to Make Resin Cores in Endodontically Treated Teeth Lacking Coronal Structure. *Oper. Dent.* **2015**, *40*, 458–461. [CrossRef]
28. Zou, X.; Zheng, X.; Liang, Y.; Zhang, C.; Fan, B.; Liang, J.; Ling, J.; Bian, Z.; Yu, Q.; Hou, B.; et al. Expert consensus on irrigation and intracanal medication in root canal therapy. *Int. J. Oral Sci.* **2024**, *16*, 23. [CrossRef] [PubMed]
29. Wenzler, J.-S.; Falk, W.; Frankenberger, R.; Braun, A. Temporary Root Canal Obturation with a Calcium Hydroxide-Based Dressing: A Randomized Controlled Clinical Trial. *Antibiotics* **2023**, *12*, 1663. [CrossRef]
30. Desai, S.; Chandler, N. Calcium hydroxide-based root canal sealers: A review. *J. Endod.* **2009**, *35*, 475–480. [CrossRef]
31. Mohammadi, Z.; Dummer, P.M. Properties and applications of calcium hydroxide in endodontics and dental traumatology. *Int. Endod. J.* **2011**, *44*, 697–730. [CrossRef]
32. Moradi, S.; Moushekhian, S.; Karazhyan, R.; Ebrahimi, A. Ex vivo evaluation of the efficacy of depotphoresis method in root canal disinfection. *Dent. Res. J.* **2023**, *20*, 76. [CrossRef] [PubMed]
33. Aminsobhani, M.; Ketabi, M.A.; Soleimani, M.; Zareian, A.; Baharlou, B.; Azizlou, E. Comparing antimicrobial effect of cupral and calcium hydroxide paste with electrophoresis in apical part of root canals blocked by separated instrument. *J. Iran. Dent. Assoc.* **2022**, *34*, 76–82.
34. Meto, A.; Colombari, B.; Castagnoli, A.; Sarti, M.; Denti, L.; Blasi, E. Efficacy of a Copper-Calcium-Hydroxide Solution in Reducing Microbial Plaque on Orthodontic Clear Aligners: A Case Report. *Eur. J. Dent.* **2019**, *13*, 478–484. [CrossRef]
35. Enginalev, A.; Gura, E. Elektrochemische Aufbereitung und Versorgung aller Wurzelkanäle durch Depot-Phorese mittels des Galvanischen Stiftelementes [Electrochemical preparation and treatment of the root canals using Depot-phoresis materials as galvanic post elements]. *ZWR* **1985**, *94*, 145–147. [PubMed]
36. Knappwost, A. Physikalisch Chemische High Tech fireine Neue Endodontie am Beispiei der Kupfer-Calciumhydroxid-Depotphorese. *DZW* **1998**, *11*, 33.

37. Zhdanov, E.V.; Gerasimenko, M.I.; Miroshnikov, O.V.; Samorodova, O.V.; Pastukhova, N.P. Opyt primeneniia depoforeza gidrookisi medi-kal'tsiia dlia lecheniia neprokhodimykh i trudnodostupnykh kornevykh kanalov [The use of depot phoresis of copper-calcium hydroxide for the treatment of impassable and hard to reach root canals]. *Stomatologiia* **2002**, *81*, 61–63. [PubMed]
38. Rumiantsev, V.A.; Rodionova, E.G.; Denis, A.G.; Ol'khovskaia, A.V.; Tsaturova, I.V. [Electronic microscopy in endodontic electrophoresis efficiency assessment]. *Stomatologiia* **2013**, *92*, 4–8. [PubMed]
39. Aminsobhani, M.; Bolhari, B.; Dorost, B.; Eslambol Nassaj, A.; Azizlou, E. Measurement of Copper ion Extrusion from the Apex of Human Teeth with Single Canals Following of Electrophoresis. *Eur. Endod. J.* **2021**, *6*, 226–229. [CrossRef] [PubMed]
40. Humanchemie GmbH. Depotphorese® System Original II Instructions. Available online: https://www.manualslib.de/manual/725776/Humanchemie-DepotphoreseOriginal-Ii.html (accessed on 10 June 2023).
41. Li, Z.; Cao, L.; Fan, M.; Xu, Q. Direct Pulp Capping with Calcium Hydroxide or Mineral Trioxide Aggregate: A Meta-analysis. *J. Endod.* **2015**, *41*, 1412–1417. [CrossRef] [PubMed]
42. Silva, E.J.N.L.; Pinto, K.P.; Riche, F.N.S.J.; Carestiato, M.G.H.; Martins, J.N.R.; Duncan, H.F.; Versiani, M.A.; De-Deus, G. A meta-analysis of calcium silicate-based cements and calcium hydroxide as promoters of hard tissue bridge formation. *Int. Endod. J.* **2025**, *58*, 685–714. [CrossRef] [PubMed]
43. Mahapatra, J.; Nikhade, P.P.; Patel, A.; Mankar, N.; Taori, P. Comparative Evaluation of the Efficacy of TheraCal LC, Mineral Trioxide Aggregate, and Biodentine As Direct Pulp Capping Materials in Patients With Pulpal Exposure in Posterior Teeth: A Triple-Blinded Randomized Parallel Group Clinical Trial. *Cureus* **2024**, *16*, e55022. [CrossRef] [PubMed]
44. Asgary, S. Bio-obturation: A Novel Approach in Root Canal Treatment Using Endodontic Biomaterials. *Iran. Endod. J.* **2025**, *20*, e15. [CrossRef] [PubMed]

6. Conclusions: Tips and Concepts for Success in Endodontics

6.1. Endodontics in Contemporary Dental Care

Endodontics has become a cornerstone of modern dental care, enabling the preservation of natural teeth that would otherwise be lost to infection or trauma. Preserving the dentition safeguards mastication, phonetics, esthetics, and occlusal stability while preventing the cascade of complications associated with tooth loss, contributing to systemic health and overall well-being [1,2].

Successful root canal therapy depends on respecting the fundamental biological principles of infection control and structural preservation. Decades of evidence confirm that, when these principles are met, long-term outcomes remain predictably high, with cumulative survival rates reported at approximately 93% at 10 years, 85% at 20 years, and over 80% even after three decades [3,4].

Careful case selection is paramount: teeth chosen for primary treatment or retreatment must be structurally restorable, periodontally stable, and supported by favorable systemic health to maximize healing potential [1,5]. When these criteria are met, non-surgical primary therapy achieves success rates exceeding 90% under standard radiographic criteria [3], and generally maintains durable function for decades [4].

For previously treated teeth, non-surgical retreatment often provides better medium- to long-term outcomes than surgical intervention, despite lower initial success during the first two years. Longitudinal analyses show that retreatment success approaches 83% at 4–6 years, whereas surgical outcomes, initially higher at two years (≈78%), may decline to ~72% by the same interval [6,7]. When non-surgical approaches fail to resolve persistent periapical infection, modern microsurgical techniques, using CBCT guidance, ultrasonic root-end preparation, and bioactive retrofilling, achieve 85–95% short-term success with improved healing of periapical tissues [8–10].

Preserving tooth structure throughout treatment remains essential. Excessive dentin removal compromises root strength, predisposing the tooth to vertical fracture and shortening its functional lifespan, whereas conservative shaping with flexible nickel-titanium instruments and proper glide path creation maintains structural integrity without sacrificing effective disinfection [11].

Advances in imaging and adjunctive disinfection technologies have transformed both diagnostic accuracy and microbial control. CBCT detects apical pathology and untreated canals with higher sensitivity than traditional radiography, allowing more precise treatment planning and reducing iatrogenic complications [12]. Guided endodontic access, dynamic navigation, and minimally invasive shaping protocols help conserve dentin and reduce procedural errors [13]. Adjunctive laser activation of irrigants, particularly Er:YAG and Nd:YAG, further enhances removal of biofilms and smear layer, contributing to superior canal disinfection and improved healing [9,14].

Equally crucial is the emphasis on patient-centered care. Clear communication about diagnosis, prognosis, and treatment alternatives fosters trust, reduces anxiety, and improves adherence, while attention to systemic factors such as diabetes and to the patient's expectations helps optimize healing outcomes and satisfaction [15,16].

Looking ahead, the field's progress will hinge on integrating validated innovations, such as robot-assisted instrumentation [17], regenerative adjuncts [18], and bioceramic sealing materials, into standardized, evidence-driven protocols. Expanding multicenter clinical trials and creating international outcomes registries will be vital to consolidating best practices and guiding future global guidelines [1,10].

By uniting meticulous biologic principles with selective adoption of proven technologies, clinicians can consistently achieve the central goals of endodontic care: eradicating disease, preserving natural teeth in function, and maintaining long-term oral and systemic health [2,3,6]. The future of the specialty lies in an evidence-driven yet patient-focused approach that prioritizes both tooth survival and overall well-being.

6.2. Key Concepts: Depth, Evidence, and Practice

Clinical excellence in endodontics depends not only on technical proficiency but also on understanding the biological principles that underlie every step of treatment. A central tenet of this approach is the preservation of the tooth's original anatomy, particularly the internal canal curvature and dentinal wall thickness. Maintaining the natural morphology minimizes procedural errors such as ledging, canal transportation, and perforation, issues often associated with aggressive canal shaping. Excessive dentin removal reduces the structural integrity of the root, increasing the risk of vertical root fracture and compromising long-term prognosis [19]. Evidence from a 10-year retrospective study demonstrated that teeth with well-preserved canal structure showed survival rates exceeding 90%, compared with teeth that underwent excessive enlargement [20].

In daily practice, this principle translates into meticulous the negotiation of the canal pathway, especially in cases of severe curvature. For instance, in a mandibular second molar presenting with irreversible pulpitis and a mesial curvature exceeding 30 degrees, initial glide path preparation with small K-files, followed by minimally tapered (0.04) heat-treated NiTi instruments, helps maintain curvature integrity while minimizing torsional stress. Such conservative shaping, combined with warm vertical compaction for obturation, preserves tooth structure and apical seal; three-year follow-up has shown full function without radiographic evidence of periodontal ligament damage or root fracture.

Another fundamental strategy is accurate working length determination, which reduces the risk of over-instrumentation and associated periapical inflammation. A systematic review reported that combining electronic apex locators with radiographic confirmation achieves up to 96% accuracy in locating the apical constriction, thereby improving treatment precision and reducing postoperative discomfort [21].

Technological advances have further enhanced both diagnostic and treatment capabilities. CBCT has transformed endodontic planning by providing high-resolution, three-dimensional imaging of root morphology and surrounding structures. Compared to conventional radiographs, CBCT identifies apical lesions, missed canals, and root fractures with approximately 34% greater detection rates, particularly in multi-rooted teeth [12]. Merging CBCT data with intraoral scans facilitates guided endodontics; studies report 97–100% accuracy in locating calcified canals when using 3D-printed guides [22]. Such guided access reduces unnecessary dentin removal, shortens procedure time, and increases treatment predictability.

An important innovation is the incorporation of laser-assisted disinfection into the irrigation protocol. Lasers such as Er: YAG and Nd: YAG generate photoacoustic and thermal effects that disrupt biofilms, enhance irrigant penetration, and improve smear layer removal. Research has shown that Er: YAG laser activation can achieve up to a 99.9% bacterial reduction compared with conventional irrigation alone [23], while additional studies have documented up to a 40% decrease in postoperative pain when lasers were integrated into treatment [24]. In a practical clinical case, combining mechanical preparation with the Er: YAG activation of EDTA and NaOCl resulted in the complete resolution of chronic apical periodontitis after 12 months of follow-up.

For persistent periapical pathology unresponsive to non-surgical treatment, modern periradicular microsurgery remains a reliable option. By incorporating CBCT imaging for preoperative mapping, ultrasonic retropreparation, and bioactive retrofilling materials, clinical success rates can reach as high as 94% [14], with favorable bone regeneration and soft tissue healing outcomes.

When these elements are integrated, namely, the preservation of anatomical integrity, precise working length determination, three-dimensional imaging, laser-enhanced disinfection, and advanced microsurgical techniques, the cumulative effect is a more predictable treatment pathway that improves both tooth survival and patient satisfaction. This synergy highlights the value of combining time-tested biological principles with carefully validated technological innovations to optimize long-term outcomes.

6.3. Integrating Current Technologies: From Diagnosis to Precision Therapy

The integration of advanced technologies has transformed endodontics from a predominantly manual specialty into a precision-driven discipline. High-resolution imaging, guided instrumentation, and laser-assisted disinfection now complement traditional approaches, allowing clinicians to achieve superior debridement, minimize procedural errors, and improve long-term success rates.

A major milestone in this transformation is the adoption of CBCT, which provides three-dimensional visualization of root canal morphology, periapical tissues, and surrounding anatomical landmarks. Unlike two-dimensional radiographs, CBCT enables the accurate identification of apical periodontitis, undetected accessory canals, and root fractures that often escape conventional imaging. Studies have shown that CBCT detects periapical pathology in approximately 34% more cases than periapical radiographs, particularly in multi-rooted teeth, underscoring its diagnostic advantage [12]. Preoperative CBCT has become invaluable for retreatment planning, mapping canal curvatures, and assessing lesion proximity to critical structures such as the maxillary sinus or inferior alveolar nerve.

Building on the strengths of CBCT, the fusion of 3D imaging with digital intraoral scans has enabled the development of guided endodontics. This workflow uses virtual planning and 3D-printed templates to navigate even severely calcified or atypical canals with unprecedented precision. Clinical evidence demonstrates 97–100% accuracy in canal localization using CBCT-guided templates, reducing treatment time and conserving dentin by preventing unnecessary coronal access [22]. For example, in a calcified maxillary central incisor, a digitally planned stent derived from CBCT and optical scans facilitated swift, conservative access within minutes while preserving pericervical dentin.

In parallel, laser-assisted endodontics has redefined intracanal disinfection strategies. Lasers such as Er: YAG (2940 nm) generate micro-explosive photoacoustic streaming in irrigants that disrupts biofilm and removes smear layer, while Nd: YAG (1064 nm) penetrates dentinal tubules for deeper antibacterial action. Diode lasers (810–980 nm) further support soft-tissue decontamination and reduce postoperative discomfort. Laboratory and clinical studies confirm that Er: YAG-activated irrigation achieves up to 99.9% bacterial reduction compared to conventional irrigation alone [23]. Moreover, laser-assisted treatment protocols have been linked to a 40% decrease in postoperative pain relative to standard chemomechanical approaches [24].

The synergy of these technologies is exemplified in complex retreatment cases. In a mandibular molar with persistent apical periodontitis, CBCT imaging revealed an untreated middle mesial canal with sharp apical curvature. A 3D-printed endodontic guide enabled targeted access to the canal, minimizing dentin removal. Mechanical preparation was complemented by Er: YAG-enhanced irrigation of NaOCl and EDTA, which improved disinfection and smear-layer removal. Follow-up at 12 months confirmed complete periapical healing and absence of symptoms, underscoring the clinical advantage of integrating imaging with laser activation.

Despite these advances, endodontic treatment often encounters persistent challenges. Anatomical complexity remains a frequent obstacle; for example, 42% of mandibular molars exhibit a middle mesial canal that is commonly missed without advanced imaging, potentially compromising outcomes [25]. Other difficulties include biofilm resistance, as species like *E. faecalis* can survive in dentinal tubules despite standard chemomechanical preparation [26]. Technological adjuncts, such as laser activation or ultrasonic irrigant agitation, help overcome these microbial defenses.

Non-technical challenges also affect success. Dental anxiety continues to hinder patient compliance; epidemiological data indicate that 10–20% of adults experience high dental fear, often delaying care or avoiding appointments [16]. Clear communication, the use of buffered anesthetics, and minimally invasive techniques are essential to reduce anxiety and pain perception. Another procedural hazard is instrument separation, reported in 0.4–5% of cases, especially in curved molar canals, which complicates treatment and may jeopardize prognosis [27]. Adherence to manufacturer torque limits, regular inspection of rotary files, and training in ultrasonic retrieval techniques are recommended preventive measures.

Advancing technical excellence also requires lifelong learning. Formal continuing education (CE) programs, such as those provided by the American Association of Endodontists (AAE), offer opportunities to master CBCT interpretation, guided endodontic workflows, and microsurgical skills through hands-on courses. Online learning platforms, including Dentinal Tubules and EndoAcademy, supplement clinical practice with virtual lectures and peer-reviewed case libraries. Regular participation in peer-review study clubs fosters collaborative problem-solving, while subscribing to journals such as the *International Endodontic Journal* and the *Journal of Endodontics* ensures clinicians remain updated on guideline revisions and emerging evidence.

Finally, the integration of technology must remain patient-centered. Transparent communication using CBCT images or intraoral photographs empowers patients to make informed decisions about their care. The American Dental Association reports that patients who receive comprehensive pre-treatment explanations are 2.5 times more likely to follow through with recommended therapy [28]. Discussing expected healing timelines and potential risks, such as comparing success rates of apicoectomy (85–95%) versus retreatment (~83% at 4–6 years), helps set realistic expectations [6,14,29]. For individuals with systemic conditions like diabetes, who have a 2.9-fold higher risk of persistent apical periodontitis when glycemic control is poor, treatment planning should include enhanced infection control and closer follow-up [30].

By uniting diagnostic imaging, minimally invasive guided access, laser-enhanced irrigation, and patient-centered communication, modern endodontics has moved closer to truly precision-based therapy improving healing rates, reducing postoperative symptoms, and enhancing long-term tooth retention.

6.4. Essential Strategies for Predictable Endodontic Success

Endodontics, a dental specialty focused on the dental pulp and surrounding tissues, demands precision, in-depth knowledge of theoretical principles, and mastery of practical techniques. Success in this field hinges on careful case selection, methodical treatment approaches, and strict adherence to established protocols. Below is a restructured overview of essential tips for achieving success in endodontics (Table 13) and key concepts that are critical for innovative endodontic treatment (Table 14).

Table 13. Strategies for Overcoming Challenges in Endodontics.

	Strategy	Key Insight
1	**Careful Case Selection**	Prioritize cases with a predictable outcome to minimize complications [1,3,11,20].
2	**Systematic Treatment Approach**	A deliberate and organized methodology reduces errors and enhances outcomes [1,2,5,11].
3	**Optimized Cavity Preparation**	Tailor cavity preparation to ensure effective treatment and long-term success [1,11,19].
4	**Precision in Length Determination**	Accurate measurement of tooth length prevents over-instrumentation and failure [1,21].
5	**Utilization of Advanced Instruments**	Use high-quality, pre-turned instruments for complex root canal anatomy [1,11,19,22].
6	**Master Cone Compression Techniques**	Ensure thorough apical sealing with precise cone compression [1,7,26].
7	**Judicious Use of Periradicular Surgery**	Reserve surgery for cases where less invasive methods are insufficient [6,8,10,11,14].
8	**Verification of Apical Seal**	Confirm the apical seal to prevent future complications [7,26].
9	**Comprehensive Restoration of Treated Teeth**	Protect treated teeth with appropriate restorative techniques [1,20].
10	**Continual Practice and Skill Enhancement**	Regular practice and updating skills improve proficiency in endodontics [1,11–13,28].

Source: Table by author.

Table 14. Innovations in Endodontic Treatment Techniques.

	Innovation	Key Insight
1	**Preservation of Anatomical Integrity**	Maintain the natural canal structure to prevent post-treatment complications [19,22,25,29].
2	**Advanced Mechanical and Chemical Processing**	Utilize cutting-edge tools and solutions for thorough canal cleaning [1,23,24].
3	**Modern Root Canal Obturation Techniques**	Employ the latest methods to achieve complete canal sealing [1,7,26].
4	**Role of High-Performance Canal Sealers**	Modern sealers improve the apical seal, reducing the risk of reinfection [7,26].
5	**Innovative Gutta-Percha Techniques**	Use contemporary gutta-percha methods for superior obturation results [1,7].
6	**Targeted Use of Medications and Antiseptics**	Enhance healing and reduce infection risk with appropriate chemicals [1,15,30].
7	**Laser-Assisted Endodontics**	Incorporate laser technology to improve precision and efficiency in treatment [23,24].
8	**Comprehensive Multi-Stage Treatment Planning**	Recognize and plan for the multiple stages of endodontic therapy [1,11].
9	**Understanding Root Canal Topography**	Detailed knowledge of root canal anatomy is essential for effective treatment [19,25].
10	**Barrier Techniques in Cavity and Canal Preparation**	Utilize barrier methods to prevent microbial contamination [1].
11	**Enhanced Removal of Necrotic Tissue**	Advanced techniques ensure complete removal of necrotic tissue, reducing failure rates [23,24].
12	**Preservation of Canal Curvature**	Maintain the natural curvature of the canal to avoid weakening the tooth structure [1,19].
13	**Uniform Canal Expansion Techniques**	Achieve consistent canal expansion to accommodate effective obturation [1,19].
14	**Physiological Narrowing Preservation**	Preserve natural narrowing to maintain tooth strength [1].
15	**Creation of Reliable Apical Stoppers**	Develop precise apical stoppers for predictable obturation [1].

Table 14. *Cont.*

	Innovation	Key Insight
16	**Accurate Working Length Determination**	Utilize the latest electronic and radiographic methods for precise length measurement [12,21].
17	**Initial Instrument Stabilization**	Secure instruments at the correct working length to ensure consistent treatment [1,21].
18	**Electronic and Radiographic Innovations**	Integrate modern imaging techniques for precise diagnostics and treatment [12,13,22,29].
19	**Topographical-Anatomical Planning**	Use topographical data to enhance treatment precision and predictability [12,19,25].
20	**Tabular Method Refinements**	Utilize updated tabular methods to determine working lengths based on comprehensive data [19,21].
21	**Instrument and Radiography Synergy**	Combine instruments and radiography to optimize working length determination [12,19,21,22].

Source: Table by author.

By addressing these strategies and leveraging innovations, dental professionals can overcome common challenges in endodontic treatment, improve patient outcomes, and stay at the forefront of modern endodontic practice. This ensures not only successful procedures but also long-term patient satisfaction and dental health.

6.5. Conclusions and Future Directions

Endodontic success rests on the seamless integration of evidence-based strategies, technological innovation, and patient-centered care. At its core, predictable treatment outcomes depend on meticulous case selection, precise working length determination, optimized cavity preparation, proficient obturation techniques, and the delivery of high-quality coronal restorations. These fundamentals continue to serve as the foundation for sustaining tooth structure, preventing reinfection, and ensuring long-term function.

The last decade has seen rapid advancements in diagnostic and therapeutic tools that have reshaped modern endodontic practice. The adoption of CBCT, guided endodontics, laser-assisted canal disinfection, and advanced bioactive sealing materials has enhanced treatment precision and reduced procedural complications. These innovations not only improve debridement and obturation quality but also contribute to superior healing rates and greater tooth survival. Central to these developments is a clinical mindset that prioritizes continuous skill refinement, evidence-based decision-making, and effective communication with patients, qualities that foster trust, compliance, and satisfaction.

Looking forward, several research avenues hold promise for transforming clinical protocols and expanding therapeutic potential. The development of next-generation obturation and sealing materials, particularly bioceramics with enhanced antimicrobial properties and nanotechnology-based sealers capable of deeper dentinal tubule penetration, may improve long-term sealing efficacy. Innovations in biofilm management, including antimicrobial peptides, photodynamic therapy, and advanced irrigation systems, are being explored to address persistent infections in anatomically complex cases. Regenerative endodontics continues to advance with stem cell-based approaches and the application of growth factors to reconstitute the pulp–dentin complex, though long-term evidence on functional recovery remains a priority.

Digital integration also represents a frontier for endodontic care. Artificial intelligence (AI) has the potential to improve diagnostic accuracy through advanced CBCT interpretation, enhance treatment planning, and even predict outcomes based on patient-specific data. Similarly, the rise of chairside digital navigation systems promises real-time guidance for clinicians performing intricate procedures in challenging anatomies. As personalized medicine becomes more prevalent, genomic and microbiome profiling may help customize treatment protocols to individual patient biology, while better incorporating systemic health factors into healing and success predictions.

Ultimately, the future of endodontics will be shaped by those who pair technical mastery with the discernment to adopt validated innovations responsibly. Clinicians who remain grounded in rigorous evidence, committed to lifelong learning, and sensitive to the holistic needs of their patients will be best positioned to preserve natural dentition and elevate the standard of care. By uniting sound scientific principles with emerging technologies and patient-centered approaches, endodontics can continue to advance its primary mission: safeguarding teeth and enhancing quality of life for patients worldwide.

References

1. European Society of Endodontology. Quality guidelines for endodontic treatment: Consensus report of the European Society of Endodontology. *Int. Endod. J.* **2006**, *39*, 921–930. [CrossRef]
2. Wu, M.K.; Wesselink, P.; Shemesh, H. New terms for categorizing the outcome of root canal treatment. *Int. Endod. J.* **2011**, *44*, 1079–1080. [CrossRef]
3. Ng, Y.L.; Mann, V.; Gulabivala, K. Outcome of secondary root canal treatment: A systematic review of the literature. *Int. Endod. J.* **2008**, *41*, 1026–1046. [CrossRef] [PubMed]
4. Karamifar, K.; Tondari, A.; Saghiri, M.A. Endodontic Periapical Lesion: An Overview on the Etiology, Diagnosis and Current Treatment Modalities. *Eur. Endod. J.* **2020**, *5*, 54–67. [CrossRef]
5. Messer, H.H.; Yu, V.S. Terminology of endodontic outcomes. *Int. Endod. J.* **2013**, *46*, 289–291. [CrossRef] [PubMed]
6. Torabinejad, M.; Corr, R.; Handysides, R.; Shabahang, S. Outcomes of nonsurgical retreatment and endodontic surgery: A systematic review. *J. Endod.* **2009**, *35*, 930–937. [CrossRef]

7. Sabeti, M.A.; Karimpourtalebi, N.; Shahravan, A.; Dianat, O. Clinical and Radiographic Failure of Nonsurgical Endodontic Treatment and Retreatment Using Single-cone Technique With Calcium Silicate-based Sealers: A Systematic Review and Meta-analysis. *J. Endod.* **2024**, *50*, 735–746.e1. [CrossRef]
8. Tsesis, I.; Rosen, E.; Taschieri, S.; Telishevsky Strauss, Y.; Ceresoli, V.; Del Fabbro, M. Outcomes of surgical endodontic treatment performed by a modern technique: An updated meta-analysis of the literature. *J. Endod.* **2013**, *39*, 332–339. [CrossRef] [PubMed]
9. Yahata, Y.; Handa, K.; Ohkura, N.; Okamoto, M.; Ohshima, J.; Itoh, S.; Kawashima, N.; Tanaka, T.; Sato, N.; Noiri, Y.; et al. Autologous concentrated growth factor mediated accelerated bone healing in root-end microsurgery: A multicenter randomized clinical trial. *Regen. Ther.* **2023**, *24*, 377–384. [CrossRef]
10. Wang, H.; Xu, X.; Bian, Z.; Liang, J.; Chen, Z.; Hou, B.; Qiu, L.; Chen, W.; Wei, X.; Hu, K.; et al. Expert consensus on apical microsurgery. *Int. J. Oral Sci.* **2025**, *17*, 2. [CrossRef]
11. Ng, Y.L.; Gulabivala, K. Factors that influence the outcomes of surgical endodontic treatment. *Int. Endod. J.* **2023**, *56*, 116–139. [CrossRef]
12. Patel, S.; Brown, J.; Semper, M.; Abella, F.; Mannocci, F. European Society of Endodontology position statement: Use of cone beam computed tomography in Endodontics: European Society of Endodontology (ESE) developed by. *Int. Endod. J.* **2019**, *52*, 1675–1678. [CrossRef]
13. Di Spirito, F.; Gasparro, R.; Di Palo, M.P.; De Benedetto, G.; Giordano, F.; Amato, M.; Bramanti, A. Dynamic Navigation in Endodontic Surgery: A Systematic Review. *Healthcare* **2025**, *13*, 2151. [CrossRef]
14. Lieblich, S.E. Current Concepts of Periapical Surgery: 2020 Update. *Oral. Maxillofac. Surg. Clin. N. Am.* **2020**, *32*, 571–582. [CrossRef]
15. Kuzekanani, M.; Mollamohamadi Kermani, S. Latest Concepts in Endodontic and Periodontal Management of Diabetic Patients. *Cureus* **2024**, *16*, e52145. [CrossRef]
16. Carter, A.E.; Carter, G.; Boschen, M.; AlShwaimi, E.; George, R. Pathways of fear and anxiety in dentistry: A review. *World J. Clin. Cases* **2014**, *2*, 642–653. [CrossRef]
17. Qin, L.; Qiao, W.; Chen, C.; Lin, Y.; Zhang, X.; Meng, L. Robot-Assisted Endodontic Retreatment: A Case Report with Clinical Considerations. *J. Endod.* **2025**, *51*, 521–527. [CrossRef] [PubMed]
18. Turjanski, D.; Lisjak, D.; Bučević Sojčić, P.; Valpotić, J.; Borojević Renić, T.; Goršeta, K.; Glavina, D. Advanced Platelet-Rich Fibrin Plus Sealed Exclusively with Glass Ionomer Cement: Setting a New Standard for Healing, Aesthetics and Predictive Modelling in Regenerative Endodontics. *Materials* **2025**, *18*, 4421. [CrossRef] [PubMed]
19. Fidler, A.; Plotino, G.; Kuralt, M. A Critical Review of Methods for Quantitative Evaluation of Root Canal Transportation. *J. Endod.* **2021**, *47*, 721–731. [CrossRef]
20. Fonzar, F.; Fonzar, A.; Buttolo, P.; Worthington, H.V.; Esposito, M. The prognosis of root canal therapy: A 10-year retrospective cohort study on 411 patients with 1175 endodontically treated teeth. *Eur. J. Oral Implantol.* **2009**, *2*, 201–208. [PubMed]
21. La Rosa, G.R.M.; Angjelova, A.; Jovanova, E.; Apostolska, S.; Santos, J.M.; Pedullà, E. Integrated electronic apex locators for determining working length: A systematic review of in-vitro studies. *Odontology* **2025**, *113*, 918–929. [CrossRef]

22. Ren, S.; Wang, W.; Cheng, M.; Tang, W.; Zhao, Y.; Miao, L. Guided endodontics in the application of personalized mini-invasive treatment in clinical cases: A literature review. *Saudi Dent. J.* **2025**, *37*, 20. [CrossRef] [PubMed]
23. Habshi, A.Y.; Aga, N.; Habshi, K.Y.; Hassan, M.E.M.; Choudhry, Z.; Ahmed, M.A.; Syed, A.U.Y.; Jouhar, R. Efficacy of Smear Layer Removal at the Apical One-Third of the Root Using Different Protocols of Erbium-Doped Yttrium Aluminium Garnet (Er:YAG) Laser. *Medicina* **2023**, *59*, 433. [CrossRef]
24. McGillivray, A.; Dutta, A. The influence of laser-activated irrigation on post-operative pain following root canal treatment: A systematic review. *J. Dent.* **2024**, *144*, 104928. [CrossRef]
25. Manik, K.; Ikhar, A.; Patel, A.; Chandak, M.; Bhopatkar, J.; Rathod, P.; Bhojwani, P.R. Anatomical Variations in Mandibular Molars: Focus on Midmesial Canals. *Cureus.* **2024**, *16*, e61711. [CrossRef]
26. Mokhtari, F.; Modaresi, J.; Salmasi, A.H.; Khamisi, N.; Zandi, H.; Lesani, K. In vitro comparison of Enterococcus Faecalis survival in dentinal tubules following root canal therapy with AH plus, endoseal MTA, and cold ceramic sealers. *BMC Oral Health* **2024**, *24*, 1488. [CrossRef] [PubMed]
27. Manteca-Fernández, L.; Meniz-García, C.; Fernández-Cáliz, F.; Barona-Dorado, C.; Santos-Marino, J.; Martínez-Rodríguez, N. Influence of Premedication and Dental Anxiety on Anesthetic Efficacy in Patients Undergoing Root Canal for Symptomatic Irreversible Pulpitis in Upper and Lower Molars: A Comparative Study of Articaine and Bupivacaine. *Dent. J.* **2025**, *13*, 199. [CrossRef]
28. American Dental Association, Health Policy Institute. Annual Dental Industry Report 2020. 2020. Available online: https://ebusiness.ada.org/productcatalog/75168/HPI-Industry-Reports/2020-Annual-Dental-Industry-Report/AD2020 (accessed on 8 June 2021).
29. Samiei, M.; Sabanik, P.; Tavakkoli Avval, S. Guided Endodontics for Non-surgical Root Canal Retreatment: A Systematic Review. *Iran. Endod. J.* **2025**, *20*, e3. [CrossRef] [PubMed]
30. Pérez-Losada, F.L.; López-López, J.; Martín-González, J.; Jané-Salas, E.; Segura-Egea, J.J.; Estrugo-Devesa, A. Apical periodontitis and glycemic control in type 2 diabetic patients: Cross-sectional study. *J. Clin. Exp. Dent.* **2020**, *12*, e964–e971. [CrossRef]

MDPI AG
Grosspeteranlage 5
4052 Basel
Switzerland
Tel.: +41 61 683 77 34

MDPI Books Editorial Office
E-mail: books@mdpi.com
www.mdpi.com/books

www.ingramcontent.com/pod-product-compliance
Lightning Source LLC
Chambersburg PA
CBHW040852230926
51850CB00012BA/2933
* 9 7 8 3 7 2 5 8 2 1 9 6 9 *